ABBREVIATIONS

Age

NB – newborn
A – adult
C – child

Time/Frequency

s – second
min – minute
h – hour
d – day
wk – week
mo – month
y – year
q.d. – every day
q.o.d. – every other day
b.i.d. – twice a day
t.i.d. – three times a day
q.i.d. – four times a day
q4–6h (for example) – every 4–6 hours
h.s. – hour of sleep (at bedtime)
a.c. – before meal
p.c. – after meal
a.m. – morning
p.m. – evening
PRN – whenever necessary

Routes

IM – intramuscularly
IO – intraosseous
IV – intravenously
PO – by mouth (oral)
PR – per rectum (rectally)
SC – subcutaneously
SL – sublingual
vag – vaginally

Drug Form

amp – ampule
amt – amount
cap – capsule/caplet
conc – concentration
elix – elixir
gt(t) – drop(s)
inf – infusion
inhal – inhalation
inj – injectable
liq – liquid
maint – maintenance
max – maximum
oint – ointment
sol – solution
supp – suppository
susp – suspension
tab – tablet

Measurements

oz – ounce
lb – pound
in – inches
g – gram
mg – milligram
μm – microgram
U – unit
mEq – milliequivalent
L – liter
mL – milliliter
dL – deciliter
kg – kilogram
m^2 – square meter
bpm – beats per minute
× – times
> – more than
< – less than
≥ – more than or equal to
≤ – less than or equal to
– – to (range of one value to another value)

Miscellaneous

UK – unknown
CSS – Controlled Substance Schedule
ACE – angiotensin-converting enzyme
ADD – attention deficit disorder
AMI – acute myocardial infarction
C&S – culture and sensitivity (test)
CHF – congestive heart failure
CNS – central nervous system
Cl$_{cr}$ – creatine clearance
D$_5$W – 5% dextrose in water
ECG – electrocardiogram; electrocardiographic; electrocardiography
ETT – endotracheal tube
GERD – gastroesophageal reflux disease
GI – gastrointestinal
GU – genitourinary
I – imipenem
ICP – increased intracranial pressure
IOP – increased ocular pressure
IPPB – intermittent positive pressure breathing
LD – loading dose
LR – lactated Ringer's
MAOIs – monoamine oxidase inhibitors
MDI – metered dose inhaler
NA – not applicable
NGT – nasogastric tube
NSAIDs – nonsteroidal anti-inflammatory drugs
NSS – normal saline solution
OTC – over-the-counter
PB – protein-binding
Preg Cat – pregnancy category
RBC(s) – red blood cell(s)
RD – respiratory distress
RDA – recommended daily allowance
SR – sustained release (tab/cap)
TDM – therapeutic drug monitoring
t½ – half-life
VS – vital signs
♦ – Canadian drug names

POCKET COMPANION FOR

PHARMACOLOGY
A Nursing Process Approach

POCKET COMPANION FOR
PHARMACOLOGY
A Nursing Process Approach

SECOND EDITION

Joyce LeFever Kee, RN, MS
Associate Professor Emerita
College of Nursing
Department of Nursing Science
University of Delaware
Newark, Delaware

Evelyn R. Hayes, RN, PhD
Professor
College of Nursing
Department of Nursing Science
University of Delaware
Newark, Delaware

W.B. SAUNDERS COMPANY
A Division of Harcourt Brace & Company
Philadelphia London Toronto Montreal Sydney Tokyo

W.B. SAUNDERS COMPANY
A Division of Harcourt Brace & Company

The Curtis Center
Independence Square West
Philadelphia, Pennsylvania 19106

Library of Congress Cataloging-in-Publication Data

Hayes, Evelyn R.
　Pocket companion for pharmacology: a nursing process approach / Evelyn R. Hayes, Joyce LeFever Kee. — 2nd ed.
　　p.　cm.
　Rev. ed. of: Pharmacology pocket companion for nurses. c1996.
　Includes bibliographical references and index.

　ISBN 0–7216–5957–8

　1. Pharmacology—Handbooks, manuals, etc.　2. Nursing—Handbooks, manuals, etc.　I. Kee, Joyce LeFever.　II. Pharmacology pocket companion for nurses.　III. Title.
　[DNLM: 1. Drugs—nurses' instruction—handbooks.　2. Drug Therapy—nurses' instruction—handbooks.　QV 39 H418pa　1997]
　RM301.12.H39　1997

　615'.1—dc21

DNLM/DLC   96-43504

POCKET COMPANION FOR PHARMACOLOGY:
A NURSING PROCESS APPROACH, 2nd Edition　　ISBN 0–7216–5957–8

Copyright © 1997, 1996 by W.B. Saunders Company.

All rights reserved. No part of this publication may be reproduced or transmitted in any form or by any means, electronic or mechanical, including photocopy, recording, or any information storage and retrieval system, without permission in writing from the publisher.

Printed in the United States of America.

Last digit is the print number:　9　8　7　6　5　4　3　2　1

*To Jennifer, Justin, and Rebecca,
who are very special to me*

Evelyn R. Hayes

*To my husband, Edward D. Kee,
for his love and support*

Joyce L. Kee

CONSULTANTS

Michele Bockrath-Welch, RNC, MSN
Senior Clinical Scientist
Wyeth-Ayerst Laboratories
Philadelphia, Pennsylvania

Betty B. Laliberte, RN, MSN
Assistant Professor
School of Nursing
University of Connecticut
Storrs, Connecticut

Anne E. Lara, RN, MS, OCN, CS
Nurse Manager
Radiation Oncology
Medical Center of Delaware
Wilmington, Delaware

Linda Laskowski-Jones, RN, MS, CCRN, CEN
Trauma Nurse Specialist
Trauma Service
Medical Center of Delaware
Wilmington, Delaware

Ronald J. Lefever, RPh
Pharmacy Services
Medical College of Virginia
Richmond, Virginia

Lois W. Lowry, PhD, RN
Associate Professor
University of Southern Florida
Tampa, Florida

Nancy G. M. Miner, RNC, MSN
Director
Bridgeport Community Mental Health Center
Bridgeport, Connecticut

Donna Obra, PharmD
Director of Medical Information
Zeneca Inc.
Wilmington, Delaware

Joseph Peoples, RPh
Clinical Pharmacist
Alfred I. Du Pont Institute
Wilmington, Delaware

Lisa Plowfield, PhD, RN
Assistant Professor
College of Nursing
University of Delaware
Newark, Delaware

Nancy Sharts-Hopko, PhD, RN
Professor
Villanova University
Villanova, Pennsylvania

Robert Thornton, RPh, BSc
Director of Pharmacy Services
St. Francis Hospital and Medical Center
Wilmington, Delaware

Judith A. Torpey, RN, MSN
Assistant Director
Visiting Nurse Association of Manchester
Manchester, Connecticut

Jennifer Trey
Senior Student
College of Nursing
University of Delaware
Newark, Delaware

Marcus D. Wilson, PharmD
Assistant Professor
Philadelphia College of Pharmacy
Philadelphia, Pennsylvania
Clinical Pharmacy Coordinator
HMO of Delaware
Wilmington, Delaware

Roni Zarge
Senior Student
College of Nursing
University of Delaware
Newark, Delaware

PREFACE

Welcome to a unique pharmacology pocket companion for nurses. This book was designed for both nurses in clinical practice and student nurses to provide complex information on prototype drugs complete with the nursing process and extensive drug tables. The easy-to-read format allows valuable information to be readily available to the reader.

More than 90 prototype drugs are illustrated in a unique graphic format that includes drug name (generic, brand, and Canadian); drug and pregnancy categories; drug forms, routes, and dosages; contraindications; drug, food, and laboratory interactions; pharmacokinetics and pharmacodynamics; therapeutic effects and uses and mode of action; and side effects and adverse reactions.

The nursing process—assessment, nursing diagnosis, planning, nursing interventions, client and family teaching, and evaluation—is integrated throughout the pocket reference. Two potential nursing diagnoses apply to each drug, including knowledge deficit and noncompliance. The most common nursing diagnoses related to the specific drug therapy are identified. The challenges of client and family teaching are described, and helpful teaching tips are offered. Client teaching focuses on general information, skills, diet, and side effects related to the drugs.

More than 1500 drugs are described in approximately 100 drug tables that include generic and brand names, common dosages, pregnancy category, drug interactions, protein-binding capacity, half-life, and onset, peak, and duration of action. Refer to the prototype for a description of the side effects and adverse reactions.

The drug tables present essential information in a quick, easy-to-read format. This format enables the reader not only to pay attention to a single drug but also to compare and contrast aspects of the drug with those of related agents.

Complete abbreviation and laboratory test keys and a description of the drug pregnancy categories are given inside the front cover. Additional references are grouped at the beginning of the book, including sample dosage calculations, nomogram for body surface area, guide for calculation of intravenous flow rates, drugs that affect the color of urine and stool, therapeutic drug monitoring, table of metric and apothecary conversion, and additional prototype forms to be developed as needed.

Canadian drugs are listed in the Appendix according to: US generic drug names with corresponding Canadian brand drug names (A), Canadian brand drug names with corresponding US generic drug names (B); fat-soluble and water-soluble vitamins: RDA, dosages for vitamin deficiencies, and therapeutic serum range (C), and hints for medication use in the community setting (D).

FDA drug approval is an ongoing process. Thus, a supplement of recently approved drugs is included at the end of the book.

Nurses in clinical practice and student nurses have an ongoing need for such a reference because of their responsibility for the administration of medications and evaluation of client response. This pocket reference details valuable information in a quick, easy-to-read format for clinical application.

ACKNOWLEDGMENTS

Sincere appreciation is given to the many professionals who assisted in the development of this reference. The perspectives of the reviewers were most helpful, and we gratefully thank them for their insightful suggestions: Michele Bockrath-Welch, RNC, MSN; Betty B. Laliberte, RN, MSN; Anne E. Lara, RN, MS, OCN, CS; Linda Laskowski-Jones, RN, MS, CCRN, CEN; Ronald J. Lefever, RPh; Lois W. Lowry, PhD, RN; Nancy G.M. Miner, RNC, MSN; Donna Obra, PharmD; Joseph Peoples, RPh; Lisa Plowfield, PhD, RN; Nancy Sharts-Hopko, PhD, RN; Robert Thornton, RPh, BSc; Judith A. Torpey, RN, MSN; and Marcus D. Wilson, PharmD. We extend special thanks also to senior students Jennifer Trey and Roni Zarge.

We extend appreciation to Patricia Beauchesne, Katherine Dougherty, and Sandy Grim for their ongoing computer expertise.

Thanks are also due to the staff at W.B. Saunders Company, especially Maura E. Connor, Editor, Nursing Books, and Stephanie Klein, Administrative Assistant.

We extend our appreciation and love to our families for their ongoing support.

NOTICE

Pharmacology is an ever-changing field. Standard safety precautions must be followed, but as new research and clinical experience broaden our knowledge, changes in treatment and drug therapy become necessary or appropriate. The editors of this work have carefully checked the generic and brand names and verified drug dosages to ensure that the dosage information in this work is accurate and in accord with the standards accepted at the time of publication. Readers are advised, however, to check the product information currently provided by the manufacturer of each drug to be administered to be certain that changes have not been made in the recommended dose or in the contraindications for administration. This is of particular importance in regard to new or infrequently used drugs. It is the responsibility of the treating physician or health care provider, relying on experience and knowledge of the patient, to determine dosages and the best treatment for their patient. The editors cannot be responsible for misuse or misapplication of the information in this work.

CONTENTS

ORIENTATION, xix
  Introduction to Using the Drug Prototype, xix
  Prototype, xx
  Metric and Apothecary Conversion, xxi
  Drug Calculation Formulas, xxi, xxiii
  Discoloration of Urine Due to Drugs, xxiv
  Discoloration of Feces Due to Drugs, xxv

THERAPEUTIC DRUG MONITORING (TDM), xxvii

VITAMINS, MINERALS, AND ELECTROLYTES, 1
  Vitamin A, Fat-Soluble, 2
  Antianemia, Mineral: Iron, 6
  Electrolyte:
    Potassium, 8
    Calcium, 12

CENTRAL NERVOUS SYSTEM STIMULANTS AND DEPRESSANTS, 15
  Central Nervous System Stimulant, 16
  Sedative-Hypnotic:
    Barbiturate, 22
    Benzodiazepine, 28
  Analgesic:
    Aspirin, 32
    Acetaminophen, 34
  Narcotic:
  Opiate: Morphine Sulfate, 38
  Nonopiate: Meperidine, 40
  Agonist-Antagonist: Pentazocine Lactate, 44

ANTICONVULSANTS, 49
  Barbiturates, 52
  Benzodiazepines, 53
  Hydantoins, 54
  Iminostilbenes, 55
  Oxazolidones, 55
  Succinimides, 55
  Valproate, 56
  Miscellaneous, 56

ANTIPSYCHOTICS, ANXIOLYTICS, AND ANTIDEPRESSANTS, 59
  Antipsychotic, 60
    Phenothiazine, 64
    Nonphenothiazine, 66
  Anxiolytics, 72
  Antidepressants, 76
  Antimanic, 82

NEUROLOGIC AND NEUROMUSCULAR AGENTS, 85
  Adrenergic Agonist, 86
  Adrenergic Blocker, 94
  Cholinergic, 98
  Anticholinergic, 104
  Antiparkinsonism, 112
    Anticholinergic, 112
    Dopaminergic, 116
  Myasthenia Gravis, 120
  Muscle Relaxant, 124

ANTI-INFLAMMATORY AGENTS, 131
  Nonsteroidal Anti-inflammatory Drugs, 132
  Gold Preparations, 140
  Antigout Drugs, 144

ANTI-INFECTIVE AGENTS, 147
  Antibacterials:
    Penicillins, 148
    Cephalosporins, 156
    Erythromycin, 162
    Tetracyclines, 166
    Aminoglycosides, 170
    Quinolones, 174
    Unclassified, 177
    Sulfonamides, 178
    Peptides, 183
  Antitubercular Drugs, 184
  Antifungals, 188

Antimalarials, 192
Antivirals, 194
Topical Anti-infectives:
  Burns, 198
  Acne Vulgaris, 200
  Psoriasis, 200

URINARY AGENTS, 203

Urinary Anti-infectives, 204
Urinary Analgesic, 210
Urinary Stimulant, 212
Urinary Antispasmodics, 212

ANTINEOPLASTIC AGENTS, 215

Alkylating Drugs, 216
Antimetabolites, 222
Miscellaneous Anticancer Drugs, 226
Biologic Response Modifiers, 232
  Epoetin Alfa, 232
  Granulocyte Colony–Stimulating Factor, 234
  Granulocyte Macrophage Colony–Stimulating Factor, 236
  Interferons, 238

RESPIRATORY AGENTS, 241

Antihistamines, 242
Antitussive and Expectorants, 248
Decongestants, 252
Bronchodilators:
  Adrenergic, 254
  Methylxanthine, 260

CARDIOVASCULAR AGENTS, 265

Cardiac Glycosides, 266
Antianginals, 270
Antidysrhythmics, 276
Diuretics:
  Thiazides, 282
  Loop (High Ceiling), Osmotic, and Carbonic Anhydrase Inhibitors, 286
  Potassium Sparing, 290
Antihypertensives, 294
  Beta Blockers and Central Alpha$_2$ Agonist, 296
  Sympatholytics: Alpha-Adrenergic, Alpha-Beta, and Peripherally Acting Blockers; and Direct-Acting Vasodilators, 300
  Angiotensin Antagonists and Calcium Blockers, 306
Anticoagulants, Antiplatelets, and Anticoagulant Antagonists, 312, 315
Thrombolytics, 318
Antilipemics, 322
Vasodilators (Peripheral), 328

GASTROINTESTINAL AGENTS, 333

Antiemetics:
  Phenothiazines, 334
  Cannabinoids and Miscellaneous, 337
  Drugs for Motion Sickness, 339
Emetics, 340
  Emetics and Adsorbent, 342
Antidiarrheals:
  Opiates, Opiate-Related, and Adsorbents, 346
  Miscellaneous and Combinations, 348
Laxatives, 350
  Osmotic and Contact, 352
  Bulk Forming, Emollients, and Evacuant, 354
Antiulcers:
  Antacids, 358
  Anticholinergics, 362
  Histamine$_2$ Blockers, 364
  Pepsin Inhibitor, Gastric Acid Secretion Inhibitor, and Prostaglandin Analog, 368

OPHTHALMIC AND OTIC AGENTS, 371

Ophthalmic:
  Miotics: Cholinergics and Beta-Adrenergic Blockers, 372
  Carbonic Anhydrase Inhibitors (CAIs), 377
  Osmotics, 378
  Mydriatics and Cycloplegics, 379
  Anti-Infectives, 381
  Anti-Inflammatories, 383

Otic:
    Anti-Infective, 384

ENDOCRINE AGENTS, 387

Pituitary Hormones, 388
Thyroid Hormone Replacements and Antithyroid Agents, 394
Parathyroid Hormones: Replacements and Supplements, 400
Adrenal Hormones:
    Glucocorticoids, 404
Antidiabetics:
    Insulin, 410
    Sulfonylureas, 414

REPRODUCTIVE AND GENDER-RELATED AGENTS, 419

Beta-Adrenergic Agonists, 420
Oxytocins, 424
Estrogen Replacements, 428
Oral Contraceptives, 432
Androgens, 434
Ovulations Stimulants, 440

AGENTS FOR EMERGENCY TREATMENT, 443

Cardiac States, 444
Neurosurgical States, 448
Poisoning, 452
Shock, 456
Hypertensive Crisis, 460

Bibliography, 463
Appendix A, 465
Appendix B, 471
Appendix C, 479
Appendix D, 481
Supplement of FDA Approved Drugs, 483
Index, 499

ORIENTATION

INTRODUCTION TO USING THE DRUG PROTOTYPE

Comprehensive information is provided for each of the prototype drugs, including generic, brand, and Canadian drug names; dosage; forms available; pregnancy category; contraindication and cautions for use; drug, food, and laboratory interactions; pharmacokinetics; pharmacodynamics; therapeutic effects and mode of action; side effects; and adverse reactions.

Drug, food, and laboratory interactions are important and can be complex. For example, the interactions for hydrochlorothiazide are that the drug will:

Increase digitalis toxicity with digitalis and hypokalemia; *increase* potassium loss with steroids; *decrease* antihypoglycemic effect; *decrease* thiazide effect with cholestyramine and colestipol

Lab: Decrease serum potassium, sodium, and magnesium levels; *increase* serum calcium, glucose, and uric acid levels

Thus, it is evident that hydrochlorothiazide affects the action of other drugs and is affected by other drug actions.

The nursing process relates to the prototype drug as well as to other drugs within the category. In addition, comprehensive drug tables detail essential data about the most commonly prescribed drugs in that category.

The prototype drug chart is presented on the following page.

Drug Category

Drug Generic Name

Drug Generic Name
Drug Brand Name(s)
🍁 Drug Canadian Name(s)

Pregnancy Category:
Drug Forms:

Dosage

Contraindications

Caution:

Drug-Lab-Food Interactions

Pharmacokinetics

Absorption:
Distribution:
Metabolism:
Excretion:

Pharmacodynamics

Onset:
Peak:
Duration:

Therapeutic Effects/Uses:

Mode of Action:

Side Effects

Adverse Reactions

Life-threatening:

NOTE: On back, include the nursing process for the drug.

Metric and Apothecary Conversion

Metric		Apothecary
Gram (g)	Milligram (mg)	Grain (gr)
1	1000	15
0.5	500	7½
0.3	300 (325)	5
0.1	100	1½
0.06	60 (64)	1
0.03	30 (32)	½
0.015	15 (16)	¼
0.010	10	⅙
0.0006	0.6	1/100
0.0004	0.4	1/150
0.0003	0.3	1/200

Liquid Conversion

30 mL (cc) = 1 oz (fl ℥) = 2 tbsp (T)
 = 6 tsp (t)
15 mL (cc) = ½ oz = 1 T = 3 t
1000 mL (cc) = 1 quart (qt) = 1 liter (L)
500 mL (cc) = 1 pint (pt)
5 mL (cc) = 1 tsp (t)
4 mL (cc) = 1 fl dr (fl ℥)
1 mL (cc) = 15 (16) minims (♏)
 = 15 (16) drops (gtt)

Drug Calculations: Basic Formula

$\dfrac{D \text{ (desired)}}{H \text{ (on hand)}} \times V \text{ (vehicle, drug form)}$

Example:
Order: Amoxicillin 100 mg PO q6h
Available: Amoxicillin 250 mg/5 mL

$\dfrac{D}{H} \times V = \dfrac{100 \text{ mg}}{250 \text{ mg}} \times 5 \text{ mL}$

$= \dfrac{500}{250} = 2 \text{ mL amoxicillin}$

Drug Calculations: Ratio and Proportion

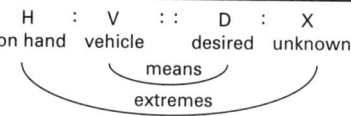

Example:
Order: Amoxicillin 100 mg PO q6h
Available: Amoxicillin 250 mg/5 mL

H : V :: D : X
250 mg : 5 mL :: 100 mg : X mL

250 X = 500
X = 2 mL amoxicillin

Body Weight (Kilograms)

To change pounds to kilograms, divide by 2.2.

Example:
Change 44 pounds to kilograms (kg)
44 ÷ 2.2 = 20 kg

Dosage/kg/d = dosage/d
(dosage × kg = dose/d)

Example:
Order: Drug 6 mg/kg/d in four divided doses

6 mg × 20 kg × 1 d = 120 mg/d
120 ÷ 4 = 30 mg per dose

Dimensional Analysis (Factor Labeling)

$= \dfrac{V \text{ (vehicle)} \times C(H) \times D \text{ (desired)}}{H \text{ (on hand)} \times C(D) \times 1}$
 (drug label) (conversion factor) (drug order)

Conversion factor: 1 g = 1000 mg
 1 g = 15 gr
 1 gr = 60 mg

Order: Amoxicillin 0.1 g, PO q6h
Available: Amoxicillin 250 mg/5 mL
How many mLs would you give?

$\dfrac{5 \text{ mL} \times \cancel{1000}^{4} \cancel{\text{mg}} \times 0.1 \cancel{g}}{\cancel{250}_{1} \cancel{\text{mg}} \times 1 \cancel{g} \times 1} =$

5 mL × 4 × 0.1 = 2 mL of amoxicillin

xxi

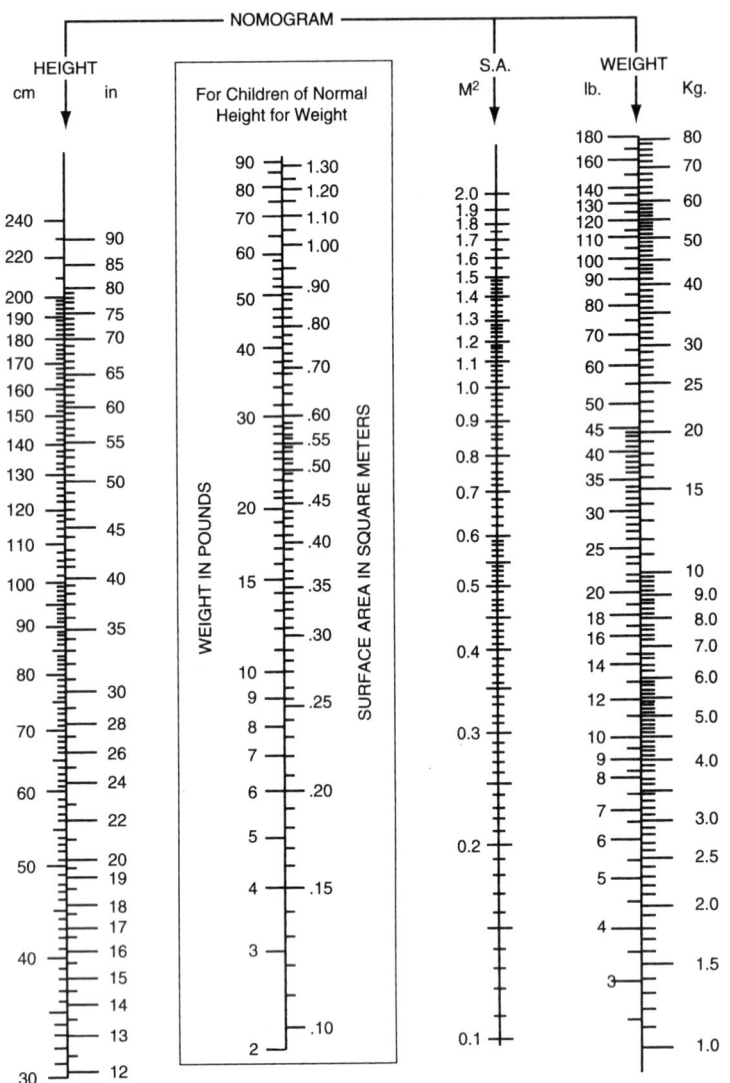

West nomogram: for infants and children. *Directions*: (1) Find height. (2) Find weight. (3) Draw a straight line connecting the height and the weight, and where the line intersects on the SA column is the body surface area (m²). Modified from data of E. Boyd and C. D. West, in Behrman, R. E., and Vaughan, V. C.: *Nelson Textbook of Pediatrics*, (14th ed). Philadelphia, W.B. Saunders Co., 1992.

IV Flow Rate: Continuous

a. amount of fluid ÷ hours to administer = mL/h

b. $\dfrac{\text{mL/h} \times \text{gtt/mL (IV set)}}{60 \text{ min/h}}$ = gtt/min

Example:
Order: 1,000 mL, D_5/½ NSS in 8 h.
IV set: Macrodrip: 10 gtt/mL.

a. 1,000 mL ÷ 8 h = 125 mL/h

b. $\dfrac{125 \text{ mL/h} \times \cancel{10}^{1} \text{ gtt/mL}}{\underset{6}{\cancel{60}} \text{ min/h}}$ = 21 gtt/min

---

IV Flow Rate: Intermittent Secondary Sets: Buretrol and Add-a-Line

$\dfrac{\text{Amount of solution} \times \text{gtt/mL (set)}}{\text{Minutes to administer}}$ = gtt/min

Order: Administer 5 mL of drug solution in 50 mL of D_5W in 30 min
IV set: Buretrol (60 gtt/mL)

$\dfrac{55 \text{ mL} \times \cancel{60}^{2} \text{ gtt/mL}}{\underset{1}{\cancel{30}} \text{ min}}$ = 110 gtt/min

---

IV Flow Rate: Intermittent Volumetric Pump

Amount of solution ÷ $\dfrac{\text{minutes to administer}}{60 \text{ min/h}}$ = mL/h

Order: Administer 5 mL of drug solution in 100 mL of D_5W in 45 min

$$105 \text{ mL} \div \dfrac{45 \text{ min}}{60 \text{ min/h}} \quad \text{(Invert divisor and multiply)}$$

$$= 105 \times \dfrac{\cancel{60}^{4}}{\underset{3}{\cancel{45}}} = 140 \text{ mL/h}$$

Set volumetric pump at 140 mL/h to deliver 105 mL in 45 min.

Discoloration of Urine Due to Drugs

Black
Cascara
Ferrous salts
Iron dextran
Levodopa
Methocarbamol
Methyldopa
Naphthalene
Phenacetin
Phenols
Quinine
Sulfonamides

Blue
Anthraquinone
Indigo blue
Indigo carmine
Methocarbamol
Methylene blue
Nitrofurans
Triamterene

Blue-Green
Amitriptyline
Anthraquinone
Indigo blue
Indigo carmine
Methylene blue

Brown
Anthraquinone dyes
Cascara
Levodopa
Methocarbamol
Methyldopa
Metronidazole
Nitrofurans
Nitrofurantoin
Phenacetin
Primaquine
Quinine
Rifampin
Senna
Sodium diatrizoate
Sulfonamides

Brown-Black
Quinine

Yellow-Brown
Cascara
Chloroquine
Methylene blue
Metronidazole
Nitrofurantoin
Primaquine
Quinacrine
Senna
Sulfonamides

Dark
Cascara
Levodopa
Metronidazole
Nitrites
Primaquine
Quinine
Senna

Green
Anthraquinone
Indigo blue
Indigo carmine
Indomethacin
Methocarbamol
Methylene blue
Nitrofurans
Phenols

Green-Yellow
Methylene blue

Milky
Phosphates

Orange
Chlorzoxazone
Dihydroergotamine mesylate
Heparin sodium
Rifampin
Sulfasalazine
Warfarin

Orange-Red
Chlorzoxazone
Doxidan
Rifampin

Orange-Yellow
Fluorescein sodium
Rifampin
Sulfasalazine

Pink
Anthraquinone dyes
Danthron
Deferoxamine
Phenolphthalein
Phenothiazines
Phenytoin
Salicylates

Yellow-Pink
Cascara
Senna

Red
Anthraquinone
Cascara
Daunorubicin
Dimethylsulfoxide
DMSO
Doxorubicin
Heparin
Ibuprofen
Methyldopa
Oxyphenbutazone
Phenacetin
Phenolphthalein
Phenothiazines
Phenylbutazone
Phenytoin
Rifampin
Senna

Red-Brown
Cascara
Methyldopa
Oxyphenbutazone
Phenacetin
Phenolphthalein
Phenothiazines
Phenylbutazone
Phenytoin
Quinine

Red-Purple
Chlorzoxazone
Ibuprofen
Phenacetin
Senna

Rust
Cascara
Chloroquine
Metronidazole
Nitrofurantoin
Phenacetin
Riboflavin
Senna
Sulfonamides

Yellow
Nitrofurantoin
Phenacetin
Sulfasalazine

Adapted from *Drugdex®—Drug Consults, Micromedex, vol 62.* Denver, CO: Rocky Mountain Drug Consultation Center, November 1989. Published by Lexi-Comp Inc. for Medical Center of Delaware: *Formulary and Drug Therapy Guide, 1993–1994.* With permission.

Discoloration of Feces Due to Drugs

Black
Acetazolamide
Alcohols
Alkalies
Aminophylline
Amphetamine
Amphotericin
Antacids
Anticoagulants
Aspirin
Betamethasone
Charcoal
Chloramphenicol
Chlorpropamide
Clindamycin
Corticosteroids
Cortisone
Cyclophosphamide
Cytarabine
Dicumarol

Blue
Chloramphenicol
Methylene blue

Dark Brown
Dexamethasone

Gray
Colchicine

Green
Indomethacin
Iron
Medroxyprogesterone

Green-Gray
Oral antibiotics
Oxyphenbutazone
Phenylbutazone

Light Brown
Anticoagulants

Digitalis
Ethacrynic acid
Ferrous salts
Floxuridine
Fluorouracil
Halothane
Heparin
Hydralazine
Hydrocortisone
Ibuprofen
Indomethacin
Iodine drugs
Iron salts
Levarterenol
Levodopa
Manganese
Melphalan
Methylprednisolone
Methotrexate

Orange-Red
Phenazopyridine
Rifampin

Pink
Anticoagulants
Aspirin
Heparin
Oxyphenbutazone
Phenylbutazone
Salicylates

Red
Anticoagulants
Aspirin
Heparin
Oxyphenbutazone
Phenolphthalein
Phenylbutazone
Salicylates
Tetracycline syrup

Methylene blue
Oxyphenbutazone
Paraldehyde
Phenacetin
Phenolphthalein
Phenylbutazone
Phenylephrine
Phosphorus
Potassium salts
Prednisolone
Procarbazine
Reserpine
Salicylates
Sulfonamides
Tetracycline
Theophylline
Thiotepa
Triamcinolone
Warfarin

Red-Brown
Oxyphenbutazone
Phenylbutazone
Rifampin

Tarry
Ergot preparations
Ibuprofen
Salicylates
Warfarin

White/Speckling
Aluminum hydroxide
Antibiotics (oral)
Indocyanine green

Yellow
Senna

Yellow-Green
Senna

Adapted from *Drugdex®—Drug Consults, Micromedex, vol 62*. Denver, CO: Rocky Mountain Drug Consultation Center, November 1989. Published by Lexi-Comp Inc. for Medical Center of Delaware: *Formulary and Drug Therapy Guide, 1993–1994*. With permission.

THERAPEUTIC DRUG MONITORING (TDM)*

Selective drugs are monitored by serum and urine for the purpose of achieving and maintaining therapeutic drug effect and for preventing drug toxicity. Drugs with a wide therapeutic range (window), the difference between effective dose and toxic dose, are not usually monitored. Drug monitoring is important in maintaining a drug concentration-response relationship, especially when the serum drug range (window) is narrow, such as with digoxin and lithium. Therapeutic drug monitoring (TDM) is the process of following drug levels and adjusting drug doses to maintain a therapeutic level. Not all drugs can be dosed and/or monitored by their blood levels alone.

Drug levels are obtained at peak time and trough time after a steady state of the drug has occurred in the client. Steady state is reached after four or five half-lives of a drug; thus, the steady state can be reached sooner if the drug has a short half-life. Once steady state is achieved, serum drug level is checked at the peak level (maximum drug concentration) and/or at trough/residual level (minimum drug concentration). If the trough or residual level is at the high therapeutic point, toxicity might occur. Careful assessment is needed by both physical and laboratory means.

TDM is required for drugs with a narrow therapeutic range (window): when other methods for monitoring drugs are noneffective, such as blood pressure (BP) monitoring; for determining when adequate blood concentrations are reached; for evaluating client's compliance to drug therapy; for determining whether other drugs have altered serum drug levels (increased or decreased) that could result in drug toxicity or lack of therapeutic effect; and for establishing new serum-drug level when dosage is changed.

Drug groups for TDM include analgesics, antibiotics, anticonvulsants, antineoplastics, bronchodilators, cardiac drugs, hypoglycemics, sedatives, and tranquilizers. To effectively conduct TDM, the laboratory must be provided with the following information: the drug name and daily dosage, time and amount of last dose, time blood was drawn, route of administration, and client's age. Without complete information, serum drug reporting might be incorrect.

---

*Revised by Ronald J. Lefever, RPh, Pharmacy Services, Medical College of Virginia, Richmond, VA.

Drug	Therapeutic Range	Peak Time	Toxic Level
Acetaminophen (Tylenol)	10–20 μg/mL	1–2.5 h	>50 μg/mL Hepatotoxicity: >200 μg/mL
Acetohexamide (Dymelor)	20–70 μg/mL (should be dosed according to blood glucose levels)	2–4 h	>75 μg/mL
Alcohol	Negative		Mild toxic: 150 mg/dL Marked toxic: >250 mg/L
Alprazolam (Xanax)	10–50 ng/mL	1–2 h	>75 ng/mL
Amikacin (Amikin)	Peak: 20–30 μg/mL Trough: ≤10 μg/mL	IV: ½ hour IM: 0.5–1.5 h	Peak: >35 μg/mL Trough: >10 μg/mL
Aminocaproic acid (Amicar)	100–400 μg/mL	1 h	>400 μg/mL
Aminophylline (see Theophylline)			
Amiodarone (Cordarone)	0.5–2.5 μg/mL	2–10 h	>2.5 μg/mL
Amitriptyline (Elavil)	125–200 ng/mL	2–12 h	>500 ng/mL
Amobarbital (Amytal)	1–5 μg/mL	2 h	>15 μg/mL Severe toxicity: >30 μg/mL
Amoxapine (Asendin)	200–400 ng/mL	1.5 h	>500 ng/mL
Amphetamine: Serum	20–30 ng/mL		0.2 μg/mL
Urine		Detectable in urine after 3 h; positive for 24–48 h	>30 μg/mL urine
Aspirin (see Salicylates)			
Atenolol (Tenormin)	200–500 ng/mL	2–4 h	>500 ng/mL
Bromide	20–80 mg/dL		>100 mg/dL
Butabarbital (Butisol)	1–2 μg/mL	3–4 h	>10 μg/mL
Caffeine	Adult: 3–15 μg/mL Infant: 8–20 μg/mL	0.5–1 h	>50 μg/mL
Carbamazepine (Tegretol)	4–12 μg/mL	6 h (Range 2–24 h)	>9–15 μg/mL
Chloral hydrate (Noctec)	2–12 μg/mL	1–2 h	>20 μg/mL

continued

Drug	Therapeutic Range	Peak Time	Toxic Level
Chloramphenicol (Chloromycetin)	10–20 mg/L		>25 mg/L
Chlordiazepoxide (Librium)	1–5 µg/mL	2–3 h	>5 µg/mL
Chlorpromazine (Thorazine)	50–300 ng/mL	2–4 h	>750 ng/mL
Chlorpropamide (Diabinese)	75–250 µg/mL	3–6 h	>250–750 µg/mL
Clonidine (Catapres)	0.2–2.0 ng/mL (hypotensive effect)	2–5 h	>2.0 ng/mL
Clorazepate (Tranxene)	0.12–1.0 µg/mL	1–2 h	>1.0 µg/mL
Cimetidine (Tagamet)	Trough: 0.5–1.2 µg/mL	1–1.5 h	Trough: >1.5 µg/mL
Clonazepam (Klonopin)	10–60 ng/mL	2 h	>80 ng/mL
Codeine	10–100 ng/mL	1–2 h	>200 ng/mL
Dantrolene (Dantrium)	1–3 µg/mL	5 h	>5 µg/mL
Desipramine (Norpramin)	125–300 ng/mL	4–6 h	>400 ng/mL
Diazepam (Valium)	0.5–2 mg/L 400–600 ng/mL Therapeutic	1–2 h	>3 mg/L >3000 ng/mL
Digitoxin (Rarely administered)	10–25 ng/mL	Noticeable: 2–4 h Peak: 12–24 h	>30 ng/mL
Digoxin	0.5–2 ng/mL	PO: 6–8 h IV: 1.5–2 h	2–3 ng/mL
Dilantin (see Phenytoin)			
Diltiazem (Cardizem)	50–200 ng/mL	2–3 h	>200 ng/mL
Disopyramide (Norpace)	2–4 µg/mL	2 h	>4 µg/mL
Doxepin (Sinequan)	150–300 ng/mL	2–4 h	>500 ng/mL
Ethchlorvynol (Placidyl)	2–8 µg/mL	1–2 h	>20 µg/mL
Ethosuximide (Zarontin)	40–100 µg/mL	2–4 h	>150 µg/mL
Flecainide (Tambocor)	0.2–1.0 µg/mL	3 h	>1.0 µg/mL
Flurazepam (Dalmane)	20–110 ng/mL		>1500 ng/mL
Gentamicin (Garamycin)	Peak: 6–12 µg/mL Trough: <2 µg/mL	IV: 15–30 min	Peak: >12 µg/mL Trough: >2 µg/mL
Glutethimide (Doriden)	2–6 µg/mL	1–2 h	>20 µg/mL

continued

Drug	Therapeutic Range	Peak Time	Toxic Level
Haloperidol (Haldol)	5–15 ng/mL	2–6 h	>50 ng/mL
Hydromorphone (Dilaudid)	1–30 ng/mL	0.5–1.5 h	>100 ng/mL
Ibuprofen (Motrin, etc)	10–50 µg/mL	1–2 h	>100 µg/mL
Imipramine (Tofranil)	150–300 ng/mL	PO: 1–2 h IM: 0.5 h	>500 mg/mL
Isoniazid (INH, Nydrazid)	1–7 µg/mL (Dose usually adjusted based on liver function tests)	1–2 h	>20 µg/mL
Kanamycin (Kantrex)	Peak: 15–30 µg/mL Trough: 1–4 µg/mL	PO: 1–2 h IM: 0.5–1 h	Peak: >35 µg/mL Trough: >10 µg/mL
Lead	<20 µg/dL Urine: >80 µg/24 h		>80 µg/dL Urine: >125 µg/24 h
Lidocaine (Xylocaine)	1.5–5 µg/mL	IV: 10 min	>6 µg/mL
Lithium	0.8–1.2 mEq/L	0.5–4 h	1.5 mEq/L
Lorazepam (Ativan)	50–240 ng/mL	1–3 h	>300 ng/mL
Maprotiline (Ludiomil)	200–300 ng/mL	12 h	>500 ng/mL
Meperidine (Demerol)	0.4–0.7 µg/mL	2–4 h	>1.0 µg/mL
Mephenytoin (Mesantoin)	15–40 µg/mL	2–4 h	>50 µg/mL
Meprobamate (Equanil, Miltown)	15–25 µg/mL	2 h	>50 µg/mL
Methadone (Dolophine)	100–400 ng/mL	0.5–1 h	>2,000 ng/mL or >0.2 µg/mL
Methyldopa (Aldomet)	1–5 µg/mL	3–6 h	>7 µg/mL
Methyprylon (Noludar)	8–10 µg/mL	1–2 h	>50 µg/mL
Metoprolol (Lopressor)	75–200 ng/mL	2–4 h	>225 ng/mL
Mexiletine (Mexitil)	0.5–2 µg/mL	2–3 h	>2 µg/mL
Morphine	10–80 ng/mL	IV: Immediately IM: 0.5–1 h SC: 1–1.5 h	>200 ng/mL
Netilmicin (Netromycin)	Peak: 0.5–10 µg/mL Trough: <4 µg/mL	IV: 0.5 h	Peak: >16 µg/mL Trough: >4 µg/mL
Nifedipine (Procardia)	50–100 ng/mL	0.5–2 h	>100 ng/mL
Nortriptyline (Aventyl)	50–150 ng/mL	8 h	>200 ng/ml
Oxazepam (Serax)	0.2–1.4 µg/mL	1–2 h	—
Oxycodone (Percodan)	10–100 ng/mL	0.5–1 h	>200 ng/mL

continued

Drug	Therapeutic Range	Peak Time	Toxic Level
Pentazocine (Talwin)	0.05–0.2 µg/mL	1–2 h	>1.0 µg/mL Urine: >30 µg/mL
Pentobarbital (Nembutal)	1–5 µg/mL	0.5–1 h	>10 µg/mL Severe toxicity: >30 µg/mL
Phenmetrazine (Preludin)	5–30 µg/mL (urine)	2 h	>50 µg/mL (urine)
Phenobarbital (Luminal)	15–40 µg/mL	6–18 h	>40 µg/mL Severe toxicity: >80 µg/mL
Phenytoin (Dilantin)	10–20 µg/mL	4–8 h	>20–30 µg/mL Severe toxicity: >40 µg/mL
Pindolol (Visken)	0.5–6.0 ng/mL	2–4 h	>10 ng/mL
Primidone (Mysoline)	5–12 µg/mL	2–4 h	>12–15 µg/mL
Procainamide (Pronestyl)	4–10 µg/mL	1 h	>10 µg/mL
Procaine (Novocain)	<11 µg/mL	10–30 min	>20 µg/mL
Prochlorperazine (Compazine)	50–300 ng/mL	2–4 h	>1,000 ng/mL
Propoxyphene (Darvon)	0.1–0.4 µg/mL	2–3 h	>0.5 µg/mL
Propranolol (Inderal)	>100 ng/mL	1–2 h	>150 ng/mL
Protriptyline (Vivactil)	50–150 ng/mL	8–12 h	>200 ng/mL
Quinidine	2–5 µg/mL	1–3 h	>6 µg/mL
Ranitidine (Zantac)	100 ng/mL	2–3 h	>100 ng/mL
Reserpine (Serpasil)	20 ng/mL	2–4 h	>20 ng/mL
Salicylates (Aspirin)	10–30 mg/dL	1–2 h	Tinnitus: >20–40 mg/mL Hyperventilation: >35 mg/dL Severe toxicity: >50 mg/dL
Secobarbital (Seconal)	2–5 µg/mL	1 h	>15 µg/mL Severe toxicity: >30 µg/mL
Theophylline (Thodur, Aminodur)	10–20 µg/mL	PO: 2–3 h IV: 15 min (Depends on smoking or nonsmoking)	>20 µg/mL
Thioridazine (Mellaril)	100–600 ng/mL 1.0–1.5 µg/mL	2–4 h	>2,000 ng/mL >10 µg/mL

continued

Drug	Therapeutic Range	Peak Time	Toxic Level
Timolol (Blocadren)	3–55 ng/mL	1–2 h	>60 ng/mL
Tobramycin (Nebcin)	Peak: 5–10 µg/mL Trough: 1–1.5 µg/mL	IV: 15–30 min IM: 0.5–1.5 h	Peak: >12 µg/mL Trough: >2 µg/mL
Tocainide (Tonocard)	4–10 µg/mL	0.5–3 h	>12 µg/mL
Tolbutamide (Orinase)	80–240 µg/mL	3–5 h	>640 µg/mL
Trazodone (Desyrel)	500–2500 ng/mL	1–2 wk	>4,000 ng/mL
Trifluoperazine (Stelazine)	50–300 ng/mL	2–4 h	>1,000 ng/mL
Valproic acid (Depakene)	50–100 µg/mL	0.5–1.5 h	>100 µg/mL Severe toxicity: >150 µg/mL
Vancomycin (Vanocin)	Peak: 20–40 µg/mL Trough: 5–10 µg/mL	IV: Peak: 5 min IV: Trough: 12 h	Peak: >80 µg/mL
Verapamil (Calan)	100–300 ng/mL	PO: 1–2 h IV: 5 min	>500 ng/mL
Warfarin (Coumadin)	1–10 µg/mL (Dose usually adjusted by 1 to 2.5 × control)	1.5–3 d	>10 µg/mL

Source: Kee, J. L. (1995): *Laboratory and Diagnostic Tests With Nursing Implications* (4th ed). Norwalk, CT: Appleton and Lange. (Used with permission.)

POCKET COMPANION FOR
PHARMACOLOGY
A Nursing Process Approach

VITAMINS, MINERALS, AND ELECTROLYTES

Vitamin A, Fat-Soluble

Antianemia, Mineral: Iron

Electrolyte:
  Potassium
  Calcium

Prototype: Vitamin A, fat-soluble

Vitamin A

Vitamin A
  (Acon, Aquasol A)
Fat-soluble vitamin
Pregnancy Category: A
Drug Forms:
Liquid (gtt) 5,000 U / 0.1 mL
Cap 50,000 U
Inj 50,000 U/mL

Dosage

A & C > 8 y: PO: 100,000–500,000 IU daily × 3 d; then 50,000 daily × 14 d
Maintenance: 10,000–20,000 IU q.d. × 60 d
C 1–8 y: IM: 17,000–35,000 IU daily × 10 d
Maintenance:
4–8 yr: 15,000 daily × 60 d
1–<4 y: 10,000 IU daily × 60 d

Contraindications

Hypervitaminosis A, pregnancy (massive doses)

Drug-Lab-Food Interactions

Decreased absorption of mineral oil, cholestyramine, oral contraceptives, corticosteroids

Pharmacokinetics

Absorption: PO: 1 h
Distribution: PB: UK
Metabolism: t 1/2: weeks–months
Excretion: Urine and feces

Pharmacodynamics

PO: Onset: 1–2 h
  Peak: 4–5 h
  Duration: UK

Therapeutic Effects/Uses: To treat vitamin A deficiency, prevent night blindness, treat skin disorders, promote bone development
Mode of action: Essential for growth, bone and teeth development, vision, integrity of skin and mucous membrane, and reproduction

Side Effects

Headache, fatigue, drowsiness, irritability, anorexia, vomiting, diarrhea, dry skin, visual changes

Adverse Reactions

Evident only with toxicity: leukopenia, aplastic anemia, papilledema, increased intracranial pressure, hypervitaminosis A

KEY: For complete abbreviation key, see inside front cover.

■ NURSING PROCESS: Vitamin A

ASSESSMENT
- Assess the client for vitamin A deficiency before start of and regularly throughout therapy. Explore such areas as inadequate nutrient intake, debilitating disease, and GI disorders.
- Assess 24–48-h diet history for foods rich in vitamin A.

POTENTIAL NURSING DIAGNOSIS
- Altered nutrition; less than body requirements

Vitamin A, fat-soluble

PLANNING
- Client will eat a well-balanced diet that includes the foods and servings recommended in the food pyramid.
- Client with vitamin deficiency will take vitamin supplements as prescribed.

NURSING INTERVENTIONS
- Administer vitamin A with food to promote absorption.
- Store drug in light-resistant container.
- When administering drop form, use the supplied calibrated dropper for accurate dosage. Solution may be administered mixed with food or dropped into the mouth.
- Administer IM primarily for clients unable to take by PO route (e.g., GI malabsorption syndrome).
- Recognize need for vitamin E supplements for infants receiving vitamin A to avoid hemolytic anemia.

CLIENT TEACHING
General
- Instruct client to take the prescribed amount of drug.
- Discourage the client from taking megavitamins over a long period unless these are prescribed for a specific purpose by the health care provider. To discontinue long-term megavitamin therapy, a gradual decrease in vitamin intake is advised to avoid a vitamin deficiency. Megadoses of vitamin A can be toxic.
- Inform the client that missing vitamins for 1 or 2 d is not a cause for concern because deficiencies do not occur for some time.
- Advise the client to check the expiration dates on vitamin containers before purchasing and taking them. Potency of the vitamin is reduced after the expiration date.
- Instruct the client to avoid taking mineral oil with vitamin A on a regular basis because it interferes with the absorption of the vitamin. If needed, take mineral oil at bedtime.

Diet
- Advise the client to eat a well-balanced diet that includes the recommended amounts and types of food detailed in the food pyramid. Vitamin supplements are not necessary if the person is healthy and receives proper nutrition on a regular basis.
- Instruct the client about foods rich in vitamin A, including whole milk, butter, eggs, leafy green and yellow vegetables, fruits, and liver.

Side Effects
- Instruct the client that nausea, vomiting, headache, loss of hair, and cracked lips (symptoms of hypervitaminosis A) should be reported to health care provider.

EVALUATION
- Evaluate the effectiveness of the client's diet for the inclusion of the appropriate amounts and types of food from the food pyramid. Have client keep periodic diet chart for a complete week.
- Determine if the client with malnutrition is receiving appropriate vitamin therapy.

Vitamins, Functions, Suggested Food Sources, and Selected Deficiency Conditions

Vitamin (Adult RDA)	Function	Food Sources	Deficiency Conditions
A (800–1000 µg)	Required to develop and maintain healthy eyes, gums, teeth, skin, hair, and selected glands. Needed for fat metabolism.	Whole milk, butter, eggs, leafy green and yellow vegetables,* fruits, liver	Dry skin, poor tooth development, night blindness
B_1 (thiamine) (1.0–1.5 mg)	Promotes use of sugars (energy). Required for good function of nervous system and heart.	Enriched breads and cereals, yeast, liver, pork, fish, milk	Sensory disturbances, retarded growth, fatigue, anorexia
B_2 (riboflavin) (1.2–1.7 mg)	Promotes body's use of carbohydrates, proteins, and fats by releasing energy to cells. Required for tissue integrity.	Milk, enriched breads and cereals, liver, lean meat, eggs, leafy green vegetables†	Visual defects, such as blurred vision and photophobia; cheilosis; rash on nose; numbness of extremities
B_3 (pyridoxine) (1.6–2 mg)	Important in metabolism, synthesis of proteins, and formation of RBCs	Lean meat, leafy green vegetables, whole-grain cereals, yeast, bananas	Neuritis, convulsions, dermatitis, anemia, lymphopenia
B_{12} (cobalamin) (2.0 mg)	Functions as a building block of nucleic acids and to form RBCs. Facilitates functioning of nervous system.	Liver, kidney, fish, milk	Gastrointestinal disorders, poor growth, anemias
Biotin (no RDA)	Synthesis of fatty acids and energy production from glucose. Required by body chemical systems.	Eggs, milk, leafy green vegetables, liver, kidney.	Natural deficiency unknown in humans

C (ascorbic acid) (60 mg)	Helps tissue repair and growth. Required in formation of collagen.	Citrus fruits, tomatoes, leafy green vegetables, potatoes	Poor wound healing, bleeding gums, scurvy, predisposition to infection
D calciferol (5 µg)	Promotes use of phosphorus and calcium. Important for strong teeth and bones.	Vitamin D-fortified milk, egg yolk, tuna, salmon	Rickets, deficit of phosphorus and calcium in blood
E tocopherol (8–10 mg)	Protects fatty acids and promotes the formation and functioning of RBCs, muscle, and other tissues.	Whole-grain cereals, wheat germ, vegetable oils, lettuce	Breakdown of RBCs
Folic acid[‡] (180–200 µg)	Helps in formation of genetic materials and proteins for the cell nucleus. Assists with intestinal functioning and prevents selected anemias.	Leafy green vegetables, yellow fruits and vegetables, yeast, meats	Decreased WBC count and clotting factors, anemias, intestinal disturbances, depression
K (60–80 µg)	Essential for blood clotting.	Leafy green vegetables, liver, cheese, egg yolk	Increased clotting time, leading to increased bleeding and hemorrhage
Niacin (13–19 mg)	In all body tissues. Necessary for energy-producing reactions. Assists nervous system.	Eggs, meat, liver, beans, peas, enriched bread, and cereals	Retarded growth, pellegra, headache, memory loss, anorexia, insomnia
Pantothenic acid (no RDA)	Promotes body's use of carbohydrates, fats, and proteins. Essential for formation of specific hormones and nerve-regulating substances.	Eggs, leafy green vegetables, nuts, liver, kidney, skimmed milk	Natural deficiency unknown in humans

---

RDAs are daily nutrient allowances recommended for healthy adults by the National Research Council, American Institute for Cancer Research.
* Yellow fruits and vegetables include apricots, cantaloupe, carrots, rutabaga, pumpkin, squash, and sweet potatoes.
† Leafy green vegetables include brussel spouts, chard, broccoli, kale, spinach, and turnip and mustard greens.
‡ Women of childbearing age should consume 400 µg/d of folic acid.

Prototype: Antianemia, Mineral: Iron

Iron

Ferrous sulfate (Feosol, Fer-Iron)
Ferrous gluconate (Fergon, Fetinic)
Ferrous fumarate (Feostat, Fumerin)
Mineral
Pregnancy Category: A
Drug Forms:
Sulfate
Tab 195, 300, 325 mg
Tab, enteric-coated 325 mg
Tab, extended-release 525 mg
Cap, time-release 525 mg

Dosage

A: PO: 300–325 mg q.i.d.: increase to 650 mg q.i.d. as needed and/or tolerated
Pregnancy: PO: 300–600 mg/d
C ≥2 y: PO: 8 mg/kg q.d. in divided doses

Contraindications

Hemolytic anemia, peptic ulcer, ulcerative colitis

Drug-Lab-Food Interactions

Increased effect of iron with vitamin C; *decreased* effect of tetracycline, antacids, penicillamine

Pharmacokinetics

Absorption: PO: 5–30% intestines
Distribution: PB: UK
Metabolism: t 1/2: UK
Excretion: Urine, feces, bile

Pharmacodynamics

PO: Onset: 4 d
　　Peak: 7–14 d
　　Duration: 3–4 mon

Therapeutic Effects/Uses: To prevent and treat iron deficiency anemia
Mode of Action: Enables RBC development and oxygen transport via hemoglobin

Side Effects

Nausea, vomiting, diarrhea, constipation, epigastric pain; elixir may stain teeth

Adverse Reactions

Pallor, drowsiness
Life-threatening: Cardiovascular collapse, metabolic acidosis

KEY: For complete abbreviation key, see inside front cover.

■ NURSING PROCESS: Antianemia, Mineral: Iron

ASSESSMENT
- Obtain a history of anemia or health problems that may lead to anemia.
- Assess the client for signs and symptoms of iron deficiency anemia, such as fatigue, malaise, pallor, shortness of breath, tachycardia, and cardiac dysrhythmia.
- Assess the client's RBC count, hemoglobin, hematocrit, iron level, and reticulocyte count before start of and throughout drug therapy.

POTENTIAL NURSING DIAGNOSIS
- Fatigue
- Altered nutrition; less than body requirements

Antianemia, Mineral: Iron

PLANNING
- Client will consume foods rich in iron.
- Client with iron deficiency anemia or with low hemoglobin will take iron replacement as recommended by the health care provider, resulting in laboratory results within the desired range.

NURSING INTERVENTIONS
- Encourage the client to eat a nutritious diet to obtain sufficient iron. Iron supplements are not needed unless the person is malnourished or pregnant.
- Store drug in light-resistant container.
- Administer IM injection of iron by the Z-track method to avoid leakage of iron into the subcutaneous tissue and skin because it irritates and stains the skin.

CLIENT TEACHING

General
- Instruct the client to take the tablet or capsule between meals with at least 8 oz of juice or water to promote absorption. If gastric irritation occurs, instruct to take with food.
- Advise client to swallow whole the tablet or capsule.
- Instruct client to maintain sitting upright position for 30 min to prevent esophageal corrosion from reflux.
- Do not administer the drug within 1 h of ingesting antacid or milk.
- Advise client to increase fluids, activity, and dietary bulk to avoid or relieve constipation. Slow-release iron capsules decrease constipation and gastric irritation.
- Instruct adults not to leave iron tablets within reach of children. If a child swallows many tablets, induce vomiting and immediately call the local poison control center; the telephone number is in the front of most telephone books (include this number on emergency reference list).
- Instruct client to take prescribed amount of drug to avoid iron poisoning.
- Be alert that iron content varies among iron salts; therefore, do not substitute one for another.
- Advise client that drug treatment for anemia is generally less than 6 mo.

Diet
- Counsel the client to include iron-rich foods in diet, such as liver, lean meats, egg yolk, dried beans, green vegetables, and fruit.

Side Effects
- Instruct the client taking the liquid iron preparation to use a straw to prevent discoloration of teeth enamel.
- Alert the client that the drug turns stools a harmless black or dark green.
- Instruct client about signs and symptoms of toxicity, including nausea, vomiting, diarrhea, pallor, hematemesis, shock, and coma, and report occurrence to health care provider.

EVALUATION
- Evaluate the effectiveness of the drug therapy by determining that the client is not fatigued or short of breath and that the hemoglobin is within the desired range.

Prototype: Electrolyte: Potassium

Potassium

Potassium chloride
  (Kaochlor, Kaon-Cl, Kay Ciel, Micro-K, K-Dur)
Potassium replacement
Pregnancy Category: A
Drug Forms:
Tablet, SR cap, elixir, liq mEq/5 mL
  Inj (mEq/mL): All in various doses

Dosage

A: *Hypokalemia (maintenance):*
PO: 20 mEq in 1–2 divided doses
Hypokalemia (correction):
PO: 40–80 mEq in 3–4 divided doses
IV: 20–40 mEq diluted in 1L of IV solution

Contraindications

Renal insufficiency or failure, Addison's disease, hyperkalemia, severe dehydration, acidosis, potassium-sparing diuretics
Caution:
Cardiac disorders, burns

Drug-Lab-Food Interactions

Increase serum potassium level with ACE inhibitors, potassium-sparing diuretics
Lab: May *increase* serum potassium level (>5.5 mEq/L)

Pharmacokinetics

Absorption: PO: rapidly absorbed, 95% in body fluids
Distribution: PB: UK
Metabolism: t 1/2: UK
Excretion: 80–90% in urine; 10% in feces

Pharmacodynamics

PO: Onset: 30 min
  Peak: 1–2 h
  Duration: UK
IV: Onset: Rapid
  Peak: 1–1.5 h
  Duration: UK

Therapeutic Effects/Uses: To correct potassium deficit; strengthen cardiac and muscular activities

Mode of action: Transmits and conducts nerve impulses; contracts skeletal, smooth, and cardiac muscles

Side Effects

Nausea, vomiting, diarrhea, abdominal cramps, irritability, rash (rare)

Adverse Reactions

Oliguria, ECG changes (peaked T waves, widened QRS complex, prolonged PR interval), GI ulceration
Life-threatening: Cardiac dysrhythmias, respiratory distress, cardiac arrest

KEY: For complete abbreviation key, see inside front cover.

Electrolyte: Potassium

■ NURSING PROCESS: Electrolyte: Potassium

ASSESSMENT
- Assess for signs and symptoms of hypokalemia (decreased serum potassium) and hyperkalemia (elevated serum potassium). Symptoms of hypokalemia include nausea, vomiting, cardiac dysrhythmias, abdominal distension, and soft flabby muscles. Symptoms of hyperkalemia include oliguria, nausea, abdominal cramps, and tachycardia and, later, bradycardia, weakness, and numbness or tingling in the extremities.
- Assess serum potassium level; normal serum potassium level is 3.5–5.3 mEq/L. Report serum potassium deficit or excess to the physician or health care prescriber.
- Obtain baseline VS and ECG readings. Report abnormal findings. The VS and ECG results can be compared with future VS and ECG readings.
- Assess the client for signs and symptoms of digitalis toxicity when receiving a digitalis preparation (digoxin) and a potassium-wasting diuretic (chlorohydrothiazide, furosemide) or a cortisone preparation (prednisone). A decreased serum potassium level enhances the action of digitalis. Signs and symptoms of digitalis toxicity are nausea, vomiting, anorexia, bradycardia (pulse rate <60 or markedly decreased), cardiac dysrhythmias, and visual disturbances.

POTENTIAL NURSING DIAGNOSIS
- Altered nutrition, less than body requirements.
- Impaired tissue integrity.

PLANNING
- Client's serum potassium level will be within normal range in 2–4 d.
- Client with hypokalemia will eat foods rich in potassium, such as fruits, fruit juices, and vegetables. Client with hyperkalemia will avoid potassium-rich foods.

NURSING INTERVENTIONS
- Give oral potassium with a sufficient amount of water or juice (at least 6–8 oz) or at mealtime. Potassium is extremely irritating to the gastric mucosa.
- Dilute IV potassium chloride in the IV bag and invert the bag several times to promote thorough mixing of potassium with IV fluids. Potassium CANNOT be given IM. **Potassium should never be given as an IV bolus or push.** Giving IV potassium directly into the vein causes cardiac dysrhythmias and cardiac arrest.
- Monitor the amount of urine output. If the client is receiving potassium and the urine output is <25 mL/h or <600 mL/d, potassium accumulation occurs. Remember, 80–90% of potassium is excreted in the urine. Report results to the health care provider.
- Monitor the serum potassium level. Hypokalemia occurs if the serum potassium value is <3.5 mEq/L; hyperkalemia occurs when the serum potassium value is >5.3 mEq/L.
- Monitor the ECG. With hypokalemia, the T wave is flat or inverted, the ST segment is depressed, and the QT interval is prolonged. With hyperkalemia, the T wave is narrow and peaked, the QRS complex is spread, and the PR interval is prolonged.
- Check the IV site for infiltration if the client is receiving potassium in the IV fluids. Potassium can cause tissue necrosis if it infiltrates into the fatty

Electrolyte: Potassium

tissue (subcutaneous tissue). The IV fluid with potassium should be discontinued when infiltration occurs.
● Monitor clients receiving various medications for hyperkalemia, such as sodium bicarbonate, calcium gluconate, insulin and glucose, and Kayexalate and sorbitol, for signs and symptoms of continuing hyperkalemia or of developing hypokalemia.
● Prepare and administer Kayexalate orally or by retention enema. Prepare according to the drug circular. The client should have a cleansing enema before the retention enema.

CLIENT TEACHING
General
● Advise the client to have serum potassium level checked at regular intervals when taking drugs that are potassium supplements or that decrease potassium levels.
● Instruct the client to drink a full glass of water or juice when taking oral potassium supplements. Potassium preparations can be taken during or after a meal. Explain to the client that potassium is very irritating to the stomach.
● Instruct the client to comply with the prescribed potassium dose, regular laboratory tests, and medical follow-up related to the health problem and drug regimen.

Diet
● Instruct the client who is taking a potassium-wasting diuretic or a cortisone preparation to eat potassium-rich foods, including citrus fruit juice, fruits (bananas, plums, oranges, canteloupes, raisins), vegetables, and nuts.

Side Effects
● Instruct the client to report signs and symptoms of hypokalemia and hyperkalemia. See assessment for the list. When taking large amounts of potassium supplements, hyperkalemia could result.

EVALUATION
● Evaluate the client's serum potassium level and ECG. Report to the health care provider if the level remains abnormal. Potassium replacements and diet may need modification.

Electrolyte: Potassium

Selected Potassium Supplements

Preparation	Drug
PO liquid	Potassium chloride: 10% = 20 mEq/15 mL, 20% = 40 mEq/15 mL. Kaochlor 10% (potassium chloride) Kaon-Cl 20% (potassium chloride) Kay Ciel (potassium chloride) Potassium triplex (potassium acetate, bicarbonate, citrate). Rarely used.
PO tablet or capsule	Kaochlor (potassium chloride) Kaon (potassium gluconate) Kaon-Cl (potassium chloride) K-Dur (potassium chloride) K-Lyte (potassium bicarbonate, effervescent tablet) K-Lyte/Cl (potassium chloride) K-Tab (potassium chloride) Micro-K (potassium chloride) Potassium chloride (enteric-coated tablet) Slow-K (potassium chloride, 8 mEq) Ten-K (potassium chloride)
IV potassium	Potassium chloride in clear liquid in multidose vial or ampule (2 mEq/mL)

Prototype: Electrolyte: Calcium

Calcium

Calcium chloride (IV)
Calcium carbonate
  (Os-Cal, Tums, Caltrate, Mega-Cal)
Calcium gluconate (Kalcinate)
Calcium lactate
Calcium replacement
Pregnancy Category: C
Drug Forms: Tab, cap, liq, inj

Dosage

Antacid use:
A: PO: 0.5–1 g q4–6h (dose varies according to the calcium salt)
Osteoporosis:
A: PO: 1–2 g b.i.d.
  IV: 0.5–1 g q.d., q.o.d.
Tetany:
A: IV 4–16 mEq
C: IV: 0.5–0.7 mEq/kg t.i.d., q.i.d.
Hypocalcemia
C: PO: 500 mg/d in divided doses

Contraindications

Hypercalcemia, renal calculi, digitalis toxicity, ventricular fibrillation
Caution:
Renal or respiratory disorders, GI hypomotility

Drug-Lab-Food Interactions

Increase digitalis toxicity: digoxin; *Decrease* calcium effect: saline solution; *decrease* effect of calcium channel blockers, verapamil; *decrease* absorption of tetracycline; *increase* serum calcium level: thiazide diuretics

Pharmacokinetics

Absorption: PO: 35% absorbed, requires vitamin D
Distribution: PB: UK
Metabolism: t 1/2: UK
Excretion: 20% in urine; 70% in feces, some in saliva

Pharmacodynamics

PO: Onset: UK
  Peak: UK
  Duration: 2–4 h
IV: Onset: Rapid
  Peak: UK
  Duration: 2–3 h

Therapeutic Effects/Uses: To correct calcium deficit or tetany symptoms, prevent osteoporosis

Mode of Action: Transmits nerve impulses, contracts skeletal and cardiac muscles, maintains cellular permeability; promotes strong bone and teeth growth

Side Effects

Nausea, vomiting, constipation, pain, drowsiness, headache, muscle weakness

Adverse Reactions

Hypercalcemia, ECG changes (shortened QT interval), metabolic alkalosis, heart block, rebound hyperacidity
Life-threatening: Renal failure, cardiac dysrhythmias, cardiac arrest

KEY: For complete abbreviation key, see inside front cover.

Electrolyte: Calcium

■ NURSING PROCESS: Electrolyte: Calcium

ASSESSMENT

- Assess the client for signs and symptoms of hypocalcemia (decreased serum calcium), such as tetany (twitching of the mouth, tingling and numbness of the fingers, facial spasms, spasms of the larynx, and carpopedal spasm), muscle cramps, bleeding tendencies, and weak cardiac contractions.
- Check the serum calcium levels (normal, 4.5–5.5 mEq/L or 8.5–10.5 mg/dL) for hypocalcemia and hypercalcemia. Report abnormal test results. Serum ionized calcium (iCa) indicates free circulating calcium and is more accurate for determining calcium imbalance.
- Obtain VS and ECG readings. Report abnormal findings. VS and ECG results can be compared with future VS and ECG readings.
- Obtain a current drug history for the client. Calcium enhances the effect of digoxin. An elevated serum calcium level (due to excess calcium), when taken with digoxin, can cause digitalis toxicity. Signs and symptoms of digitalis toxicity include nausea, vomiting, anorexia, bradycardia (pulse rate <60 or markedly decreased), cardiac dysrhythmias, and visual disturbances. Thiazide diuretics can increase the serum calcium level. Drugs that decrease the effect of calcium are calcium channel blockers, tetracycline, and sodium chloride.

POTENTIAL NURSING DIAGNOSIS

- Altered nutrition, less than body requirements.
- Impaired tissue integrity.

PLANNING

- Client's serum calcium level will be within normal range by 3–7 d.
- Tetany symptoms will cease. Client will eat foods rich in calcium or take calcium supplements as ordered.
- Client with hypercalcemia will avoid foods rich in calcium, such as milk products.

NURSING INTERVENTIONS

- Monitor VS. Report abnormal findings. Compare with baseline VS. Monitor pulse rate if the client is taking digoxin. Bradycardia is a sign of digitalis toxicity.
- Administer IV fluids slowly with 10% calcium gluconate or chloride. Calcium should be administered with D_5W and not saline solution because sodium promotes calcium loss. Calcium should not be added to solutions containing bicarbonate because rapid precipitation occurs.
- Check IV site for infiltration if the client is receiving calcium in IV fluids. Calcium can cause tissue necrosis (sloughing of the tissue) if it infiltrates into the subcutaneous tissue. Calcium gluceptate is the only calcium preparation that can be given IM.
- Monitor the serum calcium and iCa levels. Hypocalcemia occurs if the serum calcium value is <4.5 mEq/L or <8.5 mg/dL or if iCa is <2.2 mEq/L. Hypercalcemia occurs if the serum calcium value is >5.5 mEq/L or >10.5 mg/dL or if iCa is >2.5 mEq/L.
- Monitor ECGs. With hypocalcemia, the ST segment is lengthened and the QT interval is prolonged. With hypercalcemia, the ST segment is decreased and the QT interval is shortened.

Electrolyte: Calcium

CLIENT TEACHING

General

- Instruct the client to avoid overuse of antacids and to prevent the habit of chronic use of laxatives. Excessive use of certain antacids may cause alkalosis, decreasing calcium ionization. Chronic use of laxatives decreases calcium absorption from the GI tract. Suggest fruits and foods rich in fiber for improving bowel elimination.
- Instruct the client taking calcium supplements to check that the calcium tablet is absorbable. To do this, put 1 tablet into 1 oz of white vinegar. Stir every 3 min. The tablet should break up or dissolve within 30 min.
- Take oral calcium supplements with meals or after meals to increase absorption.

Diet

- Suggest that the client consume foods high in calcium, such as milk, milk products, and protein-rich foods. Protein and vitamin D are needed to enhance calcium absorption.

Side Effects

- Instruct the client to report symptoms related to calcium excess or hypercalcemia, including flabby muscles, pain over bony areas, ECG changes, and kidney (calcium form) stones.

EVALUATION

- Evaluate the client's serum calcium level. Report if calcium imbalance continues.
- Determine if side effects due to previous untreated hypocalcemia are absent.

CENTRAL NERVOUS SYSTEM STIMULANTS AND DEPRESSANTS

Central Nervous System Stimulant

Sedative-Hypnotic:
Barbiturate
Benzodiazepine

Analgesic:
Aspirin
Acetaminophen

Narcotic:
Opiate: Morphine Sulfate
Nonopiate: Meperidine
Agonist-Antagonist: Pentazocine Lactate

Prototype: Central Nervous System Stimulant

Methylphenidate HCl

Methylphenidate HCl (Ritalin, Ritalin SR)
Cerebral stimulant
CSS II
Pregnancy Category: C
Drug Forms:
Tab 5, 10, 20 mg
Tab SR 20 mg

Dosage

Attention deficit disorder:
C > 6 y: PO: 5 mg before breakfast and lunch; if necessary increase dosage weekly by 5–10 mg; max: 60 mg/d
SR not recommended for initial treatment
Narcolepsy:
A: PO: 10 mg b.i.d./t.i.d. 30 min before meals

Contraindications

Hypersensitivity, hyperthyroidism, anxiety, history of seizures or Tourette syndrome
Caution: Hypertension, depression, pregnancy

Drug-Lab-Food Interactions

Hypertensive crises within 14 days of MAOIs
Decrease effects of decongestants, antihypertensives, barbiturates
Increase effects of oral anticoagulants, anticonvulsants, tricyclic antidepressants

Food: Caffeine (coffee, tea, colas, chocolate)

Pharmacokinetics

Absorption: PO: well absorbed; SR: delayed
Distribution: PB: UK
Metabolism: t 1/2: 1–3 h
Excretion: In urine 40% unchanged

Pharmacodynamics

PO: Onset: 0.5–1 h
    Peak: 1–3 h
    Duration: 4–6 h
PO: Onset: UK
    Peak: UK
    Duration: 4–8 h

Therapeutic Effects/Uses: Adjunct to treatment to correct hyperactivity caused by attention deficit disorder (ADD), to increase attention span, to treat fatigue, and to control narcolepsy.

Mode of Action: Respiratory and CNS stimulation; exact drug action unknown.

Side Effects

Anorexia, restlessness, nervousness, headache, dizziness, irritability, insomnia, vomiting, diarrhea, talkativeness

Adverse Reactions

Tachycardia, palpitations, transient loss of weight gain in children, growth suppression, increased hyperactivity
Life-threatening: Exfoliative dermatitis, uremia, thrombocytopenia

---

KEY: For complete abbreviation key, see inside front cover.

■ NURSING PROCESS: Central Nervous System Stimulant: Methylphenidate HCl (Ritalin)

ASSESSMENT

- Determine if there is a history of heart disease, hypertension, hyperthyroidism, or glaucoma; in such cases, drug is usually contraindicated.

Central Nervous System Stimulant

- Assess vital signs to be used for future comparisons. Pay close attention to clients with cardiac disease as drug may reverse effects of antihypertensives.
- Assess the client's mental status: e.g., mood, affect, aggressiveness.
- Assess height, growth, and weight of children.
- Assess CBC, differential WBCs, and platelets before and during therapy.

POTENTIAL NURSING DIAGNOSES
- Behavior disorders (impulsiveness, short attention span, and distractibility) that interfere with peer relationships, learning, and discipline.
- Potential for family crisis related to dysfunctional behavior.

PLANNING
- Client will be free of hyperactivity.
- Client will not experience side effects or adverse reactions to therapy. Child will increase attention span and ability to organize.

NURSING INTERVENTIONS
- Monitor vital signs. Report irregularities.
- Monitor height, weight, and growth of child.
- Monitor the client for withdrawal symptoms, e.g., nausea, vomiting, weakness, headache.
- Monitor the client for side effects, e.g., insomnia, restlessness, nervousness, tremors, irritability, tachycardia, or elevated blood pressure. Report findings.

CLIENT TEACHING
General
- Instruct the client to take drug before meals.
- Instruct the client to avoid alcohol consumption.
- Encourage the use of sugarless gum to relieve dry mouth.
- Instruct the client to monitor weight 2×/wk and to report weight loss.
- Instruct the client to avoid driving and using hazardous equipment when experiencing tremors, nervousness, or increased heart rate.
- Instruct the client not to abruptly discontinue the drug; the dose must be tapered off to avoid withdrawal symptoms. Consult the health care provider before modifying the dose.
- Encourage the client to read the labels on OTC products because many contain caffeine. A high caffeine plasma level could be fatal.
- Instruct the nursing mother to avoid taking all CNS stimulants. These drugs pass into the breast milk and can cause the infant to be "jittery."
- Encourage the family to seek counseling for children with attention deficit disorder. Drug therapy alone is not an appropriate therapy program. Notify school nurse of drug therapy regimen.
- Explain to client/family that long-term use may lead to drug abuse.

Diet
- Instruct the client to avoid caffeine-containing foods.
- Instruct parents to provide children with a good-quality breakfast because drug may have anorexic effects.

Side Effects
- Instruct the client about drug side effects and the need to report tachycardia and palpitations. Monitor children for onset of Tourette syndrome.

EVALUATION
- Evaluate the effectiveness of drug therapy. The client is not hyperactive and does not have adverse effects from drug.
- Monitor weight, sleep patterns, and mental status.

Amphetamines and Amphetamine-like Drug

Generic (Brand)	Route and Dosage	Preg Cat	Interaction	t 1/2	PB	Onset	Peak	Duration
Amphetamines Amphetamine sulfate CSS II	Narcolepsy: A: PO: 5–20 mg q.d.–t.i.d.; max: 60 mg/d C >6–12 y: PO: 5 mg daily ADD: C 3–5 y: PO: 2.5 mg/d C 6–12 y: PO: 5 mg/d max: 40 mg/d	C	*Decrease* effects of tricyclic antidepressants, barbiturates; hypertensive crisis within 14 d of MAOIs	10–30 h	UK	30–45 min	1–3 h	4–20 h
Dextroamphetamine sulfate (Dexedrine) CSS II	Same as amphetamine sulfate	C	Similar to amphetamine sulfate	10–30 h	UK	30 min	1–3 h	4–20 h
Methamphetamine HCl (Desoxyn) CSS II	C: PO: 2.5–5 mg daily; increase to 20 mg as needed in 2 divided doses	C	Similar to amphetamine sulfate	UK	UK	UK	6–12 h	3–6 h
Amphetamine-like Drugs Methylphenidate (Ritalin) CSS II	See Prototype Drug Chart					ADD: days–weeks CNS stimulants: UK		
Pemoline (Cylert) CSS IV	C >6 y: PO: 37.5 mg daily and increase weekly; average: 50–75 mg/d; max: 112.5 mg/d	B	*Increase* effects with other CNS stimulants	9–12 h	50%		2–3 wk	days
							2–4 h	8 h

Anorexiants							
Benzphetamine HCl (Didrex) CSS III	A: PO: 25–50 mg q.d.–t.i.d.	X	Hypertensive crisis may result if given within 14 d of MAOIs *Increase* effects with tricyclic antidepressants	6–12 h	UK	30 min	1–4 h	4–20 h
Dextroamphetamine sulfate (Dexedrine) CSS II	A: PO: 5–30 mg daily in divided doses 30–60 min ac of 5–10 mg	C	*Decrease* effects of tricyclic antidepressants, barbiturates; may have hypertensive crisis within 14 d of MAOIs	30–34 h	UK	30 min	1–3 h	4–20 h
Diethylpropion HCl (Dospan, Tenuate, Tepanil) CSS IV	A: PO: 25 mg t.i.d.; SR: 75 mg daily	B	Hypertensive crisis with MAOIs	2–3 h	UK	UK	UK	4 h SR: 12 h
Fenfluramine HCl (Pondimin) CSS IV	A: PO: 20 mg t.i.d.; max: 120 mg/d; may increase weekly	C	Hypertensive crisis with MAOIs *Increase* effects with antacids, bicarbonates *Decrease* effects with tricyclic antidepressants	20 h	UK	1–3 min	2–4 h	4–6 h
Mazindol (Mazanor, Sanorex) CSS IV	Initial: 2 mg/d A: PO: 1 mg t.i.d. ac or 2 mg daily	C	Similar to fenfluramine	2.5–9 h	UK	30–60 min	UK	10–15 h
Phendimetrazine tartrate (Anorex, Adipost, Bacarate) CSS III	A: PO: 17.5–35 mg 1 h ac b.i.d.–t.i.d.; max: 70 mg t.i.d.	C	Similar to fenfluramine	2–10 h	UK	30 min	1–3 h	4–16 h

continued

Amphetamines and Amphetamine-like Drug— *Continued*

Generic (Brand)	Route and Dosage	Preg Cat	Interaction	t 1/2	PB	Onset	Peak	Duration
Phenmetrazine HCl (Preludin) CSS II	A: PO: 25 mg b.i.d.–t.i.d.; SR: 75 mg daily; max: 75 mg daily	C	Similar to fenfluramine	UK	UK	UK	5–12	12 h
Phentermine HCl (Adipex-P, Fastin, Ionamin) CSS IV	A: PO: 8 mg t.i.d.; ac or 15–37.5 mg/d	C	Similar to fenfluramine; diabetics may require less insulin	20 h	UK	UK	UK	10–14 h
Phenylpropanolamine HCl (Acutrim, Control, Dexatrim, Prolamine)	A: PO: 25 mg ac t.i.d.; or SR: 75 mg/d in morning	C	*Increase* effects with beta blockers; hypertensive crisis with MAOIs *Decrease* effects of antihypertensives	4–7 h	UK	UK	1–2 h	3 h SR: 12 h
Analeptics: Methylxanthines Caffeine (Nō Dōz, Tirend, Vivarin)	*Neonatal apnea:* Infants and C: PO: IM-IV: 5–10 mg/kg on day 1; then 2.5–5 mg/d *Therapeutic range:* 5–20 mg/mL	C	*Increase* CNS stimulation with theophylline and beta-adrenergic agonists	Neonate: 40–144 h A: 3–5 h	25– 35%	UK	15–45 min	UK

Theophylline	Infants: NGT: 5 mg/kg on day 1; then 2 mg in divided doses	C	See Prototype Drug Chart			
CNS Stimulant for Migraine Sumatriptan succinate (Imitrex)	A: SC: 6 mg single dose; may repeat in 1 h; max: 12 mg/d	C	*Increase* effect of ergot-containing drugs	2 h	20%	10–30 min	UK	1–2 h
Respiratory Stimulant Doxapram HCl (Dopram)	A: IV: 0.5–1 mg/kg; inf: 1–2 mg/min; max: 3 g/d *Neonatal apnea:* Initially: 0.5 mg/kg/h Maintenance: 0.5–2.5 mg/kg/h titrated to lowest effective rate	B	*Increase* pressor effect with MAOIs or sympathomimetic amines	A: 2.5–4 h Neonate: 7–10 h	UK	20–40 sec	1–2 min	6–12 min

KEY: For complete abbreviation key, see inside front cover.

Prototype: Sedative-Hypnotic: Barbiturate

Pentobarbital Sodium

Pentobarbital sodium
(Nembutal Sodium), ♦
  Novopentobarb
Short-acting barbiturate
CSS II
Pregnancy Category: D
Drug Forms:
Cap 50, 100 mg
Liq 18.2 mg/5 mL
Supp 30, 60, 120, 200 mg
Inj 50 mg/mL

Dosage

Sedative:
A: PO: 20–30 mg t.i.d.
C: PO: 2–6 mg/kg/d in 3 divided
  doses
Hypnotic:
A: PO: 100–200 mg h.s.
C: PO: 30–120 mg h.s.
Preoperative:
A: PO/IM/IV: 100 mg; repeat if
  needed

Contraindications

Respiratory depression, severe
  hepatic disease, pregnancy (fetal
  immaturity), nephrosis

Drug-Lab-Food Interactions

Decrease respiration with alcohol,
  CNS depressants; incompatible in
  solution with numerous drugs
  such as codeine, insulin, penicillin
  G, hydrocortisone, phenytoin

Pharmacokinetics

Absorption: PO: 90% absorbed slowly
Distribution: PB: 35–45%
Metabolism: t 1/2: 4 h (first phase);
  30–50 h (second phase)
Excretion: In urine as metabolites

Pharmacodynamics

PO: Onset: 15–30 min
     Peak: 0.5–1 h
     Duration: 3–6 h
IM: Onset: 10–15 min
     Peak: 0.5–1 h
     Duration: 3–6 h
IV: Onset: Immediate
     Peak: 2–5 min
     Duration: 15–60 min

Therapeutic Effects/Uses: To treat insomnia; used for sedation, preoperative medication, barbiturate coma (for controlling increased intracranial pressure).

Mode of Action: Depression of the CNS, including the motor and sensory activities.

Side Effects

Nausea, vomiting, diarrhea, lethargy,
  drowsiness, hangover, dizziness,
  rash

Adverse Reactions

Drug dependence or tolerance,
  urticaria, hypotension (rapid IV)
Life-threatening: Respiratory distress,
  laryngospasm

KEY: For complete abbreviation key, see inside front cover.

Sedative-Hypnotic: Barbiturate

■ NURSING PROCESS: Sedative-Hypnotic: Barbiturate

ASSESSMENT
- Obtain baseline vital signs for future comparison.
- Determine if there is a history of insomnia or sleep disorder.
- Assess renal function. Urine output should be >600 mL/d. Renal impairment could prolong drug action by increasing the half-life of the drug.
- Assess potential for fluid volume deficit, which would potentiate hypotensive effects.

POTENTIAL NURSING DIAGNOSIS
- Sleep pattern disturbance

PLANNING
- Client will receive adequate sleep without hangover when taking the hypnotic.

NURSING INTERVENTIONS
- Recognize that continuous use of a barbiturate might result in drug abuse.
- Monitor vital signs, especially respirations and blood pressure.
- Raise bedside rails of older adults and clients receiving a hypnotic for the first time. Confusion may occur, and injury may result.
- Observe the client, especially an older adult or a debilitated client, for adverse reactions to the pentobarbital; see prototype.
- Check the client's skin for rashes. Skin eruptions may occur in clients taking barbiturates.
- Observe the client for withdrawal symptoms when pentobarbital has been taken over a prolonged period of time and then discontinued.
- Administer IV pentobarbital at a rate of less than 50 mg/min. Do NOT mix pentobarbital with other medications. IM injection should be given deep in a large muscle such as the gluteus medius.

CLIENT TEACHING
General
- Instruct the client to use nonpharmacological ways to induce sleep, such as enjoying a warm bath, listening to music, drinking warm fluids, and avoiding drinks with caffeine after dinner.
- Instruct the client to avoid alcohol and antidepressant, antipsychotic, and narcotic drugs while taking the barbiturate. Respiratory distress may occur when these drugs are combined.
- Advise the client not to drive a motor vehicle or operate machinery. Caution is always encouraged.
- Instruct the client to take the hypnotic 30 min before bedtime. Short-acting hypnotics such as pentobarbital take effect within 15–30 min.
- Encourage the client to check with the health care provider about OTC sleeping aids. Drowsiness may result from taking these drugs, and therefore caution in driving is advised.

Side Effects
- Advise the client to report adverse reactions, such as hangover, to the health care provider. Drug selection or dosage might need to be changed.
- Instruct the client that hypnotics such as pentobarbital should be gradu-

ally withdrawn, especially if it has been taken for several weeks. Abrupt cessation of the hypnotic may result in withdrawal symptoms (tremors, muscle twitching).

EVALUATION
- Evaluate the effectiveness of pentobarbital. Usually, this drug is given before surgery.
- Evaluate respiratory status to ensure that respiratory distress has not occurred.

Sedative-Hypnotics: Barbiturates and Others— *Continued*

Generic (Brand)	Route and Dosage	Preg Cat	Interaction	t1/2	PB	Onset	Peak	Duration
Barbiturates: Short Acting Pentobarbital sodium (Nembutal Sodium)	See Prototype Drug Chart							
Secobarbital sodium (Seconal Sodium) CSS II	*Preoperative sedative:* A: PO: 100–300 mg before surgery C: PO: 50–100 mg; max: 100 mg *Hypnotic:* A: PO/IM: 100–200 mg h.s. C: IM: 3–5 mg/kg; max: 100 mg *Status epilepticus:* A: IV: 5.5 mg/kg; repeat in 3–4 h *With spinal anesthesia:* A: IV: 50–100 mg; infuse over 30 s; max: 250 mg/dose	D	*Increase* CNS depression with alcohol, narcotics, other sedatives, MAOIs *Decrease* effect of anticoagulants, glucocorticoids, quinidine	15–30 h	UK	PO: 15–30 min IM: 10–15 min IV: 1–5 min	PO: 30 min IM: 20 min IV: 1–3 min	PO: 1–4 h IM: 1–4 h IV: 30–60 min
Ethchlorvynol (Placidyl) CSS IV	*Sedative:* A: PO: 100–200 mg, b.i.d./t.i.d. *Hypnotic:* A: PO: 0.5–1 g, h.s. for 1 wk only	C	*Increase* CNS depression with alcohol, MAOIs, tricyclic antidepressants, and other CNS depressants	10–20 h	UK	30–60 min	1–2 h	5 h

continued

Sedative-Hypnotics: Barbiturates and Others—Continued

Generic (Brand)	Route and Dosage	Preg Cat	Interaction	t 1/2	PB	Onset	Peak	Duration
Barbiturates:								
Intermediate Acting Amobarbital sodium (Amytal Sodium)	*Sedative:* A: PO: 30–50 mg b.i.d.–t.i.d. C: PO: 2 mg/kg/d in 3–4 divided doses *Hypnotic:* A: PO/IM: 65–200 mg h.s. C: IM: 2–3 mg/kg A and C: IV: 65–200 mg	D	*Increase* CNS depression with alcohol, narcotics, other sedatives, antidepressants, some antihistamines. *Decrease* effect of beta blockers, glucocorticoids, phenothiazines, oral contraceptives, anticoagulants, estrogen	20–30 h	50–60%	PO: 45 min–1 h IV: 5 min	PO: UK IV: UK	PO: 6–8 h IV: 3–6 h
Aprobarbital (Alurate)	*Sedative:* A: PO: 40 mg t.i.d. *Hypnotic* A: PO: 40–160 mg h.s.	D	Same as amobarbital	15–40 h	<50%	45 min–1 h	UK	3–5 h
Butabarbital sodium (Butisol Sodium) CSS III	*Sedative:* A: PO: 15–30 mg t.i.d.,q.i.d. *Hypnotic* A: PO: 50–100 mg h.s. Preoperative sedative: A: PO: 50–100 mg, 1–1.5 h before surgery	D	Same as amobarbital	100 h	<50%	45 min–1 h	3–4 h	6–8 h

Other Sedative-Hypnotics

Drug	Route and Dosage		Uses and Considerations	$t_{1/2}$	PB	Onset	Peak	Duration
Chloral hydrate CSS IV	*Sedative:* A: PO: 250 mg t.i.d. pc C: PO: 8 mg/kg t.i.d. pc; max: 1,000 mg/d *Hypnotic:* A: PO: 500 mg–1 g h.s. (15–30 min before sleep) C: PO: 50 mg/kg h.s.; max: 1,000 mg	C	*Increase* CNS depression with alcohol, barbiturates, paraldehyde, other CNS depressants; *Increase* effect of loop diuretics, oral anticoagulants	8–10 h	70–80%	30–60 min	1–3 h	4–8 h
Paraldehyde (Paral) CSS IV	*Sedative:* A: PO: 5–10 mL q4–6 h PRN in water or juice; max: 30 mL C: PO: 0.3 mL/kg *Hypnotic:* A: PO: 10–30 mL h.s.	C	Same as chloral hydrate; *increase* urine crystals with sulfonamides	7.5 h	UK	10–15 min	1–2 h	6–8 h

KEY: For complete abbreviation key, see inside front cover.

Prototype: Sedative-Hypnotic: Benzodiazepine

Flurazepam HCl

Flurazepam HCl
  (Dalmane), ✦ Apo-Flurazepam,
  Nonoflupam
Benzodiazepine hypnotic
CSS IV
Pregnancy Category: X
Drug Forms:
Cap 15, 30 mg

Dosage

A: PO: 15–30 mg h.s.
Elderly: PO: 15 mg h.s.

Contraindications

Hypersensitivity to benzodiazepine, pregnancy, lactation, intermittent porphyria
Caution: Renal, liver, or mental disorders; elderly, debilitation

Drug-Lab-Food Interactions

May *increase* effect with cimetidine
Decrease effect with antacids, smoking
Decrease CNS function with alcohol, CNS depressants, anticonvulsants
Lab: Increase AST, ALT, ALP, bilirubin
False negatives: Clinistix, Diastix

Pharmacokinetics

Absorption: PO: well absorbed
Distribution: PB: 97%
Metabolism: t 1/2: 2–3 h; metabolites: 45–100 h
Excretion: In urine as active metabolites

Pharmacodynamics

PO: Onset: 15–45 min
  Peak: 0.5–1 h
  Duration: 7–10 h

Therapeutic Effects/Uses: To treat insomnia.
Mode of Action: Depression of the CNS; neurotransmitter inhibition.

Side Effects

Drowsiness, lethargy, hangover (residual sedation), dizziness, lightheadedness, anxiety, nausea, vomiting, diarrhea, confusion, disorientation

Adverse Reactions

Tolerance, psychological and/or physical dependence, hypotension, mental depression
Life-threatening: Coma from overdose, leukopenia (rare)

KEY: For complete abbreviation key, see inside front cover.

Sedative-Hypnotic: Benzodiazepine

■ NURSING PROCESS: Sedative-Hypnotic: Benzodiazepine

ASSESSMENT
- Obtain baseline vital signs and laboratory tests (AST, ALT, bilirubin) for future comparisons.
- Obtain drug history. Taking CNS depressants with benzodiazepine hypnotics can depress respirations. Flurazepam is highly protein-bound. Report if the client is taking other highly protein-bound drugs such as warfarin (Coumadin). Drug displacement can occur with two highly protein-bound drugs, causing an increase in circulating drug(s).
- Ascertain the client's problem with sleep disturbance.

POTENTIAL NURSING DIAGNOSIS
- Sleep pattern disturbance

PLANNING
- Client will remain asleep for 6–8 h.

NURSING INTERVENTIONS
- Monitor vital signs. Check for signs of respiratory distress, such as slow, irregular breathing patterns.
- Raise bedside rails of older adults or clients receiving flurazepam for the first time. Confusion may occur, and injury may result.
- Observe the client for side effects of flurazepam, such as hangover (residual sedation), lightheadedness, dizziness, or confusion. The metabolites of flurazepam have a long half-life, so cumulative effects of the drug can occur.

CLIENT TEACHING

General
- Instruct the client to use nonpharmacological ways to induce sleep, such as enjoying a warm bath, listening to music, drinking warm fluids such as milk, and avoiding drinks with caffeine after dinner.
- Instruct the client to avoid alcohol and antidepressant, antipsychotic, and narcotic drugs while taking sedative-hypnotics. Severe respiratory distress may occur when these drugs are combined.
- Advise the client to take flurazepam before bedtime. Flurazepam takes effect within 15–45 min.
- Suggest that the client urinate before taking flurazepam to prevent sleep disruption.
- Encourage the client to check with the health care provider about OTC sleeping aids. Drowsiness may result from taking these drugs; therefore, caution in driving is advised.

Side Effects
- Instruct the client to report adverse reactions, such as hangover, to the health care provider. Drug selection or dosage may need to be changed if hangover occurs.

EVALUATION
- Evaluate the effectiveness of flurazepam in promoting sleep.
- Determine if side effects such as hangover occur after several days of taking flurazepam. Another hypnotic may be prescribed if side effects remain.

Sedative-Hypnotics

Generic (Brand)	Route and Dosage	Preg Cat	Interaction	t1/2	PB	Onset	Peak	Duration
Benzodiazepines								
Estazolam (ProSom) CSS IV	A: PO: 1–2 mg h.s. Elderly: PO: 0.5 mg h.s.	X	*Increase* estazolam effect with cimetidine, INH, oral contraceptives; *increase* CNS depression with alcohol, narcotics, anticonvulsants *Decrease* estazolam effect with theophylline, rifampin, smoking	10–24 h	93%	15–45 min	1.5–2 h	7–8 h
Flurazepam HCl (Dalmane)	See Prototype Drug Chart							
Lorazepam (Ativan) CSS IV	*Hypnotic:* A: PO: 2–4 mg h.s.	D	Similar to temazepam; *decrease* effect with oral contraceptives, valproic acid	12–14 h	85%	20–30 min	2–3 h	12–24 h
Quazepam (Doral) CSS IV	A: PO: 7.5–15 mg h.s.	X	*Increase* CNS depression with alcohol, narcotics, anticonvulsants	39 h	>95%	0.5 h	2 h	7–8 h
Temazepam (Restoril) CSS IV	*Hypnotic:* A: PO: 15–30 mg h.s.	X	*Increase* CNS depression with alcohol, anticonvulsants, CNS depressants, narcotics, other sedative-hypnotics; may *increase* phenytoin level *Decrease* absorption with antacids; may *decrease* effect of levodopa	10–20 h	96%	30–60 min	2–3 h	6–12 h

Triazolam (Halcion) CSS IV	*Hypnotic:* A: PO: 0.125–0.5 mg h.s. Elderly: PO: 0.125–0.25 mg h.s.	X	Same as temazepam	2–4 h	89%	15–30 min	1–2 h	6–8 h
Nonbenzodiazepines Methyprylon (Noludar) CSS III	*Hypnotic:* A: PO: 200–400 mg h.s. C: PO: 50 mg h.s; may increase to 200 mg	B	Similar to glutethimide	3–6 h	60%	45–60 min	1–2 h	5–8 h
Zolpidem tartrate (Ambien)	*Hypnotic:* A: PO: Initially 5 mg; maint: 5–15 mg h.s.; average: 10 mg h.s.; use for 7–10 d	B	*Increase* CNS depression with alcohol, narcotics, antipsychotics	1.5–4 h	79–92%	10–30 min	0.5–2 h	6–8 h
Piperidinediones Glutethimide (Doriden) CSS III	*Hypnotic:* A: PO: 250–500 mg h.s.; repeat in 4 h if necessary	C	*Increase* CNS depression with alcohol, CNS antidepressants, barbiturates; *increase* anticholinergic effect with tricyclic antidepressants *Decrease* anticoagulant effect with oral anticoagulants	10–20 h	50%	30 min	1–2 h	4–8 h

KEY: For complete abbreviation key, see inside front cover.

Prototype: Analgesic: Aspirin

Aspirin

Aspirin
(A.S.A., Bayer, Astrin, Ecotrin, Alka Seltzer [in some], Empirin), 🍁 Astrin, Entrophen, Novasen
Salicylate
Pregnancy Category: D
Drug Forms:
Tab 65, 325, 500, 650 mg
Cap SR 325, 500 mg
Supp 60, 120, 200, 325, 650 mg

Dosage

Analgesic:
A: PO: 325–650 mg q4h PRN; max: 4 g/d
C: PO: 40–65 mg/d in 4–6 divided doses; max: 3.5 g/d
TIA and thromboembolic condition:
A: PO: 325–650 mg/d or b.i.d.
Arthritis:
A: PO: 3.6–5.4 g/d in divided doses
TDM: 15–30 mg/dL; 150–300 µg/mL

Contraindications

Hypersensitivity to salicylates or NSAIDs, flu or virus symptoms in children, third trimester of pregnancy
Caution: Renal or hepatic disorders

Drug-Lab-Food Interactions

Increase risk of bleeding with anticoagulants; *increase* risk of hypoglycemia with oral hypoglycemic drugs; *increase* ulcerogenic effect with glucocorticoids
Lab: Decrease cholesterol and potassium, T_3, T_4 levels; *increase* PT, bleeding time, uric acid

Pharmacokinetics

Absorption: PO: 80–100%
Distribution: PB: UK; crosses placenta
Metabolism: t 1/2: 2–3 h (low dose; 2–20 h (high dose)
Excretion: 50% in urine

Pharmacodynamics

PO: Onset: 15–30 min
    Peak: 1–2 h
    Duration: 4–6 h
Rectal: Onset: 1–2 h
    Peak: 3–5 h
    Duration: 4–7 h

Therapeutic Effects/Uses: To reduce pain and inflammatory symptoms; to decrease body temperature; to inhibit platelet aggregation.

Mode of Action: Inhibition of prostaglandin synthesis, inhibition of hypothalamic heat-regulator center.

Side Effects

Anorexia, nausea, vomiting, diarrhea, dizziness, confusion, hearing loss, heartburn, rash, stomach pains, drowsiness

Adverse Reactions

Tinnitus, urticaria, ulceration
Life-threatening: Agranulocytosis, hemolytic anemia, bronchospasm, anaphylaxis, thrombocytopenia, hepatotoxicity, leukopenia

KEY: For complete abbreviation key, see inside front cover.

■ NURSING PROCESS: Analgesic: Aspirin

ASSESSMENT

- Obtain a medical history. Determine if there is any history of gastric upset, gastric bleeding, or liver disease. Aspirin can cause gastric irritation. It prolongs bleeding time by inhibiting platelet aggregation.
- Obtain a drug history. Report if a drug-drug interaction is probable.

Analgesic: Aspirin

POTENTIAL NURSING DIAGNOSIS
- High risk for injury
- Pain

PLANNING
- Client will be free of mild pain in 12–24 hours. Aspirin may be ordered for mild to severe arthritic conditions, pain relief, anti-inflammatory effects, fever reduction, and inhibition of platelet aggregation.

NURSING INTERVENTIONS
- Monitor serum salicylate (aspirin) level when the client is taking high doses of aspirin for chronic conditions such as arthritis. The normal therapeutic range is 15–30 mg/dL. Mild toxicity occurs at serum level of >30 mg/dL, and severe toxicity occurs at >50 mg/dL.
- Observe the client for signs of bleeding, such as dark (tarry) stools, bleeding gums, petechiae (round red spots), ecchymosis (excessive bruising), and purpura (large red spots) when the client is taking high doses of aspirin.

CLIENT TEACHING
General
- Advise the client not to take aspirin with alcohol or drugs that are highly protein-bound, such as the anticoagulant warfarin (Coumadin). Aspirin displaces drugs like warfarin from the protein-binding site, causing more free anticoagulant.
- Suggest that the client inform the dentist before a dental visit if the client is taking high doses of aspirin.
- With the health care provider's approval, instruct the client to discontinue aspirin 3–7 d before surgery to reduce the risk of bleeding.
- Keep aspirin bottle out of reach of small children.
- Instruct the parent to call the poison control center immediately if a child has taken a large or unknown amount of aspirin (also acetaminophen).
- Instruct the client NOT to administer aspirin for virus or flu symptoms in children. Reye's syndrome (vomiting, lethargy, delirium, and coma) has been linked with aspirin and viral infections. Acetaminophen is usually prescribed for cold and flu symptoms.
- Inform the client that old aspirin tablets can cause GI distress; discard.
- Inform the client with dysmenorrhea to take acetaminophen instead of aspirin 2 d before and 2 d during the menstrual period.

Diet
- Instruct the client to take aspirin (also ibuprofen) with food, at mealtime, or with plenty of fluids. Enteric-coated aspirin avoids GI disturbance.

Side Effects
- Instruct the client to report side effects such as drowsiness, tinnitus (ringing in the ears), headaches, flushing, dizziness, GI symptoms (bleeding, heartburn), visual changes, and seizures.

EVALUATION
- Evaluate the effectiveness of aspirin in relieving pain. If pain persists, another analgesic such as an NSAID such as ibuprofen may be prescribed.
- Determine if the client is having any side effects to aspirin.

Prototype: Analgesic: Acetaminophen

Acetaminophen

Acetaminophen
  (Tylenol, Tempra, Panadol, Datril,
  ♣ Robigesic, Atasol
Para-aminophenol analgesic
Pregnancy Category: B
Drug Forms:
Tab and cap 325, 500, 650 mg
Chewable tab 80 mg
Liq 160 mg/5 mL
Supp 120, 325, 650 mg

Dosage

A: PO: 325–650 mg q4–6h PRN;
  max: 4,000 mg/d; rectal supp:
  650 mg q.i.d.
C: 0–3 mo: PO: 40 mg 4–5×/d
  4 mo–1 y: PO: 80 mg 4–5×/d
  1–2 y: PO: 120 mg 4–5×/d
  2–3 y: PO: 160 mg 4–5×/d
  4–5 y: PO: 240 mg 4–5×/d
  6–8 y: PO: 320 mg 4–5×/d
  9–10 y: PO: 400 mg 4–5×/d
  >11 y: PO: 480 mg 4–5×/d
C: 2–5 y: Rectal: 120 mg 4–5×/d
  6–12 y: Rectal: 325 mg 4–5×/d

Contraindications

Severe hepatic or renal disease,
  alcoholism, hypersensitivity

Drug-Lab-Food Interactions

Increase effect with caffeine, diflunisal
Decrease effect with oral
  contraceptives, anticholinergics,
  cholestyramine, charcoal

Pharmacokinetics

Absorption: PO: rapidly absorbed;
  rectal: erratic
Distribution: PB: 20–50%; crosses the
  placenta, in breast milk
Metabolism: t 1/2: 1–3.5 h
Excretion: In urine as metabolites

Pharmacodynamics

PO: Onset: 10–30 min
    Peak: 1–2 h
    Duration: 3–5 h
Rectal: Onset: UK
    Peak: UK
    Duration: 4–6 h

Therapeutic Effects/Uses: To decrease pain and fever.

Mode of Action: Inhibition (weakly) of prostaglandin synthesis, inhibition of hypothalamic heat-regulator center.

Side Effects

Anorexia, nausea, vomiting, rash

Adverse Reactions

Severe hypoglycemia, oliguria,
  urticaria
Life-threatening: Hemorrhage,
  hepatotoxicity, hemolytic anemia,
  leukopenia, thrombocytopenia

KEY: For complete abbreviation key, see inside front cover.

Analgesic: Acetaminophen

■ NURSING PROCESS: Analgesic: Acetaminophen

ASSESSMENT
- Obtain a medical history of liver dysfunction. Overdosing or extremely high doses of acetaminophen can cause hepatotoxicity.
- Ascertain the severity of the pain. Nonnarcotic NSAIDs such as ibuprofen or a narcotic may be necessary for relieving pain.

POTENTIAL NURSING DIAGNOSIS
- High risk for injury
- Pain

PLANNING
- Client's pain will be relieved or controlled.

NURSING INTERVENTIONS
- Check levels of ALT, ALP, GGT, 5-NT, bilirubin for elevations, if the client is on long-term therapy.

CLIENT TEACHING
- Instruct the client to keep acetaminophen out of children's reach. Acetaminophen for children is available in flavored tablets and liquid. High doses can cause hepatotoxicity. Self-medication of acetaminophen should not be used longer than 10 d for adults and 5 d for children without the health care provider's approval.
- Instruct the parent to call the poison control center immediately if a child has taken a large or unknown amount of acetaminophen. Ipecac should be available in the home.
- Check acetaminophen dosage on package level. Do NOT exceed the recommended dosage.

Side Effects
- Instruct the client to report side effects. Overdosing can cause severe liver damage and death.
- Check the serum acetaminophen level when toxicity is suspected. The normal serum level is 5–20 mg/mL; the toxic level is >50 μg/mL, and levels of >200 μg/mL could indicate hepatotoxicity. The antidote for acetaminophen is acetylcysteine (Mucomyst). The dosage is based on the serum acetaminophen level.

EVALUATION
- Evaluate the effectiveness of acetaminophen in relieving pain. If pain persists, another analgesic may be needed.
- Determine if the client is taking the dose as recommended and no side effects are observed or reported.

Analgesics

Generic (Brand)	Route and Dosage	Preg Cat	Interaction	t1/2	PB	Onset	Peak	Duration
NSAIDs: Propionic Acid Ibuprofen (Motrin, Advil, Nuprin, Medipren)	*Pain:* A: PO: 200–800 mg q4–6h; max: 3,200 mg/d *Fever:* A: PO: 200–400 mg t.i.d.-q.i.d. C: 6 mo–12 y: PO: 5–10 mg/kg t.i.d.-q.i.d.	B	*Increase* bleeding with heparin, oral anticoagulants; *increase* effects of phenytoin, sulfonamides, warfarin *Lab:* may *increase* lithium levels	2–4 h	98%	1/2 h	1–2 h	4–6 h
Ketoprofen (Orudis)	A: PO: 75 mg t.i.d.; max: 300 mg/d SR: 200 mg daily	B	Increased bleeding time: heparin may *increase* lithium and methotrexate toxicity	1–4 h	>90%	1–2 h	1–2 h	4–6 h
Miscellaneous Methotrimeprazine HCl (Levoprome)	Sedative-analgesic: A: C: >12 y: PO: 6–25 mg/d in divided doses with meals IM: 10–12 mg q4–6h PRN (deep IM) Elderly: IM: 5–10 mg q4–6h *Postanalgesia:* A and C: >12 y: IM: 2.5–7.5 mg q4–6h PRN	C	*Increase* hypotensive effect with antihypertensives, MAOIs *Increase* CNS depression with alcohol, narcotics	20 h	UK	15–30 min	1–2 h	4 h

Salicylates
Aspirin (Bayer, Ecotrin, Astrin)

See Prototype Drug Chart

Diflunisal (Dolobid)

A: PO: Initially: 1,000 mg; maint: 500 mg q8–12h

C

May *increase* lithium levels; may *increase* bleeding with warfarin; *increase* effects of acetaminophen, anticoagulants
Decrease effect with antacids, steroids; may *decrease* effects of diuretics, antihypertensives
Lab: may *increase* AST, ALT; may *decrease* T_4

8–12 h | 99% | 1 h | 2–3 h | 8–12 h

Para-aminophenol
Acetaminophen (Tylenol, Panadol, Tempra)

See Prototype Drug Chart

KEY: For complete abbreviation key, see inside front cover.

Prototype: Narcotic: Morphine

Morphine Sulfate

Morphine sulfate
  (Duramorph, MS Contin, Roxanol SR), ❧ Epimorph, Statex
Narcotic opiate
CSS II
Pregnancy Category: B
Drug Forms:
Tab 15, 30 mg
Liq 10, 20/5 mL
Inj 2, 4, 5, 8, 10, 15 mg/mL
Supp 5, 10, 20 mg

Dosage

A: PO: 10–30 mg q4h PRN;
  SR: 30 mg, q8–12h
  IM/SC: 5–15 mg PRN
  IV: 4–10 mg q4h PRN; diluted; inject over 5 min
  Epidural: 2–10 mg over 24 h
C: IM/SC: 0.1–0.2 mg/kg PRN; max: <15 mg/dose

Contraindications

Asthma with respiratory depression, increased intracranial pressure, shock
Caution: Respiratory, renal, or hepatic diseases; myocardial infarction; elderly; very young

Drug-Lab-Food Interactions

Increase effects of alcohol, sedative-hypnotics, antipsychotic drugs, muscle relaxants
Lab: Increase AST, ALT

Pharmacokinetics

Absorption: PO: varies; IV: rapid
Distribution: PB: UK; crosses placenta, in breast milk
Metabolism: t 1/2: 2.5–3 h
Excretion: 90% in urine

Pharmacodynamics

PO: Onset: variable
       Peak: 1–2 h
       Duration: 4–5 h; SR: 8–12 h
SC/IM: Onset: 15–30 min
       Peak: SC: 50–90 min
           IM: 0.5–1 h
       Duration: 3–5 h
IV: Onset: rapid
       Peak: 20 min
       Duration: 3–5 h

Therapeutic Effects/Uses: To relieve severe pain.

Mode of Action: Depression of the CNS, depression of pain impulses by binding with the opiate receptor in the CNS.

Side Effects

Anorexia, nausea, vomiting, constipation, drowsiness, dizziness, sedation, confusion, urinary retention, rash, blurred vision, bradycardia, flushing, euphoria, pruritus

Adverse Reactions

Hypotension, urticaria, seizures
Life-threatening: Respiratory depression, increased intracranial pressure

KEY: For complete abbreviation key, see inside front cover.

Narcotic: Morphine

■ NURSING PROCESS: Narcotic Analgesic: Morphine Sulfate

ASSESSMENT
- Obtain a medical history. Contraindications to use of morphine include severe respiratory disorders, increased intracranial pressure (ICP), and severe renal disease. Morphine may increase ICP and seizures.
- Obtain a drug history. Report if a drug-drug interaction is probable. Morphine increases the effects of alcohol, sedatives or hypnotics, antipsychotic drugs, and muscle relaxants and might cause respiratory depression.
- Assess vital signs and urinary output. Note the depth and rate of respirations. Morphine can cause urinary retention.

POTENTIAL NURSING DIAGNOSIS
- Pain related to surgery, injury
- Ineffective breathing patterns related to excess morphine dosage

PLANNING
- Client will be free of pain, or the intensity of pain will be lessened.

NURSING INTERVENTIONS
- Administer the narcotic before pain reaches its peak to maximize the effectiveness of the drug.
- Monitor vital signs at frequent intervals to detect respiratory changes. Respirations of <10/min can indicate respiratory distress.
- Monitor the client's urine output; urine output should be at least 600 mL/d.
- Check bowel sounds for decreased peristalsis, a cause of constipation due to morphine. Mild laxative or dietary change might be needed.
- Check for pupil changes and reaction. Pinpoint pupils can indicate morphine overdose.
- Have naloxone (Narcan) available as an antidote if morphine overdose occurs.
- Check child's dose of morphine before its administration; dose is 0.1–0.2 mg/kg.

CLIENT TEACHING

General
- Instruct the client not to take alcohol or CNS depressants with any narcotic analgesics such as morphine. Respiratory depression can result.
- Suggest nonpharmacological measures to relieve pain as client is recuperating from surgery. If necessary, a nonnarcotic analgesic may be prescribed.

Side Effects
- Alert the client that with continuous use, narcotics such as morphine can become addicting. If addiction occurs, inform the client about methadone treatment programs and other resources in the area.
- Instruct the client to report dizziness or difficulty in breathing while taking morphine. Dizziness could be due to orthostatic hypotension. Advise the client to ambulate with caution or only with assistance.

EVALUATION
- Evaluate the effectiveness of morphine in lessening or alleviating the pain.
- Evaluate the stability of vital signs. Report any decrease in blood pressure.

Prototype: Narcotic: Meperidine

Meperidine HCl

Meperidine HCl
  (Demerol), ✽ Pethadol,
  Pethidine HCl
Synthetic narcotic
CSS II
Pregnancy Category: B
Drug Forms:
Tab 50, 100 mg
Liq 50 mg/5 mL
Inj 25, 50, 75, 100 mg/mL

Dosage

A: PO/SC/IM/IV: 50–150 mg q3–4h PRN
C: PO/IM/IV: 1 mg/kg q4–6h; max: <100 mg q4h

Contraindications

Alcoholism; head trauma; increased intracranial pressure; severe hepatic, renal, and pulmonary diseases; MAO inhibitors

Drug-Lab-Food Interactions

Increase CNS depression with alcohol, sedative-hypnotics, and other CNS depressants
Lab: Increase serum amylase, AST, ALT, bilirubin

Pharmacokinetics

Absorption: PO: 50% absorbed; IM: well absorbed
Distribution: PB: 60–70%
Metabolism: t 1/2: 3–8 h
Excretion: In urine, mostly as metabolites

Pharmacodynamics

PO: Onset: 15 min
        Peak: 1 h
        Duration: 4 h
IM/SC: Onset: 10–15 min
        Peak: 0.5–1 h
        Duration: 2–4 h
IV: Onset: 1–5 min
        Peak: 5–10 min
        Duration: 2 h

Therapeutic Effects/Uses: To relieve moderate to severe pain.

Mode of Action: Synthetic morphine-like substance, depression of pain impulses by binding to the opiate receptor in the CNS.

Side Effects

Nausea, vomiting, constipation, headache, dizziness, drowsiness, hypotension, sedation, confusion, abdominal cramps, euphoria, blurred vision, rash, tinnitus, tremors

Adverse Reactions

Bradycardia, severe hypotension, convulsion, physical and/or psychologic dependence, seizures
Life-threatening: Respiratory depression, cardiovascular collapse, increased intracranial pressure

KEY: For complete abbreviation key, see inside front cover.

Narcotic: Meperidine

■ NURSING PROCESS: Narcotic Analgesic: Meperidine (Demerol)

ASSESSMENT
- Obtain drug history from the client of drugs he or she is currently taking. Report if a drug-drug interaction is probable. CNS depressants enhance the action of meperidine; thus, respiratory depression can occur.
- Obtain baseline vital signs for future comparisons. Meperidine tends to decrease systolic blood pressure.
- Assess type of pain, location, and duration before giving meperidine.

POTENTIAL NURSING DIAGNOSIS
- Pain related to surgery or injury

PLANNING
- Client's pain will be decreased or alleviated. Drug dosing may need to be repeated.

NURSING INTERVENTIONS
- Administer meperidine before the pain reaches its peak to maximize the effectiveness of the drug.
- Monitor vital signs to compare blood pressure with baseline pressure. Hypotension is a side effect of meperidine. Note if client is having any breathing dysfunction.
- Have available naloxone (Narcan), which can reverse respiratory depression due to narcotic overdose.
- Check urine output and bowel sounds. Urinary retention and constipation are side effects of meperidine.
- Check older adults for side effects of meperidine. Confusion may occur, so use of side rails and other precautions should be taken. Dosage may need to be decreased.

CLIENT TEACHING
General
- Instruct the client not to take alcohol or CNS depressants with meperidine because of increased depression of the CNS and of respirations.
- Inform the client that drug dependence could occur with continual use of meperidine. If severe pain is still present, another narcotic analgesic or analgesic may be prescribed.

Side Effects
- Instruct the client to report side effects such as dizziness due to orthostatic hypotension, headaches, constipation, blurred vision, or decreased urine output. Report findings to the health care provider.

EVALUATION
- Evaluate the effectiveness of the narcotic analgesic in lessening or alleviating the pain. If pain persists after several days, the cause should be determined or the narcotic should be changed.
- Evaluate the stability of vital signs. Abnormal signs, such as decreased blood pressure, should be reported.

Narcotics: Opium and Synthetics

Generic (Brand)	Route and Dosage	Preg Cat	Interaction	t 1/2	PB	Onset	Peak	Duration
Codeine (sulfate, phosphate) CSS II	A: PO/SC/IM: 15–60 mg q4–6h PRN C: PO/SC/IM: 0.5 mg/kg/dose q4–6h	C	*Increase* CNS depression with alcohol, sedative-hypnotics, antipsychotics, muscle relaxants, tricyclic antidepressants	2.5–4 h	70%	15–30 min	1–1.5 h	4–6 h
Hydromorphone HCl (Dilaudid) CSS II	A: PO: 1–6 mg q4–6h PRN SC/IM/IV: 1–4 mg q4–6h PRN Rectal: 3 mg q6–8h, PRN	C	Same as codeine	1–3 h	62%	15–30 min	0.5–1.5 h	4–5 h
Levorphanol tartrate (Levo-Dromoran) CSS II	A: PO/SC/IV: Initially: 2 mg PO/SC/IV: 2–3 mg q6–8h PRN	B	Same as oxycodone	10–16 h	50–60%	PO: 1–1.5 h SC: 30 min–1 h IV: 20 min	PO: 2 h SC: 1–2 h IV: UK	PO: 6–8 h SC: 6–8 h IV: 6–8 h
Meperidine (Demerol)	See Prototype Drug Chart							
Morphine sulfate	See Prototype Drug Chart							
Oxycodone HCl with acetaminophen; (Percocet) and oxycodone terephthalate with aspirin (Percodan) CSS II	A: PO: 5 mg q4–6h PRN or 5–10 mg q6h PRN C: 6–12 y: 1.25 mg q6h PRN 12–17 y: 2.5 mg q6h PRN	B	*Increase* CNS depression with alcohol, sedative-hypnotics, other narcotics, antipsychotics, tricyclic antidepressants, muscle relaxants	2–3 h	UK	10–15 min	0.5–1 h	4–5 h

Drug	Dose	Pregnancy Category	Interactions	Onset	Peak	PB	Half-life	Duration
Propoxyphene HCl (Darvon) Propoxyphene napsylate (Darvon-N) CSS IV	A: PO: HCl: 65 mg q4h PRN; max: 390 mg/d A: PO: napsylate: 100 mg q4h PRN; max: 600 mg/d	C (short time use)	Same as oxycodone				12 h	4-6 h
Sufentanil citrate (Sufenta) CSS II	*Primary anesthetic:* A: IV: 8-30 μg/kg with 100% O_2 and muscle relaxant C: IV: 10-25 μg/kg with 100% O_2 and muscle relaxant *Adjunct to anesthesia:* IV: 1-8 μg/kg	C	*Increase* additive effect with alcohol, sedative-hypnotics, antipsychotics	1.5-3 min		93%	1-3 h	40 min
Oxymorphone HCl (Numorphan) CSS II	A: SC/IM: 1-1.5 mg q4-6h, PRN IV: 0.5 mg q4-6h PR: 5 mg q4-6h, PRN	B, (D, prolonged high dose at term)	Increased CNS depression with alcohol and other CNS depressants, MAOIs, tricyclic antidepressants	IM:10-15 min IV: 5-10 min PR:15-30 min	1-1.5 h	UK	UK	3-6 h
For Narcotic Addiction: Levomethadyl acetate HCl (ORLAAM)	A: IM: Initially: 10-40 mg 3×/wk; maint: 60-90 mg 3×/wk; max: 140 mg 3×/wk (M, W, F regimen)	UK	*Increase* CNS depression with CNS depressants	UK	UK	UK	UK	UK

KEY: For complete abbreviation key, see inside front cover.

Prototype: Narcotic: Agonist-Antagonist

Pentazocine Lactate

Pentazocine lactate
(Talwin)
Narcotic agonist-antagonist
CSS IV
Pregnancy Category: C
Drug Forms:
Tab 50 mg
Inj 30 mg/mL

Dosage

A: PO: 50–100 mg q3–4h PRN; max: 600 mg/d
IM/IV: 30 mg q3–4h PRN

Contraindications

Alcoholism; head trauma; severe respiratory, renal, and/or hepatic disease; hypersensitivity to naloxone
Caution: Severe heart disease

Drug-Lab-Food Interactions

Increase CNS depression with alcohol, sedative-hypnotics, antipsychotics, muscle relaxants

Pharmacokinetics

Absorption: PO: well absorbed
Distribution: PB: 60%
Metabolism: t 1/2: 2–3 h
Excretion: In urine (small amount excreted unchanged); in feces (small amount)

Pharmacodynamics

PO: Onset: 15–30 min
    Peak: 1–2 h
    Duration: 2–4 h
IM: Onset: 15–20 min
    Peak: 1 h
    Duration: 2–4 h
IV: Onset: minutes
    Peak: 15 min
    Duration: 3 h

Therapeutic Effects/Uses: To relieve moderate to severe pain.

Mode of Action: Inhibition of pain impulses transmitted in the CNS by binding with the opiate receptor, pain threshold is increased.

Side Effects

Nausea, vomiting, constipation, dizziness, sedation, headaches, confusion, euphoria, rash, blurred vision, dysuria

Adverse Reactions

Hallucinations, urinary retention, urticaria, tachycardia
Life threatening: Respiratory depression, shock

KEY: For complete abbreviation key, see inside front cover.

Narcotic: Agonist-Antagonist

■ NURSING PROCESS: Narcotic Analgesic: Pentazocine (Talwin)

ASSESSMENT
- Obtain a drug history from the client. Report if a drug-drug interaction is probable. When taken with pentazocine, CNS depressants can cause respiratory depression.
- Obtain baseline vital signs for future comparison.
- Assess the type of pain, duration, and location before giving the drug.

POTENTIAL NURSING DIAGNOSIS
- Pain related to surgery or trauma

PLANNING
- Client will be free of pain, or the intensity of pain will be lessened.

NURSING INTERVENTIONS
- Monitor vital signs. Note any changes in respirations.
- Check bowel sounds. Decreased peristalsis may result in constipation. A mild laxative may be necessary.
- Check urine output. Report if urine output is <30 mL/h or <600 mL/d.
- Administer IV pentazocine diluted in sterile water or undiluted. Do not mix with barbiturates.

CLIENT TEACHING
General
- Instruct the client not to consume alcohol or CNS depressants while taking pentazocine. Respiratory depression can occur.
- Suggest nonpharmacological methods for lessening pain, such as changing position or ambulation.

Side Effects
- Instruct the client to report side effects to pentazocine such as dizziness, headaches, constipation, dysuria, rash, or blurred vision. Hallucinations, tachycardia, and respiratory depression are adverse reactions that might occur.

EVALUATION
- Evaluate the effectiveness of pentazocine in relieving pain. If ineffective, another narcotic analgesic may be ordered.
- Evaluate the stability of the vital signs. Note if there is a change in respirations, pulse rate, or blood pressure. Report abnormal findings.

Narcotics: Agonist-Antagonists and Narcotic Antagonist

Generic (Brand)	Route and Dosage	Preg Cat	Interaction	t1/2	PB	Onset	Peak	Duration
Narcotic Agonist-Antagonists								
Buprenorphine HCl (Buprenex) CSS V	A: IM/IV: Initially: 0.3 mg q6h; may increase to 0.6 mg q6h PRN	C	Same as butorphanol	2–3 h	96%	IM: 15–30 min IV: 1–2 min	IM: 1 h IV: 1 h	IM: 3–5 h IV: 2–6 h
Butorphanol tartrate (Stadol)	A: IM: 1–4 mg q3–4h PRN IV: 0.5–2 mg q3–4h PRN Nasal Spray: 1 mg (1 spray) q3–4 h	C	*Increase* butorphanol effect with narcotics, sedative-hypnotics, antipsychotics, muscle relaxants	2.5–4 h	>90%	IM: 10–30 min IV: 1–2 min	IM: 0.5–1 h IV: 4–5 min	IM: 3–4 h IV: 2–4 h
Nalbuphine HCl (Nubain) CSS II	A: SC/IM/IV: 10–20 mg q3–4h PRN; max: 160 mg/d	B	Same as butorphanol	5 h	UK	IM: 15 min IV: 2–3 min	IM: UK IV: 30 min	IM: 3–6 h IV: 3–6 h
Pentazocine lactate (Talwin)	See Prototype Drug Chart							
Dezocine (Dalgan)	A: IM: 5–20 mg q3–6h PRN; max: 120 mg/d IV: 2.5–10 mg q3–6 h PRN	C	*Increase* depressive effects with alcohol, sedative-hypnotics, antipsychotics, tranquilizers, general anesthesia *Lab:* May *increase* ALP, AST	IM: 2.2 h IV: 2.6 h	UK	IM: 30 min IV: 10 min	IM: 1–1.5 h IV: 0.5 h	IM/IV: 2–4 h

Fentanyl (Duragesic, Sublimaze) CSS II		C	Similar to dezocine	3–6 h Patch: 17 h	80–89%	IM: 10–15 min IV: 1–2 min Patch: 12–18 h	IM: 20–30 min IV: 3–5 h	IM: 1–2 h IV: 0.5–1 h
	Preoperative A: IM/IV: 50–100 µg q1–2h PRN (0.05–0.1 mg) C: 2–12 y: 1.7–3.3 µg/kg A: Transdermal patch: 72-h effect							
Narcotic Antagonist Naloxone HCl (Narcan)	*Opiate overdose; Narcotic-induced respiratory distress:* A: IV: 0.4–2 mg; may repeat q2–3min; max: 10 mg C: IV: 0.1 mg/kg; may repeat q2–3min; max: 10 mg *Postoperative RD:* A: IV: 0.1–0.2 mg; may repeat q2–3min PRN C: IV/IM: 0.005–0.01 mg/kg; may repeat q2–3min PRN	B	None significant	1–1.5 h	UK	IV: 1–2 min	IV: 5–15 min	IV: 45 min–1 h

KEY: For complete abbreviation key, see inside front cover.

ANTICONVULSANTS

Barbiturates

Benzodiazepines

Hydantoins

Iminostilbenes

Oxazolidones

Succinimides

Valproate

Miscellaneous

Prototype: Anticonvulsants

Phenytoin

Phenytoin
  (Dilantin)
Anticonvulsant, hydantoin
Pregnancy Category: D
Drug Forms:
Susp: 30, 125 mg/5 mL
Tab chewable 50 mg
Cap ext 30, 100 mg
Cap prompt 30, 100 mg
Inj 50 mg/mL

Dosage

A: PO: 100 mg t.i.d.
  IV: LD: 10–15 mg/kg/d; infusion <50 mg/min; max: 300 mg/d
C: 4–8 mg/kg/d in divided doses
Therapeutic serum range: 10–20 µg/mL
Toxic level: 30–50 µg/mL

Contraindications

Hypersensitivity, heart block, psychiatric disorders, pregnancy

Drug-Lab-Food Interactions

Increase effects with cimetidine, isoniazid, chloramphenicol; *decrease* effects with cisplatin, folic acid, and vinblastine
Decrease effects of anticoagulants, oral contraceptives, antihistamines, corticosteroids, theophylline, cyclosporin, quinidine, dopamine, rifampin
Foods: Those rich in folic acid

Pharmacokinetics

Absorption: PO: slowly absorbed; IM: erratic rate of absorption
Distribution: PB: 85–95%
Metabolism: t 1/2: 6–45 h; average: 22 h
Excretion: In urine, small amount; in bile and feces, moderate amount

Pharmacodynamics

PO: Onset: 0.5–2 h
  Peak: 1.5–3 h
  Duration: 6–12 h
IV: Onset: minutes–1 h
  Peak: 2 h
  Duration: >12 h

Therapeutic Effects/Uses: To prevent grand mal and complex partial seizures.
Mode of Action: Reduces motor cortex activity by altering transport of ions.

Side Effects

Headache, diplopia, confusion, dizziness, sluggishness, decreased coordination, ataxia, slurred speech, rash, anorexia, nausea, vomiting, hypotension (IV), pink-red/brown discoloration of urine

Adverse Reactions

Leukopenia, hepatitis, depression, gingival hyperplasia, gingivitis, nystagmus, hirsutism
Life-threatening: Aplastic anemia, thrombocytopenia, agranulocytosis, Stevens-Johnson syndrome, hypotension, ventricular fibrillation

KEY: For complete abbreviation key, see inside front cover.

■ NURSING PROCESS: Phenytoin

ASSESSMENT

- Obtain a medication history from the client, including current drugs. Report if a drug-drug interaction is probable.

Anticonvulsants

- Check urinary output to determine if adequate (>600 mL/d).
- Check laboratory values related to renal and liver function. If both BUN and creatinine levels are elevated, a renal disorder should be suspected. Elevated serum liver enzymes, such as ALP, ALT, or SGPT, γ-glutamyl transferase (GGT), and/or 5′-nucleotidase indicate a hepatic disorder.

POTENTIAL NURSING DIAGNOSES
- High risk for injury
- Altered oral mucous membranes

PLANNING
- Client will be free of seizures and will adhere to anticonvulsant therapy.
- Side effects of phenytoin will be minimal and closely monitored.

NURSING INTERVENTIONS
- Monitor serum drug levels of anticonvulsant to determine overdosing or underdosing of drug; compliance to regimen.
- Protect the client from hazards in the environment, such as sharp objects and table corners, during a seizure.
- Determine if the client is receiving adequate nutrients. Phenytoin may cause anorexia, nausea, and vomiting.
- Women taking oral contraceptives and anticonvulsants may need to use an additional contraceptive method.

CLIENT TEACHING

General
- Instruct the client to shake well the suspension form before pouring.
- Instruct the client not to drive or perform other hazardous activity when beginning anticonvulsant therapy.
- Instruct the client to inform the health care provider of adverse reactions such as gingivitis, nystagmus, slurred speech, and rash.
- Alert female clients contemplating pregnancy to consult with the health care provider as phenytoin may have a teratogenic effect on the fetus.
- Inform the client that alcohol and other CNS depressants can cause an added depressive effect on the body and should be avoided.
- Advise the client to obtain an alert ID card and medic alert bracelet or tag that indicate the health problem and the drug taken.
- Instruct the client not to abruptly stop the drug therapy but rather to withdraw the prescribed drug gradually under medical supervision to prevent seizure rebound (recurrence of seizures).
- Instruct the client of the need for preventative dental check-ups.

Side Effects
- Advise the client that urine may be a harmless pinkish-red or reddish-brown.
- Instruct the client to maintain good oral hygiene; use a soft toothbrush to prevent gum irritation and bleeding.

EVALUATION
- Evaluate the effectiveness of the drug in controlling seizures.
- Continue to monitor phenytoin serum levels to determine if they are within the desired range. High serum levels of phenytoin are frequently indicators of phenytoin toxicity.

Anticonvulsants

Generic (Brand)	Route and Dosage	Preg Cat	Interaction	t½	PB	Onset	Peak	Duration
Barbiturates Amobarbital (Amytal) CSS II	*Status epilepticus* A: IM/IV: 75–500 mg; max: IM: 500 mg; IV: 1,000 mg Therapeutic serum range: 1–5 µg/mL	D	*Increase* effect with antidepressants, CNS depressants *Decrease* effect of tricyclic antidepressants, cimetidine	*Biphasic:* 1–40 min; 2–20 h	50–60%	<5 min	UK	3–6 h
Mephobarbital (Mebaral) CSS II	A: PO: 400–600 mg/d C: PO: 6–12 mg/kg/d in divided doses or C >5 y: 32–64 mg t.i.d./q.i.d. C <5 y: 16–32 mg t.i.d./q.i.d. Therapeutic serum range: 15–40 µg/mL	D	*Decrease* effects of oral anticoagulants	34 h	UK	20–60 min	UK	6–8 h
Phenobarbital (Luminal) CSS IV	*Status epilepticus* Neonate: IV: LD: 15–20 mg/kg single or divided dose A&C: IV: 15–18 mg/kg; max: 30 mg/kg *Maintenance:* Neonate: PO/IV: 3–4 mg/kg/d in 1–2 divided doses Infant: 5–6 mg/kg/d in 1–2 divided doses	D	*Increase* effects of other CNS depressants *Decrease* effects of oral contraceptives, oral anticoagulants, theophylline, phenothiazines	A: 50–140 h C: 35–75 h Neonate: 50–500 h	20–40%	PO: 30–60 min IV: <5 min	UK 30 min	6–10 h 4–10 h

Primidone (Mysoline)	C: 1–5 y: 6–8 mg/kg/d in 1–2 divided doses 6–12 y: 4–6 mg/kg/d in 1–2 divided doses A: 1–3 mg/kg/d; 100–300 mg/d Therapeutic serum range: 15–40 µg/mL A: PO: 125–250 mg b.i.d./q.i.d. C <8 y: PO: 1/2 of adult dose Therapeutic serum range: 5–10 µg/mL	D	Same as phenobarbital	10–24 h	99%	4–7 d	7–10 d	8–12 h
Benzodiazepines (anxiolytics)								
Clonazepam (Klonopin)	A: PO: 0.5–1 mg t.i.d.; gradually increase dose q3d until seizures are controlled C: PO: 0.01–0.03 mg/kg/d; gradually increase Therapeutic serum range: 20–80 ng/mL	C	*Increase* effects with CNS depressants, phenytoin	A: 20–50 h C: 24–36 h	85%	15–60 min	1–2 h	6–8 h
Clorazepate (Tranxene) CSS IV	A: PO: 7.5 mg t.i.d. C: PO: 7.5 mg b.i.d.	D	*Increase* effect of drug with CNS depressants, oral contraceptives, alcohol *Decrease* effects with rifampin, barbiturates, valproic acid	48 h	97%	1–2 h	1–2 h	24 h

continued

Anticonvulsants—Continued

Generic (Brand)	Route and Dosage	Preg Cat	Interaction	t1/2	PB	Onset	Peak	Duration
Diazepam (Valium) Lorazepam (Ativan) CSS IV	See Prototype Drug Chart for Anxiolytics *Status epilepticus:* Neonate: IV: 0.05 mg/kg over 2–5 min; Infants & C: 0.1 mg/kg over 2–5 min; max: 4 mg/single dose A: IV: 4 mg over 2–5 min; max: 8 mg; may repeat in 10–15 min for all ages Therapeutic serum range: 50–240 ng/mL	D	*Increase* effect with morphine *Decrease* effect with oral contraceptives, smoking; toxicity with MAOIs, CNS depressants, alcohol	10–16 h	85%	IV: 1–5 min	UK	UK
Hydantoins Ethotoin (Peganone)	A: PO: 1–3 g/d in divided doses C: PO: 0.5–1 g/d Therapeutic serum range: 15–50 µg/mL	D	Same as mephenytoin	3–9 h	UK	UK	UK	UK
Mephenytoin (Mesantoin)	A: PO: Initially: 50–100 mg; 100–200 mg t.i.d. C: PO: Initially: 50–100 mg; 100–400 mg/d in divided doses Therapeutic serum range: 25–40 µg/mL	C	*Increase* effects of oral contraceptives, oral anticoagulants, phenothiazines *Decrease* effects of antineoplastics	7 h Metabolite: 100–144 h	UK	30 min	1–4 h	24–48 h
Phenytoin (Dilantin)	See Prototype Drug Chart							

Iminostilbene								
Carbamazepine (Tegretol)	A: PO: 200 mg b.i.d.; increasing doses as needed C: PO: 10–20 mg/kg/d in divided doses Therapeutic serum range: 5–12 µg/mL	C	*Increase* effects of drug with verapamil, isoniazid, cimetidine, erythromycin	15–30 h	75–90%	2–4 d	2–12 h	UK
Oxazolidones								
Paramethadione (Paradione)	A: PO: 300–600 mg t.i.d./q.i.d. C: PO: 13 mg/kg t.i.d. or 335 mg/m² t.i.d. or 300–900 mg/d in divided doses	D	None significant	1–4 h	UK	15–30 min	1–2 h	4–6 h
Trimethadione (Tridione)	Same as paramethadione	D	None significant	6–12 d	<10%	UK	1/2–2 h	UK
Succinimides								
Ethosuximide (Zarontin)	A: PO: 250 mg b.i.d.; increase dose gradually C: 3–6 y: PO: 250 mg/d Therapeutic serum range: 40–100 µg/mL	C	MAOIs and antidepressants lower seizure threshold; *increase* effects with CNS depressants	A: 50–60 h C: 25–30 h	UK	UK	>4 h	12–60 h
Methsuximide (Celontin)	A&C: PO: Initially: 300 mg/d for 1 wk; may increase at intervals	C	*Decrease* effects of oral contraceptives	2–4 h	Uk	15–30 min	1–3 h	4–6 h
Phensuximide (Milontin)	A&C: PO: 0.5–1 g b.i.d./t.i.d.	C	Similar to ethosuximide	5–12 h	UK	UK	1–4 h	UK

continued

Anticonvulsants—*Continued*

Generic (Brand)	Route and Dosage	Preg Cat	Interaction	t1/2	PB	Onset	Peak	Duration
Valproate Valproic acid (Depakene, Depakote)	A&C: PO: 15 mg/kg; max: 60 mg/kg/d in divided doses Therapeutic serum range: 40–100 µg/mL	D	*Increase* effects of drug with CNS depressants, barbiturates	6–16 h	90%	15–30 min	1–4 h	4–6 h
Miscellaneous Acetazolamide (Diamox)	Commonly used with other anticonvulsants: A: PO/IM/IV: 375 mg daily; max: 250 mg q.i.d. or PO SR: 250–500 mg daily or b.i.d. C: PO: 8–30 mg/kg in divided doses; max: 1.5 g/d	C	*Increase* effects of tricyclic antidepressants, ephedrine, procainamide, amphetamines; toxicity with salicylates	2.5–6 h	90%	PO: 1h SR: 2 h IV: 2 min	2–4 h 8–18 h <1 min	8–12 h 18–24 h 4–5 h
Gabapentin (Neurontin)	*Adjunctive therapy for partial seizures:* PO: 900–1,800 mg/d in 3 divided doses; max time between doses: 12 h	C	*Decrease* effects with antacids	5–7 h	<3%	UK	UK	UK

Drug		Dosage					
Lamotrigine (Lamictal)	C	A: PO: Initially: 50 mg/d for 14 d; then 100 mg/d in 2 divided doses; maint: 300–500 mg/d in 2 divided doses *With valproic acid:* PO: 25 mg qod for 14 d, then 25 mg/d for 14 d; maint: max: 150 mg/d in 2 divided doses	Other anticonvulsants increase or decrease drug's steady state concentrations Requires close monitoring	29 h	55%	UK	Serum: 1.5–5 h	UK
Magnesium sulfate	B	*Preeclampsia or eclampsia:* A: IV: Initially: 4 g in 250 mL D$_5$W then 4 g IM; follow with 4 g IM q4h PRN or Inf: 1–4 g/h *Hypomagnesemic seizures:* A: IV: 1–2 g (19% sol) over 20 min; follow with 1 g IM q4–6 h based on blood levels	Use cautiously with anesthesia and CNS depressants to avoid additive effect *Increase* neuromuscular blockade of vecuronium tubocurarine	UK	UK	IV: Immediate IM: 1 h	UK	IV: 30 min

KEY: For complete abbreviation key, see inside front cover.

ANTIPSYCHOTICS, ANXIOLYTICS, AND ANTIDEPRESSANTS

Antipsychotics
Phenothiazine
Nonphenothiazine

Anxiolytics

Antidepressants

Antimanic

Prototype: Antipsychotics

Chlorpromazine

Chlorpromazine
(Thorazine), ✽ Chlorpromanyl
Antipsychotic neuroleptic, antiemetic (phenothiazine)

Pregnancy Category: C

Drug Forms:
Tab 10, 25, 50, 100, 200 mg
Cap SR 30, 75, 150, 200, 300 mg
Syrup 10 mg/5 mL
Conc 30, 100 mg/mL
Supp 25, 100 mg
Inj IM/IV 25 mg/mL

Dosage

Psychoses
A: PO: 10–25 mg b.i.d./q.i.d.; increase by 20–50 mg/d q3–4d to max 800 mg/d in 4 divided doses (usual dose is 200 mg/d)
IM: Initially: 25–50 mg; may repeat in 1 h; then q3–4h PRN; increase to max of 400 mg q4–6h
C: PO: 0.55 mg/kg q4–6h
C: > 6 mon: IM: 0.55 mg/kg or 15 mg/m^2 q6–8h; max: 6 mon–5 y: 40 mg/d; 5–12 y: 75 mg/d
Consult other references for dosages for nausea, vomiting, preoperative sedation, and intractable hiccups.

Contraindications

Coma; hepatic, renal, or coronary disease; cerebral insufficiency; severe hypotension; CNS depression

Drug-Lab-Food Interactions

Increase CNS depression with alcohol, CNS depressants, narcotics, sedative-hypnotics; tricyclic antidepressants *increase* hypotensive and anticholinergic effects

Decrease absorption with antacids, antidiarrheals

Lab: *Increase* AST, ALT, and alkaline phosphatase; false pregnancy test; false PKU

Decrease hematocrit, hemoglobin, leukocytes, platelets

Pharmacokinetics

Absorption: PO: Varies
Distribution: PB: 95%
Metabolism: t 1/2: 8–30 h
Excretion: In urine

Pharmacodynamics

PO: Onset: 30–60 min
Peak: 2–4 h
Duration: 4–6 h
PO SR: Onset: 30–60 min
Peak: 2–4 h
Duration: <10–12 h
Rectal: Onset: 1–2 h
Peak: 3 h
Duration: 3–4 h
IM: Onset: 15–30 min
Peak: 30 min
Duration: 4–8 h
IV: Onset: 15 min
Peak: 10 min
Duration: UK

Therapeutic Effects/Uses: To treat psychosis (mania, schizophrenia), anxiety, agitation, intractable hiccups, nausea, vomiting, preoperative sedation, behavioral problems in children

Mode of Action: Alteration in dopamine effect on CNS, depression of limbic system and cerebral cortex that controls aggression, mechanism for antipsychotic effects unknown

Antipsychotics

Side Effects	Adverse Reactions
Sedation, hypotension, dizziness, extrapyramidal symptoms (EPS), constipation, headache, dry mouth and eyes, nausea, vomiting, diarrhea, urinary retention	Anemia, tachycardia, leukopenia, tardive dyskinesia *Life-threatening:* Agranulocytosis, seizures, laryngospasm, respiratory depression, circulatory failure

KEY: For complete abbreviation key, see inside front cover.

■ NURSING PROCESS: Chlorpromazine

ASSESSMENT
- Obtain baseline vital signs for use in future comparison.
- Obtain a history from the client of present drug therapy. If client is taking an anticonvulsant, drug dose might need to be increased as antipsychotics tend to lower seizure threshold.
- Assess mental status before start of drug therapy and continue daily.

POTENTIAL NURSING DIAGNOSES
Altered thought processes
Activity intolerance
Sensory-perceptual alteration

PLANNING
- Client's psychotic behavior will be controlled by drug(s) and psychotherapy.

NURSING INTERVENTIONS
- Monitor vital signs. Orthostatic hypotension is likely to occur.
- Remain with client while he or she takes the medication. Some clients hide drugs.
- Avoid skin contact with liquid concentrates to prevent contact dermatitis. Liquid must be protected from light and should be diluted with fruit juice.
- Administer oral doses with food or milk to decrease gastric irritation.
- Administer IM phenothiazines deep into the muscle because the drug is irritating to the fatty tissue. Do NOT inject into subcutaneous tissue. Check blood pressure for marked decrease 30 min after IM phenothiazine is injected.
- Do not mix in same syringe with heparin, pentobarbital, cimetidine, or dimenhydrinate.
- Chill suppository in the refrigerator for 30 min before removing foil wrapper.
- Observe the client for extrapyramidal syndrome (EPS): acute dystonia (spasms of the tongue, face, neck, and back), akathisia (restlessness, inability to sit still, foot tapping), pseudoparkinsonism (muscle tremors, rigidity, shuffling gait), and tardive dyskinesia (lip smacking, protruding and darting tongue, and constant chewing movement). Report these promptly to the health care provider.
- Monitor for symptoms of neuroleptic malignant syndrome (NMS): increased fever, pulse, and blood pressure; muscle rigidity; increased creatine phospho-

Antipsychotics

kinase and WBC; altered mental status; acute renal failure; varying levels of consciousness; pallor; diaphoresis, tachycardia; and dysrhythmias.
• Monitor urine output. Urinary retention may result.
• Monitor serum glucose level.

CLIENT TEACHING
General

• Instruct the client to take the drug exactly as ordered. In schizophrenia and other psychotic disorders, antipsychotics do not cure the mental illness but do prevent symptoms. Many clients on medication can function outside the institution setting.
• Advise the client that medication may take 6 wk or longer to achieve full clinical effect.
• Instruct the client not to consume alcohol or other CNS depressants such as narcotics; these drugs intensify the depressant effect on the body.
• Instruct the client not to abruptly discontinue the drug. Seek advice from the health care provider before making any changes in dosage.
• Encourage the client to read labels on OTC preparations. Some are contraindicated when taking antipsychotics.
• Advise client to consult the health care provider if dry mouth persists for more than 2 wk.
• Encourage the client to talk with the health care provider regarding family planning. The effect of antipsychotics on the fetus is not fully known; however, there may be teratogenic effects on the fetus.
• Instruct the client on the importance of routine follow-up examinations.
• Encourage the client to obtain laboratory tests on schedule. WBCs are monitored for 3 mo, especially during the start of drug therapy. Leukopenia, or decreased WBCs, may occur. Be alert to symptoms of malaise, fever, and sore throat, which may be an indication of agranulocytosis, a serious blood dyscrasia. Report this promptly to the health care provider.
• Encourage the client to wear an ID bracelet indicating the medication taken.

Side Effects

• Inform the client about EPS; instruct the client to promptly report symptoms to the health care provider.
• Photosensitivity may occur; instruct the client to avoid direct sunlight or to use a sun block and protective clothing. Sunbathing can cause a skin rash.
• Advise the client of orthostatic hypotension and possible dizziness.
• Advise the client that urine might be pink or red-brown; this discoloration is harmless.
• Inform the client that changes may occur related to sexual functioning and menstruating. Women could have irregular menstrual periods or amenorrhea, and men might experience impotence and gynecomastia (enlargement of breast tissue).

EVALUATION

• Evaluate the effectiveness of the drug; the client is free of psychotic symptoms.
• The client can cope with everyday living situation.
• Identify any side effects of or adverse reactions to the drug.

NOTES:

Antipsychotics

Generic (Brand)	Route and Dosage	Preg Cat	Interaction	t 1/2	PB	Onset	Peak	Duration
Phenothiazines: Aliphatics								
Chlorpromazine HCl (Thorazine)	See Prototype Drug Chart							
Promazine HCl (Sparine)	A: PO: 10–200 mg q4–6h IM: 50–150 mg; may repeat ×1 C > 12 y: PO: 10–25 mg q4–6h	C	*Increase* effect with CNS depressants, epinephrine, anticholinergics *Lab: Increase* cholesterol, glucose	≥24 h	≥90%	PO: 30–60 min IM: 15–30 min	2–4 h 1 h	4–6 h 4–6 h
Triflupromazine* (Vesprin)	A: PO: 10–50 mg b.i.d./t.i.d. IM: 60–150 mg/d C > 2 y: PO: 0.5–2 mg/kg/d in 3 divided doses	C	Similar to promazine	≥24 h	≥90%	PO: Erratic IM: 15–30 min	2–4 h 1 h	4–6 h 12 h
Piperazines								
Fluphenazine HCl (Prolixin)	A: PO: 1–5 mg t.i.d./q.i.d. Elderly: 1–2.5 mg/d; also long-acting weekly/biweekly dosages Therapeutic serum range: 5–20 ng/mL	C	*Increase* effect of narcotics *Decrease* effect of barbiturates, lithium, levodopa *Lab: Increase* cholesterol, glucose	5–15 h	≥90%	PO/IM: 1 h	0.5–2 h	6–8 h
Perphenazine (Trilafon)	See Prototype Drug Chart							
Prochlorperazine maleate (Compazine)	A: PO: 5–10 mg t.i.d./q.i.d.; max: 40 mg/d (can be higher for psychotic behavior)	C	*Increase* effect of anticonvulsants, CNS depressants, epinephrine	23 h	≥90%	PO: 30–40 min IM: 10–20 min	2–4 h 15–30 min	3–4 h 2–12 h

Drug		Preg. Cat.	Interactions			Onset	Peak	Duration
Thiothixene HCl (Navane)	A: PO: 2 mg t.i.d.; max: 60 mg/d IM: 4 mg b.i.d./q.i.d.; Max: 30 mg/d	C	*Increase* effect of CNS depressants, hypotensive agents *Decrease* effects of levodopa *Lab: Increase* cholesterol, glucose	24–34 h	≥90%	PO: 2–7 d IM: 15–30 min	2–8 h 1–6 h	12–24 h Up to 12 h
Trifluoperazine HCl* (Stelazine)	A: PO: 1–5 mg b.i.d.; max: 40 mg/d C: PO: 1 mg daily/b.i.d.	C	*Increase* effect with CNS depressants, propranolol *Decrease* effects with anticoagulants, anticonvulsants	≥24 h	≥90%	PO: 30–40 min IM: 10–20 min	2–4 h 15–30 min	4–6 h 12 h
Piperidine								
Mesoridazine besylate (Serentill)	A: PO: 50 mg t.i.d.; gradually increase; optimum response 100–400 mg/d Elderly: 1/3–1/2 adult dose	C	*Increase* toxicity with CNS depressants *Decrease* effects with anticholinergics, anticonvulsants	24–48 h	92–99%	PO: Erratic IM: 15–30 min	2 h 20 min	4–6 h 6–8 h
Thioridazine HCl (Mellaril)	A: PO: 50–100 mg t.i.d.; max: 800 mg/d Elderly: 1/3–1/2 adult dose	C	*Increase* effect with CNS depressants, epinephrine *Decrease* effects with anticholinergics	24–30 h	≥90%	PO: 30–60 min	2–4 h	4–6 h

*Avoid spilling liquid on skin. Contact dermatitis could result.
KEY: For complete abbreviation key, see inside front cover.

Prototype: Antipsychotic: Nonphenothiazine

Haloperidol

Haloperidol
  (Haldol), ✽ Peridol
Antipsychotic, neuroleptic
  (nonphenothiazine)
Pregnancy Category: C
Drug Forms:
Tab 0.5, 1, 2, 5, 10, 20 mg
Conc 2 mg/mL
Inj 5 mg/mL
Depot 50, 100 mg/mL

Dosage

A: PO: 0.5–5 mg b.i.d./t.i.d.
  IM: decanoate: 50–100 mg q4 wk
  IM: 2–5 mg q4h PRN
C: PO: 0.15 mg/kg/d in divided
  doses (not for child <3 y)
Elderly: Decreased doses than for
  younger adult
PO: 0.5–2mg b.i.d./t.i.d.

Contraindications

Narrow-angle glaucoma; severe hepatic, renal, and cardiovascular diseases; bone marrow depression; Parkinson's disease; blood dyscrasias; CNS depression; subcortical brain damage

Drug-Lab-Food Interactions

Increase sedation with alcohol, CNS depressants
Increase toxicity with anticholinergics, CNS depressants, lithium
Decrease effects with phenobarbital, carbamazepine, caffeine

Pharmacokinetics

Absorption: PO: 60% absorbed
Distribution: PB: 80–90%
Metabolism: t 1/2: 15–35 h
Excretion: In urine and feces

Pharmacodynamics

PO: Onset: erratic
             Peak: 2–6 h
             Duration: 24–72 h
IM: Onset: 15–30 min
             Peak: 30–45 min
             Duration: 4–8 h
IM: Decanoate: Onset: UK
             Peak: 6–7 d
             Duration: 3–4 wk

Therapeutic Effects/Uses: To treat acute and chronic psychoses, for children with severe behavior problems who are combative, to suppress narcotic withdrawal symptoms, to treat schizophrenia resistant to other drugs, to treat Tourette's syndrome, to treat symptoms of dementia in elderly.

Mode of Action: Alteration of the effect of dopamine on CNS; mechanism for antipsychotic effects are unknown.

Side Effects

Sedation, extrapyramidal symptoms, orthostatic hypotension, headache, photosensitivity, dry mouth and eyes, blurred vision

Adverse Reactions

Tachycardia, seizures, urinary retention, tardive dyskinesia
Life-threatening: Laryngospasm, respiratory depression, cardiac dysrhythmias, neuromalignant syndrome (NMS)

KEY: For complete abbreviation key, see inside front cover.

Antipsychotic: Nonphenothiazine

■ NURSING PROCESS: Nonphenothiazine Antipsychotic

ASSESSMENT
- Obtain baseline vital signs for future comparison.
- Obtain a history from the client of present drug therapy. If client is taking an anticonvulsant, drug dose might need to be increased as antipsychotics tend to lower seizure threshold.
- Assess mental status before the start of drug therapy.

POTENTIAL NURSING DIAGNOSIS
Altered thought processes; potential for violence

PLANNING
- Client's psychotic behavior will be controlled by drug and psychotherapy.

NURSING INTERVENTIONS
- Monitor vital signs. Orthostatic hypotension is likely to occur.
- Remain with client while he or she takes the medication. Some clients hide drugs. If necessary, do mouth checks or give concentrate.
- Administer by IM route deep into the muscle because the drug is irritating to the fatty tissue. Do NOT inject into subcutaneous tissue. Check blood pressure for marked decrease 30 min after drug is injected.
- Do not mix in same syringe with heparin, pentobarbital, cimetidine, or dimenhydrinate.
- Administer oral doses with food or 8 oz of water or milk to decrease gastric irritation.
- Observe the client for extrapyramidal syndrome (EPS): acute dystonia (spasms of the tongue, face, neck, and back), akathisia (restlessness, inability to sit still, foot tapping), pseudoparkinsonism (muscle tremors, rigidity, drooling, shuffling gait), and tardive dyskinesia (lip smacking, protruding and darting tongue, constant chewing movement, difficulty swallowing). Report these promptly to the health care provider.
- Monitor urine output. Urinary retention may result.
- Monitor serum glucose level.

CLIENT TEACHING

General
- Instruct the client to take the drug exactly as ordered. In schizophrenia and other psychotic disorders, antipsychotics do not cure the mental illness but do prevent symptoms. Many clients on medication can function outside the institution.
- Instruct the client not to consume alcohol or other CNS depressants such as narcotics; these drugs intensify the depressant effect on the body.
- Instruct the client not to abruptly discontinue the drug. Seek advice from the health care provider before making any changes in dosage.
- Encourage the client to read labels on OTC preparations. Some are contraindicated when taking antipsychotics.
- Instruct the client on the importance of routine follow-up examination.
- Encourage the client to talk with the health care provider regarding family planning. The effect of antipsychotics on the fetus is not fully known; however, there may be teratogenic effects on the fetus.
- Encourage the client to wear an ID bracelet indicating the medication taken.

Antipsychotic: Nonphenothiazine

Side Effects

- Instruct the client to avoid potentially dangerous situations, such as driving, until drug dosing has been stabilized.
- Advise the client to change position slowly to decrease orthostatic hypotension.
- Inform clients about EPS symptoms; promptly report these to the health care provider.
- Advise the client to consult health care provider if dry mouth persists for more than 2 wk.
- Instruct the client to have daily fluid intake of eight 8-oz glasses.
- Photosensitivity may occur; instruct the client to avoid direct sunlight or to use a sun block and protective clothing. Sunbathing can cause a skin rash.
- Advise the client to avoid extremes in temperatures and increased exercise.
- Inform the client that changes related to sexual functioning and menstruation may occur. Women could have irregular menstrual periods or amenorrhea, and men might experience impotence and gynecomastia (enlargement of breast tissue).
- Encourge the client to obtain laboratory tests on schedule. Weekly blood work is a must for clozapine. WBCs are monitored for 3 mon, especially during the start of drug therapy. Leukopenia, or decreased WBCs, may occur. Be alert to symptoms of malaise, fever, and sore throat, which may be an indication of agranulocytosis, a serious blood dyscrasia. Report this promptly to the health care provider, especially with clozapine.

EVALUATION

- Evaluate the effectiveness of the drug; the client is free of psychotic symptoms at the *lowest* dose possible.
- The client can cope with everyday living situation and attend to activities of daily living.
- Determine if any side effects of or adverse reactions to the drug have occurred.

NOTES:

Antipsychotics

Generic (Brand)	Route and Dosage	Preg Cat	Interaction	t1/2	PB	Onset	Peak	Duration
Nonphenothiazines								
Butyrophenone								
Droperidol (Inapsine)	A: IM/IV: 2.5–10 mg 30–60 min before anesthesia C: IM/IV: 0.088–0.165 mg/kg	C	*Increase* CNS depression with other CNS depressants, alcohol *Decrease* effect of guanethidine	2 h	UK	5–10 min	30 min	2–12 h
Haloperidol (Haldol)	See Prototype Drug Chart							
Dibenzoxazepine								
Loxapine (Loxitane)	A: PO: Initially: 10 mg b.i.d.; then may increase to 50–100 mg/d Elderly: 1/3–1/2 regular adult dose	C	Similar to droperidol	5 h	95%	20–30 min	1–3 h	12 h
Thioxanthenes								
Clorprothixene HCl (Taractan)	A: PO: 25–50 mg t.i.d.; gradually increase to 500–600 mg/d	C	*Increase* CNS depression with CNS depressants, alcohol *Decrease* effect of guanethidine	Initial phase: 3 h Late phase: 34 h	UK	30–60 min	2–4 h	4–6 h

Thiothixene HCl (Navane)	A: PO: Initially: 2 mg t.i.d.; gradually increase to 10–25 mg/d	C	Similar to droperidol	34 h	UK	2–7 d	2–8 h	12–24 h
Others								
Clozapine (Clozaril)	A: PO/IM: Initially: <50 mg/d; if tolerated, gradually increase to 300–450 mg/d in divided doses	B	*Increase* CNS depression with antihistamines, sedative-hypnotics, narcotics	8–12 h	95%	UK	2–4 wk	4–12 h
Molindone HCl (Moban)	A: PO: 5–50 mg t.i.d./q.i.d. Elderly: 1/3–1/2 adult dose	C	*Increase* toxicity with antihypertensives, anticonvulsants, CNS depressants	1.5 h	UK	UK	1/2 h	24–30 h
Risperidone (Risperdal)	A: PO: 1–3 mg b.i.d. Elderly: 1/3–1/2 adult dose	C	*Increase* effects with CNS depressants, alcohol *Increase* toxicity with warfarin, quinidine *Lab:* must monitor for agranulocytosis with WBCs weekly	24 h	90%	UK	1–2 h	UK

KEY: For complete abbreviation key, see inside front cover.

Prototype: Anxiolytics

Diazepam

Diazepam
  (Valium), ✤ Apo-Diazepam,
  Diazemuls, Novodipam
Benzodiazepine
  CSS IV
Pregnancy Category: D
Drug Forms:
Tab 2, 5, 10 mg
Cap SR 15 mg
Oral solution 5 mg/5 mL, 5 mg/mL
Inj 5 mg/5 mL (1, 2, and 10 mL)

Dosage

Anxiety:
A: PO/IM/IV: 2–10 mg b.i.d./q.i.d.
Elderly: 2.5 mg b.i.d.
C >6 mon: 1–2.5 mg t.i.d./q.i.d.
Musculoskeletal spasm:
A: PO: 2–10 mg b.i.d./q.i.d.
  IM: 5–10 mg q3–4h
Preoperative sedation:
A: IV: 5–15 mg 15 min before event
Status epilepticus:
A: IV: 5–10 mg q10–20 min; max:
  30 mg
C <6 y: 0.2–0.5 mg/kg q15–30 min;
  max: 5 mg total dose
C >6 y: 0.2–0.5 mg/kg q15–30 min;
  max: 10 mg total dose
IV: max: 5 mg/3 min

Contraindications

Hypersensitivity, CNS depression, shock, coma, narrow-angle glaucoma, pregnancy, lactation
Caution: Hepatic or renal dysfunction; epilepsy, elderly and infants; history of drug abuse; depression, addiction-prone, or suicidal tendency

Drug-Lab-Food Interactions

Increase effects of diazepam with alcohol, oral contraceptives, CNS depressants, cimetidine, disulfiram, fluoxetine, isoniazid, ketoconazole, levodopa, metoprolol, propoxyphene, propranolol, valproic acid; toxic effects with MAOIs; *Decrease* effects with rifampin, cigarettes, and theophylline
Increase effects of digoxin, phenytoin
Do not mix or dilute with other drugs in syringe
Lab: Increase bilirubin

Pharmacokinetics

Absorption: Rapid from GI tract; erratic from IM administration; most rapid and complete from deltoid muscle
Distribution: Widely PB: 98%
Metabolism: t 1/2: 25–50 h
Excretion: In urine

Pharmacodynamics

PO: Onset: 30–60 min
    Peak: 1–2 h
    Duration: 2–3 h (varies)
IM: Onset: 15–30 min
    Peak: 1–2 h
    Duration: 1–1 1/2 h (varies)
IV: Onset: 1–5 min
    Peak: 15–30 min
    Duration: 15–60 min

Therapeutic Effects/Uses: To control anxiety, preoperative sedation, skeletal muscle relaxant, to treat status epilepticus, alcohol withdrawal, convulsive disorders, anterograde amnesia.

Mode of Action: Depression of limbic and subcortical CNS and skeletal muscle relaxation, shortens stage 4 and REM sleep.

Side Effects	Adverse Reactions
Drowsiness, dizziness, syncope, orthostatic hypotension, blurred vision, nausea, vomiting, fatigue, confusion	ECG changes, tachycardia, psychological and physical dependence with long-term use *Life-threatening:* Laryngospasm

KEY: For complete abbreviation key, see inside front cover.

■ NURSING PROCESS: Anxiolytics: Diazepam

ASSESSMENT
- Assess for suicidal ideation.
- Obtain a history of the client's anxiety reaction.
- Determine the client's support system (family, friends, groups), if any.
- Obtain the client's drug history. Report possible drug-drug interaction.

POTENTIAL NURSING DIAGNOSES
Anxiety
Mobility, impaired physical

PLANNING
- Client's anxiety and stress will be reduced through nonpharmacological methods, anxiolytic drugs, or support/group therapy.

NURSING INTERVENTIONS
- Administer by IM route in large muscle mass, and inject drug slowly.
- Observe the client for side effects of anxiolytics. Recognize that drug tolerance and physical and psychological dependency can result with most anxiolytics.
- Recognize that anxiolytic drug dosages should be less for older adults and debilitated persons than for young and middle-aged adults.
- Monitor vital signs, especially blood pressure and pulse; orthostatic hypotension may occur.
- Encourage the family to be supportive of the client.

CLIENT TEACHING

General
- Advise the client not to drive a motor vehicle or operate dangerous equipment when taking anxiolytics since sedation is a common side effect.
- Instruct the client not to consume alcohol or CNS depressants such as narcotics while taking an anxiolytic.
- Instruct the client on ways to control excess stress and anxiety, such as relaxation techniques.
- Inform the client that effective response may take 1 to 2 wk.
- Encourage the client to follow drug regimen and not to abruptly stop taking the drug after prolonged use because withdrawal symptoms can occur.

Side Effects
- Instruct the client to arise slowly from the sitting to standing position to avoid dizziness from orthostatic hypotension.

EVALUATION
- Evaluate the effectiveness of drug therapy by determining if the client is less anxious and more able to cope with stresses and anxieties.
- Determine if the client is taking anxiolytic drug as prescribed and is adhering to client teaching instructions.

Anxiolytics

Generic (Brand)	Route and Dosage	Preg Cat	Interaction	t 1/2	PB	Onset	Peak	Duration
Antihistamines								
Hydroxyzine HCl (Atarax, Vistaril)	A: PO: 50–100 mg t.i.d./q.i.d. IM: 25–100 mg C <6 y: 25 mg b.i.d. C >6 y: 25 mg b.i.d./q.i.d.	C	*Increase* effect with anticholinergic, CNS depressants *Decrease* effect with epinephrine	3–7 h	UK	PO/IM: 15–30 min	2–4 h	4–6 h
Benzodiazepines								
Alprazolam (Xanax) CSS IV	A: PO: 0.25–0.5 mg t.i.d. Elderly: 0.25 mg b.i.d./t.i.d.; max: 4 mg/d	D	*Increase* effects of drug with CNS depressants	12–15 h	80%	1–2 h	1–2 h	12–24 h
Chlordiazepoxide HCl (Librium) CSS IV	*Anxiety disorders:* A: PO: 5–25 mg t.i.d./q.i.d. C: PO: 5 mg b.i.d/q.i.d. *Acute alcohol withdrawal:* A: PO/IM/IV: 50–100 mg; max: 300 mg/d Elderly: 1/2 adult dose	D	*Increase* effect of drug with CNS depressants, oral contraceptives, alcohol, barbiturates, valproic acid *Decrease* effects of drug with rifampin	6–30 h	90–98%	PO: 15–30 min	15–30 min	2–4 h
Clorazepate dipotassium (Tranxene) CSS IV	A: PO: 15–60 mg/d in divided doses Elderly: 7.5 mg b.i.d.	D	Similar to chlordiazepoxide	48 h	80–90%	30–60 min	1–2 h	24 h
Diazepam (Valium)	See Prototype Drug Chart							

Drug		Dosage	Pregnancy Category	Drug Interactions	Half-Life	Protein Binding	Onset	Peak	Duration
Halazepam (Paxipam)		A: PO: 20–40 mg t.i.d./q.i.d. Elderly: 20 mg daily/b.i.d.	D	Same as chlordiazepoxide	14 h	97%	30–60 min	1–3 h	UK
Lorazepam (Ativan) CSS IV		A: PO: 2–6 mg/d in divided doses A: IM/IV: 2–4 mg Elderly: 1/2 adult dose	D	*Increase* effects with probenecid, CNS depressants *Decrease* effect with smoking	10–20 h	90%	15–45 min	1–6 h	36–48 h
Oxazepam (Serax)		A: PO: 10–30 mg t.i.d./q.i.d. Elderly: 10–15 mg t.i.d./q.i.d.	D	Similar to chlordiazepoxide	3.5–21 h	85–95%	45–90 min	1–2 h	6–12 h
Prazepam (Centrax) CSS IV		A: PO: 10 mg t.i.d./q.i.d. Elderly: 10–15 mg/d in divided doses	D	Same as chlordiazepoxide	30–200 h	97%	UK	7–14 d	2–3 d
Propanediols									
Meprobamate (Equanil, Miltown) CSS IV		A: PO: 400 mg t.i.d./q.i.d. C: PO: 100–200 mg b.i.d./t.i.d.	D	*Increase* effects with CNS depressants, sedative-hypnotics	6–16 h	UK	1 h	1–3 h	6–12 h
Others									
Buspirone HCl (BuSpar)		A: PO: Initial: 5 mg b.i.d./t.i.d.; 15–30 mg/d in divided doses; max: 60 mg/d Elderly: 30 mg/d	B	*Increase* effect with cimetidine; hypertensive crises may result with MAOIs; avoid alcohol *Increase* toxicity of digoxin *Lab: Increase* AST, ALT	2–3 h	95%	7–14 d	3–4 wk	UK

KEY: For complete abbreviation key, see inside front cover.

Prototype: Antidepressants

Amoxapine

Amoxapine
  (Asendin)
Antidepressant: Second-generation tricyclic
Pregnancy Category: C
Drug Forms:
Tab 25, 50, 100, 150 mg

Dosage

A: PO: 50 mg b.i.d./t.i.d.; increase dose gradually to <300 mg/d or give as single dose at h.s.; max: inpatient: 600 mg/d; max: outpatient: 400 mg/d; generally not recommended for children <16y
Elderly: PO: 25 mg b.i.d./t.i.d.; may increase to 50 mg b.i.d.
Therapeutic serum range: 200–400 ng/ml

Contraindications

Within 14 d of receiving MAOIs, myocardial infarction recovery phase
Caution: Severe depression with suicidal tendency, severe liver or kidney disease, seizures, narrow-angle glaucoma, prostatic disease

Drug-Lab-Food Interactions

Increase effect of CNS depressants, alcohol, adrenergic agents, anticholinergics; *increase* effects with phenothiazines, haloperidol, smoking
Hypertensive crisis and death may occur with MAOIs
Decrease effect of clonidine; guanethidine
Lab: Altered ECG

Pharmacokinetics

Absorption: PO: well absorbed
Distribution: PB: 90%
Metabolism: t 1/2: 8 h, 30 h as metabolite
Excretion: 80% in urine; 20% in feces

Pharmacodynamics

Antidepressant effect:
PO: Onset: 2–4 wk
    Peak: 90 min
    Duration: weeks

Therapeutic Effects/Uses: To treat depression with or without melancholia, depressive phase of bipolar disorder, depression associated with organic disease, alcoholism, mixed symptoms of anxiety and depression, or urinary incontinence.

Mode of Action: Serotonin and norepinephrine increased in nerve cells due to blockage from nerve fibers.

Side Effects

Sedation, drowsiness, dry mouth and eyes, blurred vision, urinary retention, constipation, extrapyramidal syndrome, weight gain

Adverse Reactions

Life-threatening: Cardiac dysrhythmias, agranulocytosis, thrombocytopenia, leukopenia, neuroleptic malignant syndrome (hyperpyrexia, muscle rigidity, tachycardia, cardiac dysrhythmias)

KEY: For complete abbreviation key, see inside front cover.

Antidepressants

■ NURSING PROCESS: Second-Generation Antidepressant

ASSESSMENT
- Assess the client's baseline vital signs and weight for future comparison.
- Check the client's liver and renal function by assessing urine output (> 600 mL/d), BUN, and serum creatinine and liver enzyme levels.
- Obtain a history of episodes of depression or manic-depressive behavior; assess mental status.
- Obtain the client's drug history. CNS depressants can cause an additive effect. Antidepressants cause anticholinergic-like symptoms and are contraindicated if the client has glaucoma.
- Assess for tardive dyskinesia and neuroleptic malignant syndrome (NMS), including hyperpyrexia, muscle rigidity, tachycardia, cardiac dysrhythmias.

POTENTIAL NURSING DIAGNOSES
Potential for violence and injury
Anxiety
Social isolation

PLANNING
- Client's depression or manic-depressive behavior will be decreased.

NURSING INTERVENTIONS
- Observe the client for signs and symptoms of depression: mood changes, insomnia, apathy, or lack of interest in activities.
- Check the client's vital signs. Orthostatic hypotension is common. Check for anticholinergic-like symptoms: dry mouth, increased heart rate, urinary retention, or constipation. Weight check two to three times per week.
- Monitor the client for suicidal tendencies when marked depression is present.
- If the client is taking anticonvulsant, observe the client for seizures; antidepressants lower the seizure threshold.
- Provide the client with a list of foods to avoid, especially with MAOIs.

CLIENT TEACHING

General
- Instruct the client to take the medication as prescribed.
- Inform the client that the effectiveness of the drug may not be evident until 1–2 wk after the start of therapy.
- Encourage the client to keep medical appointments.
- Instruct the client not to consume alcohol or any CNS depressants.
- Instruct the client not to drive or be involved in potentially dangerous mechanical activity until stabilization of drug dose has been established.
- Instruct the client not to abruptly stop taking drug.
- Encourage the client who is planning pregnancy to consult with the health care provider about possible teratogenic effects of the drug on the fetus.

Side Effects
- Advise the client that antidepressants may be taken at bedtime to decrease the dangers from the sedative effect.

EVALUATION
- Evaluate the effectiveness of the drug therapy.

Antidepressants

Generic (Brand)	Route and Dosage	Preg Cat	Interaction	t1/2	PB	Onset	Peak	Duration
Tricyclics								
Amitriptyline HCl (Elavil, Endep, Enovil)	A: PO: 25 mg t.i.d.; increase to 150 mg/d; dose may be given as single h.s. dose *Therapeutic serum range:* 100–200 ng/mL	D	*Increase* effects of CNS depressants, anticholinergics, warfarin, adrenergics; *increase* toxicity with MAOIs, clonidine *Decrease* effect of guanethidine *Lab:* Increase glucose	10–50 h	95%	7–21 d	2–6 wk	UK
Clomipramine HCl (Anafranil)	A: 25–100 mg/d in divided doses; max: 250 mg/d; after titration; entire dose may be given h.s. Elderly: 20–30 mg/d	C	*Decrease* effects of phenytoin, barbiturates *Increase* effects of CNS depressants, anticholinergics, alcohol Toxicity MAOIs *Lab:* Increase glucose Similar to amitriptyline	20–30 h	96–97%	1–6 wk	UK	UK
Desipramine HCl (Norpramin, Pertofrane)	A: PO: 25 mg t.i.d. or 75 mg h.s.; increase to 200 mg/d; max: 300 mg/d Elderly: 25–50 mg/d in divided doses; max: 150 mg/d *Therapeutic serum range:* 150–250 ng/mL	D		15–90 h	90–95%	2–3 wk	6 wk	UK
Doxepin HCl (Sinequan)	A: PO: 75–100 mg/d h.s. or in divided doses; max: 300 mg/d Elderly: 25–50 mg/d *Therapeutic serum range:* 30–50 ng/mL	C	Similar to amitriptyline	6–8 h	80–85%	2–3 wk	4–6 wk	UK

Imipramine HCl (Tofranil)	A: PO: 75 mg/d t.i.d.); max: 300 mg/d IM: Initially: max: 100 mg/d in divided doses Elderly: 25–100 mg in divided doses C < 12 y: PO: 25–50 mg h.s. C > 12 y: PO: 75 mg h.s. *Therapeutic serum range:* 150–250 ng/mL	D	Similar to amitriptyline	8–15 h	89–95%	1 h	≥1 wk
Nortriptyline HCl (Aventyl)	A: PO: 25 mg t.i.d./q.i.d.; max: 100 mg/d Elderly: 30–50 mg/d in divided doses *Therapeutic serum range:* 50–150 ng/mL	D	*Increase* effects of CNS depressants, alcohol, epinephrine, benzodiazepines, MAOIs *Lab:* May increase PT of patients on warfarin; increase glucose	18–28 h	90–95%	2–3 wk	6 wk
Protriptyline HCl (Vivactil)	A: PO: 15–40 mg/d in divided doses; increase gradually; max: 60 mg/d Elderly: 5 mg/d; max: 20 mg/d *Therapeutic serum range:* 70–250 ng/mL	C	Similar to amitriptyline	60–98 h	92%	15–30 min	UK
Trimipramine maleate (Surmontil)	A: PO: 75–150 mg/d in divided doses or all h.s.; max: 200 mg/d Elderly: max: 100 mg/d	C	Similar to amitriptyline	20–26 h	95%	UK	4–6 h

continued

Antidepressants—Continued

Generic (Brand)	Route and Dosage	Preg Cat	Interaction	t 1/2	PB	Action Onset	Action Peak	Action Duration
Second Generation								
Amoxapine (Asendin)	See Prototype Drug Chart							
Bupropion HCl (Wellbutrin)	A: PO: Initially: 200 mg/d as b.i.d.; increase gradually to 300 mg/d in divided doses; max: 450 mg/d	B	*Increase* toxicity with anticonvulsants, cimetidine, MAOIs, levodopa	50 h	>80%	3–4 wk	1–3 h	UK
Fluoxetine HCl (Prozac)	A: PO: 20 mg in a.m.; max: 80 mg/d in divided doses	B	*Increase* toxicity with MAOIs, L-tryptophan, highly protein-bound drugs (e.g., warfarin)	7–9 d (active metabolite)	95%	Steady state: 2–4 wk	4 wk	2 wk
Maprotiline HCl (Ludiomil)	A: PO: 75 mg h.s. or in divided doses; max: 150 mg/d Elderly: 25 mg/d; max: 75 mg/d	B	*Increase* effects of norepinephrine, MAOIs, CNS depressants *Decrease* effects with phenytoin, barbiturates	21–25 h	88%	3–7 d	2–3 wk	UK
Paroxetine HCl (Paxil)	A: PO: 20 mg/d in a.m.; max: 50 mg/d Elderly: PO: Initially: 10 mg/d; max: 40 mg/d	B	Avoid use with highly protein-bound drugs, cimetidine, MAOIs, phenobarbital, phenytoin, alcohol, digoxin	21 h Elderly: 68 h	90–95%	Steady state: 10 d	5–8 h	UK

Drug	Dosage	Pregnancy Category	Contraindications/Drug Interactions	Half-life	Protein Binding	Onset	Peak	Duration
Sertraline HCl (Zoloft)	A: PO: 50 mg daily; max: 200 mg/d	B	Avoid use with highly protein-bound drugs, within 14 days of MAOIs; alcohol; caution with CNS depressants	26 h	98%	Steady state: 7 d	2–4 wk	UK
Trazodone HCl (Desyrel)	A: PO: 75 mg h.s. or 50 mg t.i.d.; max: 600 mg/d A: PO: 225–375 mg/d in 3 divided doses	C	Increase effects of CNS depressants, phenytoin, digitalis	5–10 h	85–95%	2 wk	2–4 wk	UK
Venlafaxine HCl (Effexor)		C	Do not give with MAOIs to avoid serotonin syndrome	3–5 h	25–30%	UK	UK	UK
Monoamine Oxidase Inhibitors								
Isocarboxazid (Marplan)	A: PO: 10–20 mg/d; max: 60 mg/d	C	Increase pressor effects of amphetamines, meperidine, vasoconstrictors, levodopa, tricyclic antidepressants, ephedrine, imipramine; foods with tyramine may cause hypertensive crisis	UK	UK	1–4 wk	3–4 wk	2 wk
Phenelzine sulfate (Nardil)	A: PO: 15 mg t.i.d.; 1 mg/kg in divided doses; max: 90 mg/d Elderly: max: 45–60 mg/d	C	Similar to isocarboxazid	UK	UK	1–4 wk	2–5 wk	2 wk
Tranylcypromine sulfate (Parnate)	A: PO: 10 mg b.i.d.; max: 60 mg Elderly: max: 45 mg/d	C	Similar to isocarboxazid	UK	UK	3–5 d	2–3 wk	3–5 d
Antimanic								
Lithium carbonate; lithium citrate	See Prototype Drug Chart							

KEY: For complete abbreviation key, see inside front cover.

Prototype: Antimanic: Lithium

Lithium carbonate

Lithium carbonate
(Eskalith, Lithane, Lithonate, Lithobid), ✦ Carbolith, Lithizine
Antimanic
Pregnancy Category: D
Drug Forms:
Cap 150, 300 mg
Tab 300 mg
Tab ER 300, 450 mg
Oral solution 8 mEq/5 mL (300 mg/5 mL)

Dosage

A: PO: 300–600 mg/t.i.d.;
Maint: 300 mg, t.i.d./q.i.d.;
max: 2.4 g/d
Elderly: lower dosage
Therapeutic range: 0.5–1.5 mEq/L

Contraindications

Liver and renal disease, pregnancy, lactation, severe cardiovascular disease, severe dehydration, brain tumor or damage, sodium depletion, children <12 y
Caution: Thyroid disease

Drug-Lab-Food Interactions

May *increase* lithium level with thiazide diuretics, methyldopa, haloperidol, NSAIDs, antidepressants, carbamazepine, theophylline, aminophylline, sodium bicarbonate, phenothiazines
Food: Increase sodium intake; lithium may cause sodium depletion
Lab: Increase urine and blood glucose, protein

Pharmacokinetics

Absorption: PO: well absorbed
Distribution: PB: UK
Metabolism: t 1/2: 21–30 h; >36 h with renal impairment or elderly
Excretion: 98% in urine, mostly unchanged

Pharmacodynamics

Antimanic effects:
PO: Onset: 5–7 d
     Peak: 10–21 d
     Duration: days
PO SR: Peak: 5–7 d

Therapeutic Effects/Uses: To treat bipolar manic-depressive psychosis, manic episodes.

Mode of Action: Alteration of ion transport in muscle and nerve cells; increased receptor sensitivity to serotonin.

Side Effects

Headache, lethargy, drowsiness, dizziness, tremors, slurred speech, dry mouth, anorexia, vomiting, diarrhea, polyuria, hypotension, abdominal pain, muscle weakness, restlessness

Adverse Reactions

Urinary incontinence, clonic movements, stupor, azotemia, leukocytosis
Life-threatening: Cardiac dysrhythmias, circulatory collapse

KEY: For complete abbreviation key, see inside front cover.

Antimanic: Lithium

■ NURSING PROCESS: Lithium

ASSESSMENT
- Assess for suicidal ideation.
- Assess the client's baseline vital signs for future comparison.
- Assess client's neurological status, including gait, level of consciousness, reflexes, and tremors.
- Check the client's hepatic and renal function by assessing urine output (>600 mL/d), whether BUN, serum creatinine and liver enzyme levels are within normal range. Assess for toxicity. Draw weekly blood levels initially and then every 1–2 mon. Therapeutic serum levels for acute mania are 1.0–1.5 mEq/L; for maintenance, levels are 0.6–1.2 mEq/L. Signs and symptoms of toxicity at serum levels of 1.5–2.0 mEq/L are persistent nausea and vomiting, severe diarrhea, ataxia, blurred vision, and tinnitus; at 2.0–3.5 mEq/L, signs and symptoms are excessive output of dilute urine, increasing tremors, muscular irritability, psychomotor retardation, mental confusion, and giddiness; and at >3.5 mEq/L, levels are life threatening and may result in impaired consciousness, nystagmus, seizures, coma, oliguria/anuria, cardiac dysrhythmias, myocardial infarction, and cardiovascular collapse. Withhold medications and notify health care provider immediately if any of these occur.
- Obtain a history of episodes of depression or manic-depressive behavior.
- Obtain the client's drug history. CNS depressants can cause an additive effect. Antidepressants cause anticholinergic-like symptoms and are contraindicated if the client has glaucoma. Renal or liver disorders may result in drug accumulation.

POTENTIAL NURSING DIAGNOSES
Potential for injury or violence related to excessive hyperactivity
Ineffective individual coping
Noncompliance

PLANNING
- Client's depression or manic-depressive behavior will be decreased.

NURSING INTERVENTIONS
- Observe the client for signs and symptoms of depression: mood changes, insomnia, apathy, or lack of interest in activities.
- Check the client's vital signs. Orthostatic hypotension is common. Check for anticholinergic-like symptoms: dry mouth, increased heart rate, urinary retention, or constipation.
- When drawing blood to check for lithium levels, draw samples immediately before the next dose (8–12 h after the previous dose). Monitor for signs of lithium toxicity.
- Monitor client for suicidal tendencies when marked depression is present.
- If the client is taking an anticonvulsant, observe the client for seizures; antidepressants lower the seizure threshold. The anticonvulsant dosage might need to be increased.
- Provide the client with a list of foods and drugs to avoid.

Antimanic: Lithium

CLIENT TEACHING
General
- Instruct the client to take lithium as prescribed. Emphasize the importance of adherence to the therapy and laboratory tests. If lithium is stopped, manic symptoms will reappear.
- Instruct the client to contact the health care provider if signs of toxicity occur: diarrhea, vomiting, unsteady gait, tremor, or muscle weakness.
- Encourage the client to keep medical appointments. Have client check with the health care provider before taking OTC preparations.
- Instruct the client not to drive a motor vehicle or be involved in potentially dangerous mechanical activity until stable lithium level is established.
- Advise the client to maintain adequate fluid intake: 2–3 L/d initially and 1–2 L/d maintenance.
- Instruct the client to take the lithium with meals to decrease gastric irritation.
- Inform the client that the effectiveness of the drug may not be evident until 1–2 wk after the start of therapy.
- Encourage the client who is planning pregnancy to consult with the health care provider about possible teratogenic effects of the drug on the fetus.
- Encourage the client to wear or carry an ID tag or bracelet indicating the drug taken.

Diet
- Advise the client to avoid caffeine products because they can aggravate the manic phase of the bipolar disorder.
- Instruct the client to maintain adequate sodium intake and to avoid crash diets that affect physical and mental health.

EVALUATION
- Evaluate the effectiveness of the drug therapy. The client is free of manic-depressive behavior.
- Client verbalizes understanding of symptoms of toxicity.
- Client demonstrates a subsiding or resolution of the symptoms.

NEUROLOGIC AND NEUROMUSCULAR AGENTS

Adrenergic Agonist

Adrenergic Blocker

Cholinergic

Anticholinergic

Antiparkinsonism:
  Anticholinergic
  Dopaminergic

Myasthenia Gravis

Muscle Relaxant

Prototype: Adrenergic Agonist

Epinephrine

Epinephrine
  (Adrenalin)
Sympathomimetic
Pregnancy Category: C
Drug Forms:
Aerosol spray 0.16, 0.2, 0.25 mg
Inj 1:1000 (1 mg/mL), 1:200
  (5 mg/mL)

Dosage

Asthma anaphylaxis:
A: SC: 0.1–0.5 mL of 1:1000 PRN
   IV: 0.1–0.25 mL of 1:1000
C: SC: 0.01 mL/kg of 1:1000
   IV: 0.01 mL/kg of 1:1000

Contraindications

Cardiac dysrhythmias, cerebral arteriosclerosis, pregnancy, narrow-angle glaucoma, cardiogenic shock
Caution: Hypertension, prostatic hypertrophy, hyperthyroidism, pregnancy

Drug-Lab-Food Interactions

Decrease epinephrine effect with methyldopa, beta blockers
Lab: Increase blood glucose, serum lactic acid

Pharmacokinetics

Absorption: SC/IM/IV: Rapidly
Distribution: PB: UK; in breast milk
Metabolism: t 1/2: UK
Excretion: In urine unchanged

Pharmacodynamics

SC/IM: Onset: 3–10 min
       Peak: 20 min
       Duration: 20–30 min
IV: Onset: Immediate
       Peak: 2–5 min
       Duration: 5–10 min
Inhal: Onset: 1 min
       Peak: 3–5 min
       Duration: 1–3 h

Therapeutic Effects/Uses: To treat allergic reaction, anaphylaxis, bronchospasm, cardiac arrest.

Mode of Action: Action on one or more adrenergic sites; promotion of CNS and cardiac stimulation, and bronchodilation.

Side Effects

Anorexia, nausea, vomiting, nervousness, tremors, agitation, headache, pallor, insomnia, syncope, dizziness

Adverse Reactions

Palpitations, tachycardia, dyspnea
Life-threatening: Ventricular fibrillation, pulmonary edema

KEY: For complete abbreviation key, see inside front cover.

■ NURSING PROCESS: ADRENERGIC AGONIST: Epinephrine

ASSESSMENT

• Obtain VS for future comparison. Epinephrine stimulates the alpha$_1$ (increases blood pressure), beta$_1$ (increase heart rate), and beta$_2$ (dilates bronchial tubes) receptors. Isoproterenol (Isuprel) stimulates the beta$_1$ and beta$_2$ receptors. Albuterol (Proventil) stimulates the beta$_2$ receptor.

Adrenergic Agonist

- Assess the drugs the client is taking and report possible drug–drug interaction. Beta blockers decrease the effect of epinephrine.
- Assess the medical history. Most adrenergic drugs are contraindicated if the client has cardiac dysrhythmias, narrow-angle glaucoma, or cardiogenic shock.
- Assess the results of laboratory values and compare with future laboratory findings.

POTENTIAL NURSING DIAGNOSES
High risk for impaired tissue integrity
Decreased cardiac output

PLANNING
- Client's VS will be closely monitored and will be within normal or acceptable ranges.

NURSING INTERVENTIONS
- Monitor the client's VS. Report signs of increasing blood pressure and increasing pulse rate. If the client is receiving an alpha-adrenergic drug IV for shock, the blood pressure should be checked every 3–5 min or as indicated to avoid severe hypertension.
- Report side effects of adrenergic drugs, such as tachycardia, palpitations, tremors, dizziness, and increased blood pressure.
- Check the client's urinary output and assess for bladder distention. Urinary retention can result from high drug dose or continuous use of adrenergic drugs.
- For cardiac resuscitation, administer epinephrine 1:1000 IV (1 mg/mL), which may be diluted in 10 mL of saline solution (as prescribed).
- Check IV site frequently when administering norepinephrine bitartrate (Levarternol) or dopamine (Intropin) because infiltration of these drugs causes tissue necrosis. These drugs should be diluted sufficiently in IV fluids. An antidote for norepinephrine (Levophed) and dopamine is phentolamine mesylate (Regitine) 5–10 mg, diluted in 10–15 mL of saline infiltrated into the area.
- Offer food when giving adrenergic drugs to avoid nausea and vomiting.
- Monitor laboratory test results. Blood glucose levels may be increased.

CLIENT TEACHING

General
- Instruct the client to read labels on all OTC drugs for cold symptoms and diet pills. Many of these have properties of sympathetic (adrenergic, sympathomimetics) drugs and should not be taken if the client is hypertensive or has diabetes mellitus, cardiac dysrhythmias, or coronary artery disease.
- Instruct mothers not to take drugs containing sympathetic drugs while nursing infants. These drugs pass into the breast milk.
- Explain to the client that continuous use of nasal sprays or drops that contain adrenergics may result in nasal congestion rebound (inflamed and congested nasal tissue).

Skill
- Instruct the client and family how to administer cold medications by spray or drops in the nostrils. Spray should be used with head in upright position. The use of nasal spray lying down can cause systemic absorption. Coloration of nasal spray or drops might indicate deterioration.

Adrenergic Agonist

- Instruct the client not to use bronchodilator sprays in excess. If the client is using a nonselective adrenergic drug that affects beta$_1$ and beta$_2$ receptors, tachycardia may occur.

Side Effects
- Instruct the client to report side effects to health care provider, i.e., rapid heart rate, palpitations, or dizziness.

EVALUATION
- Evaluate the client's response to the adrenergic drug. Continue monitoring the client's VS and report abnormal findings.

Adrenergic Drugs (Alpha, Beta₁, and Beta₂)

Generic (Brand)	Route and Dosage	Preg Cat	Interaction	t 1/2	PB	Onset	Peak	Duration
Albuterol (Proventil, Ventolin) Beta₂	A: PO: 2–4 mg t.i.d./q.i.d. PO/SR: 4–8 mg q12h Inhal: 1–2 puffs q4–6h PRN C: 2–6 y: PO: 0.1 mg/kg t.i.d. 6–12 y: PO: 2 mg t.i.d./q.i.d. C: 6–12 y: Inhal: Same as adult	C	Similar to norepinephrine	PO: 2.5–5 h Inhal: 2–3 h	UK	PO: 30 min Inhal: 5–15 min	PO: 2.5 h Inhal: 0.5–2 h	PO: 4–6 h SR: 8–12 h Inhal: 3–5 h
Dobutamine HCl (Dobutrex) Beta₁	A or C: IV: 2.5–20 µg/kg/min initially; increase dose gradually; max: 40 µg/kg/min	C	*Decrease* dobutamine effect with beta blockers; others: similar to norepinephrine	2 min	UK	1–2 min	10–20 min	UK
Dopamine HCl (Intropin) Beta₁	A: IV/Inf: 1–5 µg/kg/min initially; gradually increase 5–10 µg/kg/min; max: 50 µg/kg/min C: IV: usually the same	C	Similar to norepinephrine	2 min	UK	5 min	UK	<10 min

continued

Adrenergic Drugs (Alpha, Beta₁, and Beta₂)—Continued

Generic (Brand)	Route and Dosage	Preg Cat	Interaction	t 1/2	PB	Onset	Peak	Duration
Ephedrine HCl (Efedron) Ephedrine sulfate (Efedrin) Alpha, beta₁, and beta₂	A: PO: 25–50 mg t.i.d./q.i.d. SC/IM: 25–50 mg IV: 10–25 mg PRN; max: 150 mg/24 h C >2 y: PO: 2–3 mg/kg/d or 25–100 mg/m²/d in 4–6 divided doses	C	Severely *increase* alpha-adrenergic effect with MAOIs, tricyclic antidepressants *Increase* cardiac dysrhythmic effect with digoxin, anesthetics *Decrease* effect with methyldopa, reserpine	3–6 h	UK	PO: 15–60 min IM: 10–20 min IV: 5 min	UK	PO: 2–4 h IV: 2 h
Epinephrine (Adrenaline) Alpha, beta₁, and beta₂	See Prototype Drug Chart							
Isoetharine HCl (Bronkosol) Beta₂	A: IPPB: 0.5–1.0 mL of 5% sol OR 0.5 mL of 1% sol diluted in 3 mL of NSS Inhal: 1–2 puffs	C	Similar to norepinephrine	UK	UK	Immediate	5–15 min	1–4 h
Isoproterenol HCl (Isuprel) Beta₁ and beta₂	A: SL: 10–20 mg t.i.d.; max: 60 mg/d Inhal: 1–2 puffs q4–6 h PRN IV: 2–20 μg/min via inf	C	Similar to norepinephrine	2.5–5 min	UK	SL: 15–30 min Inhal: Rapid IV: Rapid	UK	SL: 2 h Inhal: 1 h IV: 2–5 min

Drug	Dosage	Pregnancy Category	Interactions	Onset	Peak	Duration
	C: SL: 5–10 mg t.i.d. Inhal: Same as adult IV: 2.5 µg/min OR 0.1 mg/kg/min via inf					
Metaproterenol sulfate (Alupent, Metaprel) Beta₁ and beta₂	A&C: >9 y: PO: 10–20 mg t.i.d./q.i.d. C <2 y: PO: 0.4 mg/kg t.i.d./q.i.d. 2–6 y: PO: 1–2.6 mg/kg t.i.d./q.i.d. 6–9 y: PO: 10 mg t.i.d./q.i.d. A&C: >12 y: inhal: 2–3 puffs q3–4h; max: 12 puffs/d	C	Similar to norepinephrine	UK	Inhal: <1 min PO: 15 min	Inhal/PO: 1 h	Inhal/PO: 1–5 h
Norepinephrine bitartrate (Levarterenol, Levophed) Alpha and beta₁	A: IV: 4 mg in 250–500 mL of D_5W or NSS infused initially 8–12 µg/min, then 4 µg/min; monitor blood pressure	D	*Increase* norepinephrine effect with MAOIs, tricyclic antidepressants, antihistamines *Increase* cardiac dysrhythmias with anesthetics *Decrease* norepinephrine effect with alpha-adrenergics	UK	1 min	UK	2–4 min

continued

Adrenergic Drugs (Alpha, Beta₁, and Beta₂) — Continued

Generic (Brand)	Route and Dosage	Preg Cat	Interaction	t 1/2	PB	Onset	Peak	Duration
Phenylephrine HCl 12-hour spray (oxymetazoline HCl) (Neo-Synephrine) Alpha	*Nasal decongestant:* A: Instill: 2–3 sprays or gtt of 0.25–0.5% sol C <6 y: Instill: 2–3 gtt of 0.125% sol C 6–12 y: Instill: 2–3 gtt of 0.25% sol Also available IM, IV	C	*Decrease* phenylephrine effect with alpha and beta blockers; others: similar to norepinephrine	2.5 h	UK	Rapid	UK	3–6 h
Phenylpropanolamine HCl *Decongestant:* Dimetapp, Dristan, Contac 12 Hour, Triaminicol, Triaminic *Anorexiant:* Dexatrim, Dietac, Control Alpha and beta₁	*Nasal decongestant:* A: PO: 25 mg q4h PRN PO/SR: 75 mg q12h PRN C 2–6 y: PO: 6.25 mg q4h PRN C 6–12 y: 12.5 mg q4h PRN *Appetite suppressant:* A: PO/SR: 75 mg q.d. (before breakfast) PO: 25 mg t.i.d. a.c.	C	*Decrease* antihypertensive effect with antihypertensives *Decrease* effects of phenothiazines, tricyclic antidepressants	3–4 h	UK	15–30 min	PO: 1–2 h SR: 4 h	PO: 3–4 h SR: 12 h
Pseudoephedrine HCl (Sudafed, Actifed, Co-Tylenol PediaCare) Alpha and beta₁	*Nasal decongestant:* A: PO: 60 mg q.i.d./q6h PO/SR: 120 mg q12h; max: 240 mg/d C 2–6 y: PO: 15 mg q6h; max: 60 mg/d C 6–12 y: PO: 30 mg q6h; max: 120 mg/d	C	Similar to ephedrine	9–16 h	UK	PO: 15–30 min	UK	PO: 4–6 h SR: 8–12 h

Ritodrine HCl (Yutopar) Beta$_2$ and some beta$_1$	A: PO: Initially: 10 mg q2h for first 24 h; maint: 10–20 mg q4–6h; max: 120 mg/d IV: 50–100 μg/min; dose may gradually increase to 300 μg/min	C	*Decrease ritodrine effect with beta blockers; may cause pulmonary edema with corticosteroids*	1.7–2.5 h Final: >10 h	32%	UK	PO: 30 min–1 h IV: 1 h	UK
Terbutaline sulfate (Brethine, Brethaire, Bricanyl) Beta$_2$	A: PO: 2.5–5 mg t.i.d. OR q8h SC: 0.25 mg initial; no more than 0.5 mg in q4h Inhal: 2 puffs q4–6h *Premature labor:* A: PO: 2.5 mg q4–6h IV: 10 μg/min, gradually increase; max: 80 μg/min C >12 y: PO: 2.5 mg t.i.d. OR q8h	B	Similar to norepinephrine	3–11 h	25%	PO: 30 min Inhal: 5–30 min	PO: 2–3 h Inhal: 1–2 h	PO: 4–8 h Inhal: 3–5 h

KEY: For complete abbreviation key, see inside front cover.

Prototype: Adrenergic Blocker

Propranolol HCl

Propranolol HCl

(Inderal), ❧ Apo-Propranolol, Detensol, Novopranol
Sympatholytic (beta$_1$ and beta$_2$ blocker)
Pregnancy Category: C
Drug Forms:
Tab 10, 20, 40, 60, 80 mg
SR cap 80, 120, 160 mg
Liq 4, 8 mg/mL
Inj 1 mg/mL

Dosage

See Antihypertension, antianginal, and antidysrhythmics
A: PO: 20–40 mg b.i.d. titrate up to 160–240 mg/d in 2–3 divided doses
SR: 120–160 mg/d
IV: 0.5–3 mg q4h PRN
C: PO: 1–4 mg/kg/d in 4 divided doses

Contraindications

Congestive heart failure, secondary heart block, cardiogenic shock, bronchial asthma, bronchospasm
Caution: Renal or hepatic dysfunction

Drug-Lab-Food Interactions

Increase atrioventricular block with digoxin, calcium channel blockers
Increase hypotensive effect with phenothiazines, diuretics, antihypertensives
Decrease absorption with antacids
Lab: Increase serum potassium, uric acid, AST (SGOT), ALT (SGPT), ALP; *decrease* blood sugar

Pharmacokinetics

Absorption: PO: Well absorbed
Distribution: PB: 93%
Metabolism: t 1/2: 2–4 h
Excretion: 90% excreted in urine as metabolites

Pharmacodynamics

PO: Onset: 30 min
    Peak: 1–1.5 h (SR: 6 h)
    Duration: 6 h
IV: Onset: Immediate
    Peak: 5 min
    Duration: UK

Therapeutic Effects/Uses: To treat cardiac dysrhythmias, hypertension, angina pectoris, myocardial infarction.

Mode of Action: Blocks beta$_1$-(cardiac) and beta$_2$-(pulmonary) adrenergic receptor sites

Side Effects

Bradycardia, confusion, drowsiness, fatigue, vertigo, pruritus, dry mouth, nasal stuffiness, brown discoloration of the tongue (rare)

Adverse Reactions

Visual hallucinations, thrombocytopenia
Life-threatening: Laryngospasm, atrioventricular heart block, agranulocytosis

KEY: For complete abbreviation key, see inside front cover.

■ NURSING PROCESS: ADRENERGIC BLOCKER: Propranolol

Adrenergic alpha and beta blockers are also presented within the antihypertensive, antianginal, and antidysrhythmia sections.

ASSESSMENT

• Obtain baseline VS and ECG for future comparison. Bradycardia and decrease in blood pressure are common cardiac effects of adrenergic beta block-

Adrenergic Blocker

ers. Adrenergic beta blockers are frequently referred to as beta blockers, blocking beta$_1$ and beta$_2$ (nonselective) or beta$_1$ (cardiac selective).
- Assess whether the client is having respiratory problems by listening for signs of wheezing or noting dyspnea (difficulty in breathing). If the beta blocker is nonselective, not only does the pulse rate decrease but also bronchoconstriction can result. Clients with asthma should take a beta$_1$ blocker, such as metoprolol (Lopressor), and avoid nonselective beta blockers.
- Assess the drugs the client is currently taking. Report if any are phenothiazines, digoxin, calcium channel blockers, or other antihypertensives.
- Assess the client's urine output and use for future comparison.

POTENTIAL NURSING DIAGNOSES

Decreased cardiac output
Impaired tissue integrity

PLANNING

- The client will comply with the drug regimen.
- The client's VS will be within desired range.

NURSING INTERVENTIONS

- Monitor the client's VS. Report marked changes.
- Administer IV propranolol undiluted or diluted in D$_5$W.
- Report any complaints of excessive dizziness or lightheadedness.
- Report any complaint of stuffy nose. Vasodilation results from use of alpha-adrenergic blockers, and nasal congestion can occur.
- Report if the client is a diabetic and receiving an adrenergic beta blocker; insulin dose or oral hypoglycemic may need to be adjusted.

CLIENT TEACHING

General

- Advise the client to avoid abruptly stopping a beta blocker; rebound hypertension, rebound tachycardia, or an angina attack could result.
- Instruct the client to comply with the drug regimen.
- Advise clients on insulin therapy that early warning signs of hypoglycemia may be masked by the beta blocker (i.e., tachycardia, nervousness).

Skill

- Instruct the client and family how to take pulse and blood pressure.

Side Effects

- Instruct the client to avoid orthostatic (postural) hypotension, such as by slowly rising from supine or sitting to standing positions.
- Inform the client and family of possible mood changes when taking beta blockers. Mood changes can include depression, nightmares, and suicidal tendencies.
- Advise the male client that certain beta blockers, such as propranolol, metoprolol, and pindolol, and alpha blockers, such as prazosin, may cause impotence. Usually the problem is dose related.

EVALUATION

- Evaluate the effectiveness of the adrenergic blocker. VS must be stable within desired range.

Adrenergic Blockers

Generic (Brand)	Route and Dosage	Preg Cat	Interaction	t 1/2	PB	Onset	Peak	Duration
Acebutolol HCl (Sectral) Beta$_1$	A: PO: Initially: 200–400 mg/d A: PO: 400–800 mg/d in 1–2 divided doses; max: 1200 mg/d	B	Same as nadolol	3–13 h	26%	1 h	3–4 h	21–24 h
Atenolol (Tenormin) Beta$_1$	A: PO: 25–100 mg/d	C	Same as nadolol; *Increase* absorption with anticholinergics; may *increase* lidocaine levels *Decrease* hypotensive effect with NSAIDs	6–7 h	6–16%	1 h	2–4 h	24 h
Metoprolol tartrate (Lopressor) Beta$_1$	*Hypertension:* A: PO: 50–100 mg/d in 1–2 divided doses; maint: 100–450 mg/d in divided doses; max: 450 mg/d in divided doses *Myocardial infarction:* A: IV: 5 mg q2min ×3 doses, then PO: 100 mg b.i.d.	C	Same as nadolol *Increase* bradycardia with digoxin	3–4 h	12%	PO: 15 min IV: Immediate	PO: 1.5 h IV: 20 min	PO: 10–19 h IV: 5–10 h
Nadolol (Corgard) Beta$_1$ and beta$_2$	A: PO: 40–80 mg/d; max: 320 mg/d	C	*Increase* hypotensive effect with diuretics, other antihypertensives	10–24 h	30%	1 h	2–4 h	18–24 h

Drug	Dosage	Pregnancy Category	Drug Interactions	Onset	Bioavailability	Peak	Duration (IM/IV)	Duration
Phentolamine mesylate (Regitine) Alpha	A: IM/IV: 2.5–5 mg, repeat q5min until controlled, then q2–3h PRN C: IM/IV: 0.05–0.1 mg/kg, repeat if needed	C	*Increase* hypotensive effect with antihypertensives	20 min	UK	UK	IM: 20 min IV: 2 min	IM: 3–4 h IV: 15 min
Pindolol (Visken) Beta$_1$ and beta$_2$	A: PO: 5 mg b.i.d./t.i.d.; maint: 10–30 mg in divided doses; max: 60 mg/d in divided doses	B	Same as nadolol	3–4 h	40%	3 h	UK	24 h
Prazosin HCl (Minipress) Alpha	A: PO: 1 mg b.i.d./t.i.d.; maint: 3–15 mg/d; max: 20 mg/d in divided doses	C	*Increase* hypotensive effect with alcohol, antihypertensives, nitrates	3 h	95%	0.5–2 h	2–4 h	10 h
Propranolol HCl (Inderal) Beta$_1$ and beta$_2$	See Prototype Drug Chart							
Timolol maleate (Blocadren) Beta$_1$ and beta$_2$	A: PO: Initially: 10 mg b.i.d.; maint: 20–40 mg/d in 2 divided doses; max: 60 mg/d	C	Same as nadolol	3–4 h	<10%	1 h	2–4 h	12–24 h
Tolazoline (Priscoline HCl) Alpha	A: SC/IV: 10–50 mg q.i.d. *Pulmonary hypertension:* NB: IV: 1–2 mg/kg infused over 10 min, followed by 1–2 mg/kg/h	C	*Increase* tolazoline effect with alcohol, beta blockers, antihypertensives	3–10 h	UK	30 min	IM: 0.5–1 h	IM: 3–4 h

KEY: For complete abbreviation key, see inside front cover.

Prototype: Cholinergic

Bethanechol Chloride

Bethanechol Chloride

(Urecholine), ✤ Dervoid, Urecholine
Parasympathomimetic
Pregnancy Category: C
Drug Forms:
Tab 5, 10, 25, 50 mg
Inj 5 mg/mL

Dosage

A: PO: 10–50 mg b.i.d./t.i.d./q.i.d.; max: 120 mg/d
SC: 2.5–5 mg, repeat at 15–30 min intervals PRN
Do NOT give IM or IV

Contraindications

Severe bradycardia or hypotension, chronic obstructive pulmonary disease, asthma, peptic ulcer, parkinsonism, hyperthyroidism

Drug-Lab-Food Interactions

Decrease bethanechol effect with antidysrhythmics
Lab: Increase AST, bilirubin, amylase, lipase

Pharmacokinetics

Absorption: PO: Poorly absorbed
Distribution: PB: UK
Metabolism: t 1/2: UK
Excretion: In urine

Pharmacodynamics

PO: Onset: 0.5–1.5 h
 Peak: 1–2 h
 Duration: 4–6 h
SC: Onset: 5–15 min
 Peak: 0.5 h
 Duration: 2 h

Therapeutic Effects/Uses: To treat urinary retention, abdominal distention.

Mode of Action: Stimulation of the cholinergic (muscarinic) receptor. Promote contraction of the bladder; increase GI peristalsis, GI secretion, pupillary constriction, and bronchoconstriction.

Side Effects

Nausea, vomiting, diarrhea, salivation, sweating, flushing, frequent urination, rash, miosis, blurred vision

Adverse Reactions

Hypotension, bradycardia, muscle weakness
Life-threatening: Acute asthmatic attack, heart block, circulatory collapse, cardiac arrest

KEY: For complete abbreviation key, see inside front cover.

Cholinergic

■ NURSING PROCESS: CHOLINERGIC DIRECT ACTING:
Bethanechol (Urecholine)

ASSESSMENT
- Obtain baseline VS for future comparison.
- Assess urine output that should be >600 mL/d. Report decrease in urine output.
- Obtain a history from the client of health problems, such as peptic ulcer, urinary obstruction, or asthma. Cholinergics can aggravate symptoms of these conditions.

POTENTIAL NURSING DIAGNOSES
Urinary retention
Anxiety

PLANNING
- Client will have increased bladder and GI tone after taking cholinergics.
- Client will have increased neuromuscular strength.

NURSING INTERVENTIONS
Direct Acting
- Monitor the client's VS. Pulse rate and blood pressure decrease when large doses of cholinergics are taken. Orthostatic hypotension is a side effect of a cholinergic such as bethanechol.
- Monitor fluid intake and output. Decreased urinary output should be reported for it may be related to urinary obstruction.
- Give cholinergics 1 h before or 2 h after meals. If the client complains of gastric pain, the drug may be given with meals.
- Check serum enzyme values for amylase and lipase, as well as AST (SGOT) and bilirubin levels. These laboratory values may increase slightly when taking cholinergics.
- Observe the client for side effects, such as gastric pain or cramping, diarrhea, increased salivary or bronchial secretions, bradycardia, and orthostatic hypotension.
- Auscultate for bowel sounds. Report decreased or hyperactive bowel sounds.
- Auscultate breath sounds for rales (cracking sounds from fluid congestion in lung tissue) or rhonchi (rough sounds due to mucus secretions in lung tissue). Cholinergic drugs can increase bronchial secretions.
- Have IV atropine sulfate (0.6 mg) available as an antidote for overdosing of cholinergics. Early signs of overdosing include salivation, sweating, abdominal cramps, and flushing.
- Note that diaphoresis (excessive perspiration) may occur; linens should be changed as needed.

Indirect Acting
- Beware of the possibility of cholinergic crisis (overdose); symptoms include muscular weakness and increased salivation.

Cholinergic

CLIENT TEACHING

Direct Acting

General

- Instruct the client to take the cholinergic as prescribed. Compliance with the drug regimen is essential.

Side Effects

- Instruct the client to report severe side effects, such as profound dizziness or a drop in pulse rate below 60.
- Instruct the client to arise from a lying position slowly to avoid dizziness; this is most likely due to orthostatic hypotension.
- Encourage the client to maintain effective oral hygiene if excess salivation occurs.
- Advise the client to report any difficulty in breathing due to respiratory distress.

Indirect Acting: See Drugs for Myasthenia Gravis

- Instruct the client to take the drug on time to avoid respiratory muscle weakness.
- Instruct the client to assess changes in muscle strength. Cholinesterase inhibitors (anticholinesterases) increase muscle strength.

EVALUATION

- Evaluate the effectiveness of the cholinergic or anticholinesterase drug.
- Evaluate the stability of the client's VS, and note the presence of side effects or adverse reactions.

Cholinergics

Generic (Brand)	Route and Dosage	Preg Cat	Interaction	t 1/2	PB	Onset	Peak	Duration
Direct Acting Bethanechol (Urecholine)	See Prototype Drug Chart							
Carbachol (Carcholin, Miostat)	Ophthalmic: 0.75–3%, 1 gt See Drugs for the Eye		See Drugs for the Eye					
Pilocarpine HCl (Pilocar)	Ophthalmic: 0.5–4%, 1 gt See Drugs for the Eye		See Drugs for the Eye					
Cholinesterase Inhibitor *For Alzheimer's Disease:* Tacrine HCl (Cognex)	A: PO: 10 mg q.i.d., P.C.; increase dose at 6 wk intervals; max: 160 mg/d	C	*Increase* effect of theophylline *Increase* effect with cimetidine	1.5–3.5 h	50%	0.5–1.5 h	2 h	24–36 h
Velnacrine (Mentane)	A: PO: 150–225 mg/d in divided doses		Investigational drug *Lab:* May *increase* liver enzymes	2–3 h	UK	UK	1 h	UK
Indirect Acting Irreversible Anticholinesterases Demecarium bromide (Humorsol)	0.125–0.25%, 1 gt q12–48h See Drugs for the Eye		See Drugs for the Eye					

continued

101

Cholinergics—Continued

Generic (Brand)	Route and Dosage	Preg Cat	Interaction	t1/2	PB	Onset	Peak	Duration
Echothiophate iodide (Phospholine iodide)	0.03–0.25%, 1 gt q.d./b.i.d. See Drugs for the Eye		See Drugs for the Eye					
Isoflurophate (Floropryl)	0.25%, ointment q8–72h See Drugs for the Eye		See Drugs for the Eye					
Indirect Acting, Reversible Anticholinesterases								
Ambenonium Cl (Mytelease)	A: PO: 2.5–5.0 mg t.i.d./q.i.d.; dose may be increased; maint: 5–25 mg t.i.d./q.i.d.	C	Similar to neostigmine	UK	UK	30 min	UK	3–8 h
Edrophonium Cl (Tensilon)	A: IV: 2 mg; then 8 mg if no response IM: 10 mg; may repeat with 2 mg in 30 min C <34 kg: IV: 1 mg; repeat in 30–45 sec if no response; max: 5 mg C >34 kg: IV: 2 mg; repeat with 1 mg if no response; max: 10 mg	C	*Increase* bradycardia with digoxin	1.2–2 h	UK	IV: 0.5–1 min IM: 2–10 min	IV/IM: UK	IV: 6–12 min IM: 5–30 min

Neostigmine bromide (Prostigmin) Neostigmine methysulfate (injectable form)	A: PO: Initially: 15 mg t.i.d.; maint: 150 mg/d in divided doses; range: 15–375 mg/d IM/IV: 0.5–2.5 mg as needed C: PO: 2 mg/kg/d in 6 divided doses	C	*Increase* neostigmine effect with other cholinergics *Decrease* neostigmine effect with atropine, antidysrhythmics	1–1.5 h	15–25%	PO: 1–4 h IM: 15–30 min IV: 5–8 min	PO: UK IM: 20–30 min IV: UK	PO/IM: 2.5–4 h IV: 2–4 h
Physostigmine salicylate (Eserine salicylate)	0.25–0.5%, 1 gt q.d./q.i.d. See Drugs for the Eye		See Drugs for the Eye					
Pyridostigmine bromide (Mestinon)	A: PO: 60–120 mg t.i.d./q.i.d.; maint: 600 mg/d in 3–4 divided doses; max: 1.5 g/d SR: 180–540 mg daily/b.i.d. IM/IV: 2 mg q2–3h C: PO: 7 mg/kg/d in 5–6 divided doses	C	Same as neostigmine	3.5–4 h	<10%	PO: 30–45 min SR: 0.5–1 h IM: 15 min IV: 2–5 min	PO/SR/IM/IV: UK	PO: 3–6 h SR: 6–12 h IM: 2–4 h IV: 2–3 h

KEY: For complete abbreviation key, see inside front cover.

Prototype: Anticholinergic

Atropine SO$_4$

Atropine SO$_4$

(Atropine), ❋ Atropair
Atropisol (Optic)
Parasympatholytic
Pregnancy Category: C
Drug Forms:
Tab 0.4 mg
Inj 0.1, 0.4, 1 mg/mL
Ophthalmic ointment and sol (1%)

Dosage

A: PO/IM/IV: 0.4–0.6 mg q4–6h PRN
C: PO/IM/IV: 0.01 mg/kg/dose; max: 0.4 mg/dose q4–6h PRN

Contraindications

Narrow-angle glaucoma, obstructive GI disorders, paralytic ileus, ulcerative colitis, tachycardia, benign prostatic hypertrophy, myasthenia gravis

Caution: Renal or hepatic disorders, chronic obstructive pulmonary disease, congestive heart failure

Drug-Lab-Food Interactions

Increase anticholinergic effect with phenothiazines, antidepressants, MAOIs

Pharmacokinetics

Absorption: PO/IM: Well absorbed
Distribution: PB: UK; crosses the placenta
Metabolism: t 1/2: 2–3 h
Excretion: >75% excreted in urine

Pharmacodynamics

PO: Onset: 0.5–1 h
   Peak: 1–2 h
   Duration: 4 h
IM: Onset: 10–30 min
   Peak: 0.5 h
   Duration: 4 h
IV: Onset: Immediate
   Peak: 5 min
   Duration: UK
Instill: Onset: 20–30 min
   Peak: 30–40 min
   Duration: days

Therapeutic Effects/Uses: Preoperative medication to reduce salivation, increase heart rate, dilate pupils of the eye.

Mode of Action: Inhibition of acetylcholine by occupying the receptors; increase heart rate by blocking vagus stimulation; promote dilation of the pupil by blocking iris sphincter muscle.

Side Effects

Dry mouth, nausea, headache, constipation, rash, dry skin, flushing, blurred vision, photophobia

Adverse Reactions

Tachycardia, hypotension, pupillary dilatation, abdominal distention, nasal congestion

Life-threatening: Paralytic ileus, coma

KEY: For complete abbreviation key, see inside front cover.

Anticholinergic

■ NURSING PROCESS: ANTICHOLINERGIC DRUGS: Atropine

ASSESSMENT
- Obtain baseline VS for future comparison. Tachycardia is a side effect that occurs with large doses of anticholinergics such as atropine sulfate.
- Assess urine output. Urinary retention may occur.
- Check the client's medical history. Atropine and atropine-like drugs are contraindicated if the client has narrow-angle glaucoma, obstructive GI disorder, paralytic ileus, ulcerative colitis, benign prostatic hypertrophy (BPH), or myasthenia gravis.
- Obtain a history of the drugs the client is taking. Phenothiazines and antidepressants increase the effect of anticholinergics.

POTENTIAL NURSING DIAGNOSES
Urinary retention
Altered oral mucous membrane
Constipation

PLANNING
- The client's secretions will be decreased before surgery.
- Client will not have side effects that may become a health problem.

NURSING INTERVENTIONS
- Monitor the client's VS. Report if tachycardia occurs.
- Check intake and output. Encourage the client to void before taking the medication. Report decreased urine output. Anticholinergics can cause urinary retention. Maintain adequate fluid intake.
- Check bowel sounds. Absence of bowel sounds may indicate paralytic ileus due to decrease in GI motility (peristalsis).
- Check for constipation due to the decrease in GI motility. Encourage the client to ingest foods that are high in fiber, to drink adequate amounts of fluids, and to exercise if able.
- Raise bedside rails for clients who are confused, debilitated, or elderly. Atropine could cause CNS stimulation (excitement, confusion) or drowsiness.
- Administer mouth care. Atropine decreases oral secretions and can cause dryness of the mouth.
- Administer IV atropine undiluted or diluted in 10 mL of sterile water. Rate of administration is 0.6 mg/min.

CLIENT TEACHING
General
- Instruct the client with glaucoma to avoid atropine-like drugs. Anticholinergics cause mydriasis and increase the intraocular pressure. Clients should be alerted to check labels on OTC drugs to determine if they are contraindicated for glaucoma.
- Instruct the client not to drive a motor vehicle or participate in activities that require alertness. Drowsiness is common.
- Advise the client to avoid alcohol, cigarette smoking, caffeine, and aspirin at bedtime to decrease gastric acidity.
- Instruct the client with mydriasis from an eye examination to use sunglasses in bright light because of photophobia (intolerance of bright light).

Anticholinergic

- Instruct the client to avoid hot environments and excess physical exertion. Elevations in body temperature can result from diminished sweat gland activity.

Diet

- Suggest that the client's diet include foods high in fiber and increased water intake to prevent constipation.

Side Effects

- Advise the client of common side effects from long-term use of anticholinergics, such as dry mouth, decrease in urination, and constipation.
- Instruct the client to increase fluid intake to prevent constipation when taking anticholinergics for a prolonged period of time.
- Instruct the client to urinate before taking the anticholinergic. Urinary retention can be a problem. The client should report a marked decrease in urine output.
- Suggest that the client use hard candy, ice chips, or chewing gum and maintain effective oral hygiene if the client's mouth is dry. Anticholinergics decrease salivation.
- Encourage the client to use Artificial Tears (eye drops) for dry eyes due to decreased lacrimation (tearing).

EVALUATION

- Evaluate the client's response to the anticholinergic.
- Determine if constipation, urine retention, or increased pulse rate is or remains a problem.

Anticholinergics

Generic (Brand)	Route and Dosage	Preg Cat	Interaction	t 1/2	PB	Onset	Peak	Duration
Eye								
Cyclopentolate HCl (Cyclogyl)	0.5–2% sol, 1–2 gtt See Drugs for the Eye		See Drugs for the Eye					
Homatropine (Isopto Homatropine)	2–5% sol, 1–2 gtt See Drugs for the Eye		See Drugs for the Eye					
Tropicamide (Mydriacyl Ophthalmic)	0.5–1% sol, 1–2 gtt See Drugs for the Eye		See Drugs for the Eye					
Gastrointestinal Atropine sulfate	See Prototype Drug Chart							
Dicyclomine HCl (Bentyl, Antispas, Di-Spaz)	A: PO: 10–20 mg t.i.d./q.i.d. IM: 20 mg q6h C >2 y: PO: 10 mg t.i.d./q.i.d.	B	*Increase* anticholinergic effect with MAOIs, tricyclic antidepressants, antihistamines (H$_1$)	9–10 h	UK	1–2 h	UK	3–4 h

continued

Anticholinergics—Continued

Generic (Brand)	Route and Dosage	Preg Cat	Interaction	t1/2	PB	Onset	Peak	Duration
Glycopyrrolate (Robinul)	GI disorders: A: PO: 1–2 mg b.i.d./t.i.d. IM/IV: 0.1–0.2 mg t.i.d./q.i.d. Preoperative: A: IM: 4.4 µg/kg 30 min–1 h before surgery	B	Same as dicyclomine Decrease levodopa effects; may decrease antipsychotic effects of phenothiazines	1–4.6 h	UK	PO: 1 h IM: 30 min IV: 1–10 min	PO: 1–2 h IM: 0.5–1 h IV: 10 min	PO: 8–12 h IM: 3–7 h IV: 3–4 h
Hyoscyamine SO$_4$ (Cystospaz, Anaspaz, Levsin)	A: PO/SL: 0.125–0.25 mg t.i.d./q.i.d. ac & h.s. SR: 0.375–0.75 mg q12h SC/IM/IV: 0.25–0.5 mg b.i.d./q.i.d. C 2–10 y: one-half of the adult dose or individualized	C	Increase hyoscyamine effect with antihistamines, tricyclic antidepressants, amantadine Decrease effect with antacids; decrease effects of phenothiazines, levodopa	3.5 h	50–60%	PO: 20–30 min IV: 2–3 min	PO: 0.5–1 h IV: 15–30 min	PO/IV: 4–6 h
Clidinium bromide (Quarzan) *Anticholinergic*	A: PO: 2.5–5 mg, t.i.d./q.i.d. p.c. & h.s. Elderly: PO: 2.5 mg t.i.d.	UK	*Increase* adverse effects of antiparkinsonism, disopyramide, phenothiazines, antidysrhythmics, tricyclic antidepressants	UK	UK	1 h	3 h	UK

Isopropamide iodide (Darbid)	A: PO: 5 mg b.i.d. or q12h; may increase to 10 mg b.i.d.	C	Similar to glycopyrrolate	UK	UK	UK	10–12 h
Mepenzolate bromide (Cantil)	A: PO: 25–50 mg t.i.d. with meals and h.s.	C	Similar to glycopyrrolate	UK	UK	1 h	UK	3–4 h
Methscopolamine bromide (Pamine)	A: PO: 2.5–5 mg a.c., h.s. C: PO: 0.2 mg/kg q.i.d.	C	*Increase* additive effect with antihistamines, antiparkinsonism, disopyramide, phenothiazides, antihypertensives *Decrease* effect of phenothiazines, levodopa, ketoconazole	UK	UK	1 h	UK	4–8 h
Oxyphencyclimine HCl (Daricon)	A: PO: 5–10 mg b.i.d.	C	Same as methscopolamine	UK	UK	1–2 h	UK	>12 h
Propantheline bromide (Pro-Banthine)	A: PO: 15 mg a.c. t.i.d; 30 mg h.s.; max: 120 mg/d Elderly: 7.5 mg a.c. t.i.d.	C	Same as glycopyrrolate	9 h	UK	30–60 min	UK	4–6 h

continued

Anticholinergics—Continued

Generic (Brand)	Route and Dosage	Preg Cat	Interaction	t1/2	PB	Onset	Peak	Duration
Scopolamine hydrobromide (also hyoscine hydrobromide)	*Preoperative:* A: PO: 0.5–1.0 mg SC/IM/IV: 0.3–0.6 mg C: SC: 0.006 mg/kg or 0.2 mg/m^2; max: 0.3 mg *Motion sickness:* A: PO: 0.3–0.6 mg; transderm patch: 1 patch behind ear q72h	C	Same as glycopyrrolate	8 h	<30%	PO: 30 min IV: 10 min Transderm: 4 h	PO: 1 h IV: 1 h Transderm: UK	PO: 4–6 h IV: 2–4 h Transderm: 72 h
Neuromuscular (Atropine-like Agents: Antiparkinsonism Drugs) Benztropine mesylate (Cogentin) See Antiparkinsonism Drugs	*Parkinsonism:* A: PO: Initially: 0.5–1.0 mg/d in 1–2 divided doses (larger dose at h.s.); maint: 0.5–6 mg/d in 1–2 divided doses	C	*Increase* anticholinergic effect with narcotics, antipsychotics, tricyclic antidepressants, antihistamines, some antidysrhythmics *Decrease* effect of levodopa	UK	UK	PO: 1 h	UK	PO: 6–24 h

Biperiden lactate (Akineton) See Antiparkinsonism Drugs	*Parkinsonism:* A: PO: 2 mg t.i.d./q.i.d. IM/IV: 2 mg q30min for 4 doses	C	Same as benztropine	UK	UK	PO: 1 h	UK	PO: 6–24 h
Procyclidine HCl (Kemadrin) See Antiparkinsonism Drugs	*Parkinsonism:* A: PO: 2.5–5 mg pc t.i.d; maint: 10–20 mg/d	C	Same as benztropine	UK	UK	30–40 min	UK	4–6 h
Trihexyphenidyl HCl (Artane, Trihexy) See Antiparkinsonism Drugs	*Parkinsonism:* A: PO: Initially: 1–2 mg/d, increase to 6–10 mg/d in divided doses	C	Same as benztropine *Decrease* trihexyphenidyl absorption with antacids	UK	UK	PO: 1 h SR: UK	PO: 2–3 h SR: UK	PO: 6–12 h SR: 12–24 h

KEY: For complete abbreviation key, see inside front cover.

Prototype: Antiparkinsonism: Anticholinergic

Trihexyphenidyl HCl

Trihexyphenidyl HCl
 (Artane, Aphen, Hexaphen,
 Trihexane, Trihexy), ✦ Aparkane
Anticholinergic
Pregnancy Category: C
Drug Forms:
Tab 2, 5 mg
SR cap 5 mg
Elix 2 mg/5 mL

Contraindications

Narrow-angle glaucoma, GI obstruction, urinary retention, severe angina pectoris, myasthenia gravis
Caution: Tachycardia, benign prostatic hypertrophy, children, elderly, during lactation

Pharmacokinetics

Absorption: PO: Well absorbed
Distribution: PB: UK
Metabolism: t 1/2: UK
Excretion: In urine

Dosage

Parkinsonism:
A: PO: Initially 1 mg/d; increase to 6–10 mg/d in divided doses
Extrapyramidal symptoms: Drug induced:
A: PO: 1 mg/d; increase to 5–15 mg/d in divided doses

Drug-Lab-Food Interactions

Increase anticholinergic effect with phenothiazines, antihistamines, tricyclic antidepressants, quinidine
Decrease trihexyphenidyl absorption with antacids

Pharmacodynamics

PO: Onset: 1 h
        Peak: 2–3 h
        Duration: 6–12 h
SR/PO: Onset: UK
        Peak: UK
        Duration: 12–24 h

Therapeutic Effects/Uses: To decrease involuntary symptoms of parkinsonism or drug-induced parkinsonism by inhibiting acetylcholine.

Mode of Action: Blocks cholinergic (muscarinic) receptors; thus decreases involuntary movements.

Side Effects

Nausea, vomiting, dry mouth, constipation, anxiety, restlessness, headache, dizziness, blurred vision, photophobia, pupil dilation, dysphagia

Adverse Reactions

Tachycardia, palpitations, urticaria, postural hypotension, urinary retention
Life-threatening: Paralytic ileus

KEY: For complete abbreviation key, see inside front cover.

Antiparkinsonism: Anticholinergic

■ NURSING PROCESS: ANTIPARKINSONISM:
Anticholinergic: Trihexyphenidyl

ASSESSMENT
- Obtain a medical history. Report if the client has a history of glaucoma, GI dysfunction, urinary retention, angina pectoris, or myasthenia gravis. All anticholinergics are contraindicated if the client has glaucoma.
- Obtain a drug history. Report if a drug-drug interaction is probable. Phenothiazines, tricyclic antidepressants, and antihistamines increase the effect of trihexyphenidyl.
- Assess baseline VS for future comparisons. Pulse rate may increase.
- Assess urinary output for comparison. Urinary retention may occur with continuous use of anticholinergics.

POTENTIAL NURSING DIAGNOSES
Impaired physical mobility
High risk for activity intolerance

PLANNING
- Client will have decreased involuntary symptoms due to parkinsonism or drug-induced parkinsonism.

NURSING INTERVENTIONS
- Monitor VS, urine output, and bowel sounds. Increased pulse rate, urinary retention, and constipation are side effects of anticholinergics.

CLIENT TEACHING
General
- Advise the client to avoid alcohol, cigarette smoking, caffeine, and aspirin to decrease gastric acidity.

Diet
- Encourage the client to ingest foods that are high in fiber and to increase fluid intake to prevent constipation.

Side Effects
- Suggest that the client relieve dry mouth with hard candy, ice chips, or sugarless chewing gum. Anticholinergics decrease salivation.
- Suggest that the client use sunglasses in direct sun because of possible photophobia.
- Advise the client to void before taking the drug to minimize urinary retention. This is especially important if urine retention is present.
- Advise the client taking an anticholinergic to control symptoms of parkinsonism and to have routine eye examinations to determine the presence of increased intraocular pressure, which indicates glaucoma. Clients who have glaucoma should NOT take anticholinergics.

EVALUATION
- Evaluate the client's response to trihexyphenidyl to determine if parkinsonism symptoms are controlled.

Antiparkinsonism Drugs: Anticholinergics

Generic (Brand)	Route and Dosage	Preg Cat	Interaction	t1/2	PB	Onset	Peak	Duration
Benztropine mesylate (Cogentin)	*Parkinsonism:* A: PO: Initially: 0.5–1.0 mg/d in 1–2 divided doses (larger dose at h.s.); maint: 0.5–6 mg/d in 1–2 divided doses *Extrapyramidal syndrome:* A: PO: 1–4 mg/d in 1–2 divided doses IM/IV: 1–2 mg/d	C	*Increase* anticholinergic effect with narcotics, antipsychotics, tricyclic antidepressants, antihistamines, some antidysrhythmics *Decrease* effect of levodopa	UK	UK	PO: 1 h IM/IV: 15 min	UK	PO: 6–24 h IM/IV: 6–24 h
Biperiden HCl (Akineton)	*Parkinsonism:* A: PO: 2 mg t.i.d./q.i.d. IM/IV: 2 mg every 30 min to 4 doses C: IM/IV: 0.04 mg/kg or 1.2 mg/m², repeat if necessary; max: 8 mg/d	C	Same as benztropine	UK	UK	PO: 1 h IM/IV: 15 min	UK	PO/IM/IV: 6–24 h

114

Ethopropazine HCl (Parsidol)	*Parkinsonism:* A: PO: Initially: 50 mg q.d./b.i.d.; maint: 100–400 mg/d in divided doses; max: 600 mg/d in divided doses	C	Similar to benztropine	UK	0.5–1 h	4 h
Orphenadrine HCl or citrate (Disipal, Norflex, Banflex)	A: PO: 50 mg t.i.d. or 100 mg b.i.d.	C	None significant	14 h	1 h	2 h	4–6 h
Procyclidine HCl (Kemadrin)	*Parkinsonism:* A: PO: 2.5 mg p.c. t.i.d. *Extrapyramidal syndrome:* A: PO: Initially: 2.5 mg p.c. t.i.d.; maint: 2.5–5 mg p.c. t.i.d.	C	Similar to benztropine	UK	UK	PO: 30–40 min	4–6 h
Trihexyphenidyl HCl (Artane)	See Prototype Drug Chart						

KEY: For complete abbreviation key, see inside front cover.

Prototype: Antiparkinsonism: Dopaminergic

Carbidopa-Levodopa	Dosage
Carbidopa-Levodopa (Sinemet) Dopaminergic *Pregnancy Category:* C *Drug Forms:* Tab 10/100, 25/250 mg (carbidopa/levodopa)	A: PO: 1:10 ratio; initially 10 carbidopa/100 levodopa t.i.d.; maint: 25/250 mg t.i.d.

Contraindications	Drug-Lab-Food Interactions
Narrow-angle glaucoma; severe cardiac, renal, or hepatic disease *Caution:* peptic ulcer, psychiatric disorders	*Increase* hypertensive crisis with MAOIs *Decrease* levodopa effect with other anticholinergics, phenytoin, tricyclic antidepressants, pyridoxine *Lab:* May *increase* BUN, AST, ALT, ALP, LDH *Food:* Avoid foods containing pyridoxine (vitamin B_6)

Pharmacokinetics	Pharmacodynamics
Absorption: PO: Well absorbed *Distribution:* PB: Carbidopa: 36%; levodopa: UK *Metabolism:* t 1/2: 1-2 h *Excretion:* In urine as metabolites	PO: Onset: 15 min Peak: 1-3 h Duration: 5-12 h

Therapeutic Effects/Uses: To treat parkinsonism, to relieve tremors and rigidity.

Mode of Action: Transmission of levodopa to brain cells for conversion to dopamine; carbidopa blocks the conversion of levodopa to dopamine in the periphery.

Side Effects	Adverse Reactions
Anorexia, nausea, vomiting, dysphagia, fatigue, dizziness, headache, dry mouth, bitter taste, twitching, blurred vision, insomnia	Involuntary choreiform movements, palpitations, orthostatic hypotension, urinary retention, psychosis, severe depression, hallucinations *Life-threatening:* Agranulocytosis, hemolytic anemia, cardiac dysrhythmias, leukopenia

KEY: For complete abbreviation key, see inside front cover.

■ NURSING PROCESS: ANTIPARKINSONISM: Dopaminergic Agent: Carbidopa-Levodopa

ASSESSMENT
- Obtain the client's VS to use for future comparison.

Antiparkinsonism: Dopaminergic

- Assess the client for signs and symptoms of parkinsonism, including stooped, forward posture; shuffling gait; masked facies; and resting tremors.
- Obtain a history from the client of glaucoma, heart disease, peptic ulcers, kidney or liver disease, and psychosis.
- Report if drug–drug interaction is probable. Drugs that should be avoided or closely monitored are levodopa, bromocriptine, and anticholinergics.

POTENTIAL NURSING DIAGNOSES
Impaired physical mobility
High risk for activity intolerance

PLANNING
- Symptoms of parkinsonism will be decreased or absent after 1–4 wk of drug therapy.

NURSING INTERVENTIONS
- Monitor the client's VS and ECG. Orthostatic hypotension may occur during early use of levodopa and bromocriptine. Have the client rise slowly to avoid faintness.
- Check for weakness, dizziness, or faintness, which are symptoms of orthostatic hypotension.
- Administer carbidopa-levodopa (Sinemet) with low-protein foods. High-protein diets interfere with drug transport to the CNS.

CLIENT TEACHING
General
- Advise the client not to abruptly discontinue the medication. Rebound parkinsonism (increased symptoms of parkinsonism) can occur.
- Inform the client that urine may be discolored and will darken with exposure to air. Perspiration also may be dark. Explain that both are harmless but that clothes may be stained.
- Advise the diabetic client that the blood sugar should be checked with a OTC reagent strip (Hemastix or Chemstrip bG) and not done through urine testing. With Clinitest, a false-positive test result can occur; with Tes-Tape or Clinistix, a false-negative test result can occur.

Diet
- Suggest to the client that taking levodopa with food may decrease GI upset; however, food will slow the drug absorption rate.
- Advise the client to avoid vitamins that contain vitamin B_6 (pyridoxine) and foods rich in vitamin B_6, such as beans (lima, navy, kidney) and cereals that contain the vitamin.

Side Effects
- Instruct the client to report side effects and symptoms of dyskinesia. Explain to the client that it may take weeks or months before the symptoms are controlled.

EVALUATION
- Evaluate the effectiveness of the drug therapy in controlling the symptoms of parkinsonism.
- Determine that there is an absence of side effects.

Antiparkinsonism: Dopaminergics

Generic (Brand)	Route and Dosage	Preg Cat	Interaction	t 1/2	PB	Onset	Peak	Duration
Dopaminergics								
Carbidopa-Levodopa (Sinemet)	See Prototype Drug Chart							
Levodopa (or L-dopa) (Dopar, Larodopa)	A: PO: 0.5–1.0 g/d in 2–4 divided doses; increase dose gradually; average maint: 3–6 g/d with food, in divided doses; max: 8 g/d	C	*Increase* hypertensive crisis with MAOIs *Decrease* levodopa effect with anticholinergics, phenytoin, tricyclic antidepressants, pyridoxine, papaverine	1–3 h	UK	15–30 min	1–3 h	5–24 h
Dopamine Agonists								
Amantadine HCl; (Symmetrel)	*Parkinsonism:* A: PO: 100 mg b.i.d.; may increase dose; max: 400 mg/d	C	*Increase* anticholinergic effect with other anticholinergics	24 h; longer with poor renal function	60–70%	48 h	1–4 h	UK

Bromocriptine mesylate (Parlodel)	A: PO: Initially: 1.25–2.5 mg/d; may gradually increase dose; maint: 30–60 mg/d in 3 divided doses; max: 100 mg/d	C	*Increase* hypotensive effect with antihypertensive drugs *Increase* CNS depression with alcohol, narcotics, sedative-hypnotics *Decrease* bromocriptine effect with phenothiazines, amitriptyline, haloperidol, methyldopa	6–8 h Terminal phase: 50 h	90–96%	30 min–1 h	1–2 h	4–8 h
Pergolide mesylate (Permax)	A: PO: Initially: 0.05 mg/d ×2d; increase by 0.1–0.15 mg q3d ×12d; max: 5 mg/d	B	May *increase* highly protein-bound drugs May *decrease* effect with phenothiazines, thioxanthines, butyrophenones	UK	90%	UK	UK	UK
Selegiline HCl (Eldepryl)	A: PO: 10 mg/d in 2 divided doses	C	*Increase* toxicity with meperidine	2–20 h	UK	1 h	UK	UK

KEY: For complete abbreviation key, see inside front cover.

Prototype: Myasthenia Gravis (Drugs for)

Pyridostigmine Bromide

Pyridostigmine Bromide (Mestinon)
Cholinesterase inhibitor
Pregnancy Category: C
Drug Forms:
Tab 60 mg
SR tab 180 mg
Liquid 60 mg/ 5 mL
Inj 5 mg/mL

Dosage

A: PO: 60–120 mg t.i.d./q.i.d.; max: 1.5 g/d
SR: 180–540 mg q.d. or b.i.d.
IM/IV: 2 mg q2–3h
C: PO: 7 mg/kg/d in 5–6 divided doses

Contraindications

GI and GU obstruction, severe renal disease
Caution: Asthma, bradycardia, peptic ulcer, cardiac dysrhythmias, pregnancy

Drug-Lab-Food Interactions

Decrease pyridostigmine effect with atropine, muscle relaxants, antidysrhythmics, magnesium

Pharmacokinetics

Absorption: PO: Poorly absorbed; SR: 50% absorbed
Distribution: PB: UK
Metabolism: t 1/2: PO: 3.5–4 h; IV: 2 h
Excretion: In urine and by liver

Pharmacodynamics

PO: Onset: 30–45 min
Peak: UK
Duration: 3–6 h
PO SR: Onset: 0.5–1 h
Peak: UK
Duration: 6–12 h
IM: Onset: 15 min
Peak: UK
Duration: 2–4 h
IV: Onset: 2–5 min
Peak: UK
Duration: 2–3 h

Therapeutic Effects/Uses: To control and treat myasthenia gravis.

Mode of Action: Transmission of neuromuscular impulses by preventing the destruction of acetylcholine.

Side Effects

Nausea, vomiting, diarrhea, headache, dizziness, abdominal cramps, sweating, rash, miosis

Adverse Reactions

Hypotension, urticaria
Life-threatening: Respiratory depression, bronchospasm, cardiac dysrhythmias, seizures

KEY: For complete abbreviation key, see inside front cover.

Myasthenia Gravis (Drugs for)

■ NURSING PROCESS: MYASTHENIA GRAVIS (Drugs for): Pyridostigmine (Mestinon)

ASSESSMENT
- Obtain a drug history of drugs that the client is currently taking. Report if a drug-drug interaction is likely. Client should avoid atropine, atropine-like drugs, and muscle relaxants.
- Obtain baseline VS for future comparison.
- Assess the client for signs and symptoms of **myasthenia crisis**, such as muscle weakness with difficulty breathing and swallowing.

POTENTIAL NURSING DIAGNOSES
Inability to sustain spontaneous ventilation
High risk for activity intolerance
Anxiety related to possible recurrence of myasthenia crisis

PLANNING
- The client's symptoms of muscle weakness and difficulty breathing and swallowing due to myasthenia gravis will be eliminated or reduced in 2–3 d.

NURSING INTERVENTIONS
- Monitor the effectiveness of drug therapy (acetylcholinesterase [AChE] inhibitors). Muscle strength should be increased. Both depth and rate of respirations should be assessed and maintained within normal range.
- Administer IV pyridostigmine undiluted at rate of 0.5 mg/min. Do NOT add the drug to IV fluids.
- Observe the client for signs and symptoms of **cholinergic crisis** due to overdosing, including muscle weakness, increased salivation, sweating, tearing, and miosis.
- Have readily available an antidote for cholinergic crisis (atropine sulfate).

CLIENT TEACHING
General
- Instruct the client to take the drugs as prescribed to avoid recurrence of symptoms.
- Encourage the client to wear a medical ID bracelet or necklace, e.g., Medic Alert, indicating the health problem and the drug(s) taken.

Diet
- Instruct the client to take the drug before meals for best drug absorption. If gastric irritation occurs, take the drug with food.

Side Effects
- Advise the client to report to health care provider recurrence of symptoms of myasthenia gravis. Drug therapy may need to be modified.

EVALUATION
- Evaluate the effectiveness of the drug therapy. Muscle strength should be maintained.
- Determine the absence of respiratory distress.

Acetylcholinesterase Inhibitors: Myasthenia Gravis (Drugs for)

Generic (Brand)	Route and Dosage	Preg Cat	Interaction	t 1/2	PB	Onset	Peak	Duration
Ambenonium (Mytelase)	A: PO: 2.5–5.0 mg t.i.d/q.i.d.; dose may be increased; maint: 5–25 mg t.i.d./q.i.d.; max: 75 mg b.i.d./q.i.d.	C	Similar to neostigmine	UK	UK	30 min	UK	3–8 h
Edrophonium Cl (Tensilon)	A: IV: 2 mg; then 8 mg if no response IM: 10 mg, may repeat with 2 mg in 30 min C <34 kg: IV: 1 mg, repeat in 30–45 sec if no response; max: 5 mg C >34 kg: IV: 2 mg, repeat with 1 mg if no response; max: 10 mg	C	*Increase* bradycardia with digoxin	1.2–2 h	UK	IV: 30–60 s IM: 2–10 min	IV:UK IM: UK	IV: 6–12 min IM: 5–30 min

Neostigmine bromide (Prostigmin) Neostigmine methylsulfate (injectable form)	A: PO: 150 mg/d in divided doses; range: 15–375 mg/d IM/IV: 0.5–2.5 mg as needed C: PO: 2 mg/kg/d in divided doses or 10 mg/m² q4h	C	*Increase* neostigmine effect with other cholinergics *Decrease* neostigmine effect with atropine, antidysrhythmics	1–1.5 h	15–25%	PO: 1–4 h IM: 15–30 min IV: 5–8 min	PO: UK IM: 20–30 min IV: UK	PO: 2.5–4 h IM: 2.5–4 h IV: 2–4 h
Pyridostigmine (Mestinon)	See Prototype Drug Chart							

KEY: For complete abbreviation key, see inside front cover.

Prototype: Muscle Relaxant

Carisoprodol
Carisoprodol (Soma)   Skeletal muscle relaxant   *Pregnancy Category:* C   *Drug Forms:*   Tab 350 mg

Dosage
A: PO: 350 mg t.i.d. h.s.   C > 5 y: PO: 25 mg/kg/d in 4 divided doses

Contraindications
Severe renal and hepatic disease

Drug-Lab-Food Interactions
Increase CNS depression with alcohol, narcotics, sedative-hypnotics, antihistamines, tricyclic antidepressants

Pharmacokinetics
Absorption: PO: Well absorbed   *Distribution:* PB: UK; in breast milk   *Metabolism:* t 1/2: 8 h   *Excretion:* In urine

Pharmacodynamics
PO: Onset: 30 min   Peak: 3–4 h   Duration: 4–6 h

Therapeutic Effects/Uses: To relax skeletal muscles.

Mode of Action: Depression of the CNS and, thus, relaxation of skeletal muscles.

Side Effects
Nausea, vomiting, syncope, dizziness, drowsiness, weakness, insomnia, headache, depression, irritability, rash

Adverse Reactions
Tachycardia, postural hypotension, diplopia   *Life-threatening:* Asthmatic attack, leukopenia, anaphylactic shock

KEY: For complete abbreviation key, see inside front cover.

Muscle Relaxant

■ NURSING PROCESS: MUSCLE RELAXANT: Carisoprodol

ASSESSMENT
- Obtain a medical history. Carisoprodol is contraindicated if the client has severe renal or liver disease.
- Obtain baseline VS for future comparison.
- Obtain the client's history to identify the cause of muscle spasm and to determine if it is acute or chronic.
- Obtain a drug history. Report if a drug-drug interaction is probable.
- Note if there is a history of narrow-angle glaucoma or myasthenia gravis. Cyclobenzaprine and orphenadrine are contraindicated with these health problems.

POTENTIAL NURSING DIAGNOSES
Impaired physical mobility
Activity intolerance

PLANNING
- Client will be free of muscular pain within 1 wk.

NURSING INTERVENTIONS
- Monitor serum liver enzyme levels of clients taking dantrolene and carisoprodol. Report elevated liver enzymes, such as ALP, ALT, and GGPT.
- Monitor VS. Report abnormal results.

CLIENT TEACHING
General
- Inform the client that the muscle relaxant should not be abruptly stopped. Drug should be tapered over 1 wk to avoid rebound spasms.
- Advise the client not to drive or operate dangerous machinery when taking muscle relaxants. These drugs have a sedative effect and can cause drowsiness.
- Inform the client that most of the centrally acting muscle relaxants for acute spasms are usually taken for no longer than 3 wk.
- Advise the client to avoid alcohol and CNS depressants. If muscle relaxants are taken with these drugs, CNS depression may be intensified.
- Inform the client that these drugs are contraindicated during pregnancy or by lactating mothers. Check with the health care provider.

Diet
- Advise the client to take muscle relaxants with food to decrease GI upset.

Side Effects
- Instruct the client to report side effects of the muscle relaxant, such as nausea, vomiting, dizziness, faintness, headache, and diplopia. Dizziness and faintness are most likely due to orthostatic (postural) hypotension.

EVALUATION
- Evaluate the effectiveness of the muscle relaxant to determine if the client's muscular pain has decreased or disappeared.

Muscle Relaxant (Skeletal)

Generic (Brand)	Route and Dosage	Preg Cat	Interaction	t 1/2	PB	Onset	Peak	Duration
Anxiolytics Diazepam (Valium) CSS IV	A: PO: 2–10 mg b.i.d./q.i.d IM/IV: 5–10 mg; may repeat	D	*Increase* CNS depression with alcohol, narcotics, sedatives/hypnotics, anticonvulsants *Increase* phenytoin levels; increase diazepam effect with cimetidine, oral contraceptives *Decrease* diazepam effects with oral contraceptives, rifampin	20–50 h	98%	PO: 30–60 min IM: 15–30 min IV: 1–5 min	PO: 1–2 h IV: 10–15 min	PO: 3 h IV: 30–60 min
Meprobamate (Equanil, Miltown) CSS IV	A: PO: 400 mg–1.2 g/d in divided doses	D	Similar to diazepam	10–12 h	UK	1 h	1–3 h	6–12 h

Centrally Acting Muscle Relaxants

Drug	Dosage		Side Effects / Interactions		Onset	Peak	Duration
Baclofen (Lioresal)	A: PO: Initially: 5 mg t.i.d.; may increase dose; maint: 10–20 mg t.i.d./q.i.d.; max: 80 mg/d	C	*Increase* CNS depression with alcohol, narcotics, sedative/ hypnotics, tricyclic antidepressants, MAOIs, some antihistamines *Lab:* may *increase* blood glucose levels	3–4 h	30%	UK	2–3 h	8 h
Carisoprodol (Soma)	See Prototype Drug Chart							
Chlorphenesin carbamate (Maolate)	A: PO: Initially: 800 mg t.i.d.; maint: 400 mg q.i.d.	C	Same as baclofen	3–4 h	UK	1 h	1–2 h	4–6 h
Chlorzoxazone (Paraflex, Parafon Forte)	A: PO: 250–750 mg t.i.d./q.i.d.; max: 3 g/d C: PO: 20 mg/kg/d or 600 mg/m^2/d in 3–4 divided doses	C	Same as baclofen	1 h	UK	1 h	2–4 h	4–5 h
Cyclobenzaprine HCl (Flexeril)	A: PO: 10 mg t.i.d.; may increase dose; max: 60 mg/d	B	Same as baclofen; may cause hypertensive crisis with MAOIs	1–3 d	93%	1 h	3–8 h	12–24 h

continued

Muscle Relaxant (Skeletal) — Continued

Generic (Brand)	Route and Dosage	Preg Cat	Interaction	t 1/2	PB	Onset	Peak	Duration
Methocarbamol (Robaxin, Delaxin, Marbaxin)	A: PO: Initially: 1.5 g q.i.d.; maint: 1 g q.i.d. IM/IV: 0.5–1 g q8h; max: 3 g/d	C	Same as baclofen	1–2 h	UK	30 min	1–2 h	UK
Orphenadrine citrate (Norflex, Flexon)	A: PO: 100 mg b.i.d. IM/IV: 60 mg daily/b.i.d.	C	*Increase* CNS effects with other anticholinergics, oral contraceptives, propoxyphene	14 h	<20%	PO: 1 h IV: Immediate	PO: 2 h	PO: 4–6 h
Depolarizing Muscle Relaxants (adjunct to anesthesia)								
Atracurium besylate (Tracrium)	A: IV: Initially: 0.4–0.5 mg/kg bolus; then 20–45 min later: 0.08–0.1 mg/kg	C	*Increase* neuromuscular blockage with aminoglycosides, lidocaine, verapamil, clindamycin, antidysrhythmics	20 min	UK	2 min	5 min	1 h
Doxacurium C (Nuromax)	A: IV: Induction: 0.05 mg/kg bolus over 5–15 sec C: IV: Induction: IV: 0.03–0.05 mg/kg	C	Similar to atracurium besylate	1.5 h	30%	5 min	10 min	1–4 h

Pancuronium bromide (Pavulon)	A: IV: 0.04–0.1 mg/kg; then 0.01 mg/kg every 30–60 min as needed C >10 y: same as for adult	C	*Increase* neuromuscular blockade with local anesthetic, aminoglycosides, quinidine, narcotics, thiazides, lithium, bacitracin, lidocaine *Decrease* pancuronium effect with phenytoin	2 h	<10%	30–45 s	2–3 min	45–60 min
Succinylcholine Cl (Anectine Cl, Quelicin, Sucostrin)	A: IM: 2.5–4 mg/kg; max: 150 mg IV: 0.3–1.1 mg/kg; max: 150 mg C: IM/IV: 1–2 mg/kg; max: IM: 150 mg	C	Same as pancuronium	UK	UK	IM: 2–3 min IV: 1 min	IM: UK IV: 2–3 min	IM: 10–30 min IV: 6–10 min
Vecuronium bromide (Norcuron)	A or C >9 y: IV: Initially: 0.08–0.1 mg/kg/dose; maint: 0.05–0.1 mg/kg/h as needed	C	Similar to pancuronium	1–1.5 h	60–80%	30–60 min	3–5 min	25–40 min

continued

Muscle Relaxant (Skeletal)—Continued

Generic (Brand)	Route and Dosage	Preg Cat	Interaction	t1/2	PB	Onset	Peak	Duration
Muscle Relaxant Recuronium bromide (Flumadine)	*Anesthesia intubation:* A: IV: Initially: 0.45–0.6 mg/kg C: IV: 0.6 mg/kg *During surgery:* A: IV bolus: 0.9–1.2 mg/kg *Postoperative:* A: IV: 0.01–0.012 mg/kg/min	B	*Increase* effect with anesthetics	2–18 min	30%	2 min	4 min	UK
Peripherally Acting Muscle Relaxant Dantrolene sodium (Dantrium)	A: PO: Initially: 25 mg/d; increase gradually; maint: 100 mg b.i.d.–q.i.d. C: PO: Initially: 0.5 mg/kg b.i.d.; increase dose gradually by 0.5 mg/kg t.i.d./q.i.d.; max: 100 mg q.i.d.	C	*Increase* CNS depression with alcohol, narcotics, sedatives/hypnotics, tricyclic antidepressants	8.7 h	95%	1 h	5 h	8 h

KEY: For complete abbreviation key, see inside front cover.

ANTI-INFLAMMATORY AGENTS

Nonsteroidal Anti-inflammatory Drugs

Gold Preparations

Antigout Drugs

Prototype: Anti-inflammatory: Nonsteroidal Anti-inflammatory Drugs (NSAID)

Ibuprofen

Ibuprofen
 (Motrin, Advil, Nuprin, Medipren, Rufen), ✤ Amersol
NSAID: Propionic acid derivative
Pregnancy Category: B
Drug Forms:
Tab 200, 400, 600, 800 mg

Dosage

A: PO: 200–800 mg t.i.d./q.i.d.; max: <3.2 g/d (<3,200 mg/d)
C: PO: Average: 5–10 mg/kg/d; max: 40 mg/kg/d
1–4 y: 400 mg/d in divided doses
5–7 y: 600 mg/d in divided doses
>8 y: 800 mg/d in divided doses

Contraindications

Severe renal or hepatic disease, asthma, peptic ulcer
Caution: Bleeding disorders, early pregnancy, lactation, systemic lupus erythematosus (SLE)

Drug-Lab-Food Interactions

Increase bleeding time with oral anticoagulants; *increase* effects of phenytoin, sulfonamides, warfarin
Decrease effect with aspirin; may *increase* severe side effect of lithium

Pharmacokinetics

Absorption: PO: Well absorbed
Distribution: PB: 98%
Metabolism: t 1/2: 2–4 h
Excretion: In urine, mostly as inactive metabolites; some in bile

Pharmacodynamics

PO: Onset: 0.5 h
   Peak: 1–2 h
   Duration: 4–6 h

Therapeutic Effects/Uses: To reduce inflammatory process; to relieve pain; anti-inflammatory effect for arthritic conditions.

Mode of Action: Inhibition of prostaglandin synthesis, thus relieving pain and inflammation.

Side Effects

Anorexia, nausea, vomiting, diarrhea, edema, rash, purpura, tinnitus, fatigue, dizziness, lightheadedness, anxiety, confusion

Adverse Reactions

GI bleeding
Life-threatening: Blood dyscrasias, cardiac dysrhythmias, nephrotoxicity, anaphylaxis

KEY: For complete abbreviation key, see inside front cover.

Anti-inflammatory: Nonsteroidal Anti-inflammatory Drugs (NSAID)

■ NURSING PROCESS: ANTI-INFLAMMATORY: Nonsteroidal Anti-inflammatory Drug

ASSESSMENT
- Check the client's history of allergy to NSAIDs, including aspirin. If an allergy is present, notify the health care provider.
- Obtain a drug history and report any possible drug-drug interaction. NSAIDs can increase the effects of phenytoin (Dilantin), sulfonamides, and warfarin. Most NSAIDs are highly protein-bound and can displace other highly protein-bound drugs, like warfarin (Coumadin).
- Obtain a medical history. NSAIDs are contraindicated if the client has a severe renal or liver disease, peptic ulcer, or bleeding disorder.
- Assess the client for GI upset and peripheral edema, which are common side effects of NSAIDs.

POTENTIAL NURSING DIAGNOSES
Impaired tissue integrity
High risk for activity intolerance

PLANNING
- The inflammatory process will subside in 1–3 wk.

NURSING INTERVENTIONS
- Observe the client for bleeding gums, petechiae, ecchymoses, or black (tarry) stools. Bleeding time can be prolonged when taking NSAIDs, especially with a highly protein-bound drug such as warfarin (anticoagulant).
- Report if the client is having GI discomfort. Administer the NSAIDs at mealtime or with food to prevent GI upset.
- Monitor VS and check for peripheral edema, especially in the morning.

CLIENT TEACHING
General
- Instruct the client not to take aspirin with other NSAIDs and, when taking an NSAID, not to take aspirin or acetaminophen.
- Instruct the client to avoid alcohol when taking NSAIDs. GI upset or gastric ulcer may result.
- Advise the client to inform the dentist or surgeon before a procedure when taking ibuprofen or other NSAIDs for a continuous period of time.
- Advise women not to take NSAIDs 1–2 d before menstruation to avoid heavy menstrual flow. If discomfort occurs, acetaminophen is usually prescribed.
- Advise women in the third trimester of pregnancy to avoid NSAIDs. If delivery occurs, excess bleeding might occur with NSAIDs.
- Inform the client that it may take several weeks to experience the desired drug effect of some NSAIDs.

Diet
- Instruct the client to take NSAIDs with meals or food to reduce GI upset.

Anti-inflammatory: Nonsteroidal Anti-inflammatory Drugs (NSAID)

Side Effects
- Advise the client of the common side effects of NSAIDs. Nausea, vomiting, peripheral edema, GI upset, purpura or petechiae, and/or dizziness might occur. Report occurrences of side effects.

EVALUATION
- Evaluate the effectiveness of the drug therapy, such as a decrease in pain and in swollen joints and an increase in mobility.

Anti-inflammatory: Nonsteroidal Anti-inflammatory Drugs

Generic (Brand)	Route and Dosage	Preg Cat	Interaction	t 1/2	PB	Onset	Peak	Duration
Salicylates								
Aspirin (ASA, Bayer, Ecotrin)	A: PO: 325–650 mg PRN See Prototype Drug—Aspirin—Analgesic	D: Near term	*Increase* risk of bleeding with anticoagulants; *increase* ulcerogenic effect with glucocorticoids *Lab: Increase* PT, bleeding time, uric acid	2–3 h (low dose)	90%	15–30 min	1–2 h	4–6 h
Diflunisal (Dolobid)	A: PO: Initially: 1 g (1,000 mg); maint: 500 mg q8–12h	C	*Increase* effects of acetaminophen, anticoagulants; may *increase* bleeding with warfarin *Decrease* diflunisal effects with antacids, steroids; may *decrease* effect of diuretics, anticoagulants	1 h	99%	1 h	2–3 h	8–12 h

continued

Anti-inflammatory: Nonsteroidal Anti-inflammatory Drugs—*Continued*

Generic (Brand)	Route and Dosage	Preg Cat	Interaction	t1/2	PB	Onset	Peak	Duration
Para-Chlorobenzoic Acid (Indoles)								
Indomethacin (Indocin)	A: PO: 25–50 mg b.i.d./t.i.d. with food SR: 75 mg q.d./b.i.d.; max: 200 mg/d C: PO: 1–2 mg/kg/d in 2–4 divided doses; may increase to 4 mg/kg/d; max: 150–200 mg/d	B (D at near term)	May *increase* effect of digoxin, phenytoin, sulfonamides, warfarin, lithium; may *increase* bleeding time with aspirin, anticoagulants, alcohol May *decrease* effect of diuretics	3–120 h	90–99%	0.5–2 h	3 h	4–6 h
Sulindac (Clinoril)	A: PO: 150–200 mg b.i.d.	C	Same as indomethacin	7–18 h	93%	1–2 h	2 h or 4 h with food	10–12 h
Tolmetin (Tolectin)	A: PO: Initially: 400 mg t.i.d.; maint: 600–1800 mg/d in divided doses; max: 2 g/d C >2 y: PO: 20 mg/kg/d in divided doses; max: 30 mg/kg/d	B (D at near term)	Same as indomethacin *Lab: Increase* BUN, ALP, AST, hematocrit, bleeding time	1–1.5 h	99%	15–30 min	0.5–1 h	UK

Pyrazolone Phenylbutazone (Butazolidin)	A: PO: 100–400 mg/d in divided doses; max: 600 mg/d	C	May *increase* bleeding time with warfarin, aspirin, other NSAIDs, glucocorticoids; may *increase* lithium effect May *decrease* hypotensive effect of antihypertensives *Lab: Increase* AST, ALT	50–100 h	98%	UK	2 h	UK
Propionic Acid Fenoprofen calcium (Nalfon)	A: PO: 300–600 mg t.i.d./q.i.d.; max: 3.2 g/d	B (D at term)	Similar to ibuprofen	3 h	90%	30 min	1–2 h	4–6 h
Flurbiprofen sodium (Ansaid, Ocufen)	A: PO: 50–300 mg/d in 2–4 divided doses; max: 300 mg/d *Ophthalmic use:* 0.03% sol	C	*Increase* bleeding time with heparin, warfarin May *decrease* effects of aspirin, diuretics	5 h	UK	<2 h	1.5–2 h	6–8 h
Ibuprofen (Motrin, Advil, Nuprin, Medipren)	See Prototype Drug Chart							

continued

Anti-inflammatory: Nonsteroidal Anti-inflammatory Drugs—*Continued*

Generic (Brand)	Route and Dosage	Preg Cat	Interaction	t 1/2	PB	Onset	Peak	Duration
Ketoprofen (Orudis)	*Inflammatory:* A: PO: 150–300 mg/d in 3–4 divided doses *Mild-moderate pain:* A: PO: 25–50 mg q6–8h PRN; max: 300 mg/d	B, D at near term	Similar to flurbiprofen	3–4 h	99%	1 h	1.5–2 h	4–6 h
Naproxen (Naprosyn)	A: PO: 250–500 mg b.i.d. C: PO: 5–10 mg/kg/d in 2 divided doses	B	Similar to ibuprofen	10–15 h	99%	1 h	2 h	7 h
Oxaprozin (Daypro)	A: PO: Initially: 1,200 mg/d; maint: 600 mg/d; max: 1800 mg/d in divided doses	C	*Increase* GI disturbance with aspirin, alcohol, steroids; *increase* effect of aspirin, warfarin *Decrease* antihypertensive effect with antihypertensive drugs	40 h	99%	UK	Up to 2–6 wk	UK
Anthranylic Acids (Fenamates) Meclofenamate (Meclomen)	A: PO: 200–400 mg in 3–4 divided doses	B, D at term	*Increase* bleeding time with anticoagulants; may *increase* effects of phenytoin, sulfonamides, sulfonylureas	3 h	99%	0.5–1 h	1–2 h	2–6 h

Mefenamic acid (Ponstel)	A: PO: Initially: 500 mg; then 250 mg q6h PRN; max: 1 g/d	C	Same as meclofenamate	2–4 h	90%	1–2 h	2–4 h	6 h
Oxicams Piroxicam (Feldene)	A: PO: 10 mg b.i.d. or 20 mg q.d.	C	Similar to meclofenamate	30–86 h	99%	1 h	3–5 h	24–72 h
Phenylacetic Acid Diclofenac sodium (Voltaren)	A: PO: 25–50 mg t.i.d./q.i.d. or 75 mg b.i.d.	B	May *increase* digoxin levels; may *increase* bleeding time with warfarin; *increase* effects of phenytoin, sulfonamides, sulfonylurea *Decrease* antihypertensive effect with diuretics, beta blockers	2 h	90–99%	1 h	2–3 h	UK
Etodolac (Lodine)	A: PO: 200–400 mg q6–8h PRN; max: 1,200 mg/d	C	May *increase* serum levels with digoxin, lithium May *decrease* effects of diuretics, beta blockers (antihypertensive effect)	6–7 h	99%	0.5 h	1–2 h	4–12 h
Ketorolac (Toradol)	A: <50kg: IM: LD: 30 mg; maint: 15 mg q6h A: >50kg: IM: LD: 30–60 mg; maint: 15–30 mg PRN	B	Similar to diclofenac	5–6 h	99%	15–45 min	1 h	6–8 h

KEY: For complete abbreviation key, see inside front cover.

Prototype: Anti-inflammatory Agent: Gold

Auranofin

Auranofin
  (Ridaura)
Gold preparation
Pregnancy Category: C
Drug Forms:
Cap 3 mg

Dosage

A: PO: 6 mg/d in single or divided doses; may increase dose to 9 mg/d
C: Initial 0.1 mg/kg/d in 1–2 divided doses; maint: 0.15 mg/kg/d in 1–2 divided doses; max: 0.2 mg/kg/d in 1–2 divided doses

Contraindications

Severe renal or hepatic disease, colitis, systemic lupus erythematosus (SLE), pregnancy, blood dyscrasias
Caution: Diabetes mellitus, CHF

Drug-Lab-Food Interactions

With anticancer drugs, may cause bone marrow depression
Lab: Slightly *increase* liver enzyme tests

Pharmacokinetics

Absorption: PO: 25% absorbed
Distribution: PB: 60%
Metabolism: t 1/2: 26 d in blood; 40–120 d in tissue
Excretion: >60% in urine (may appear for 15 mon); in feces

Pharmacodynamics

PO: Onset: UK
 Peak: 1–2 h
 Duration: Months

Therapeutic Effects/Uses: To alleviate inflammation and pain of rheumatoid arthritis.
Mode of Action: Inhibition of prostaglandin synthesis and decreased phagocytosis.

Side Effects

Anorexia, nausea, vomiting, diarrhea, stomatitis, abdominal cramps, pruritus, dizziness, headache, metallic taste, rash, dermatitis, photosensitivity

Adverse Reactions

Corneal gold deposits, urticaria, hematuria, proteinuria, bradycardia
Life-threatening: Nephrotoxicity, agranulocytosis, thrombocytopenia, interstitial pneumonitis

KEY: For complete abbreviation key, see inside front cover.

Anti-inflammatory Agent: Gold

■ NURSING PROCESS: ANTI-INFLAMMATORY DRUGS: Gold

ASSESSMENT
- Obtain the client's health history. Usually, gold drugs such as auranofin are contraindicated if there is renal or hepatic dysfunction, marked hypertension, congestive heart failure, systemic lupus erythematosus (SLE), or uncontrolled diabetes mellitus.
- Check for proteinuria and hematuria before giving initial gold dose and during gold therapy.
- Observe the client for 30 min after gold injection for possible allergic reaction after the first and second injections. It takes approximately 10–15 min for a serious allergic reaction (anaphylaxis) to occur.
- Obtain baseline VS and hematology laboratory findings for future comparisons.

POTENTIAL NURSING DIAGNOSES
Impaired physical mobility
Pain
High risk for impaired skin integrity

PLANNING
- The client will be free of inflammation and pain while taking the gold treatment without adverse drug reaction.

NURSING INTERVENTIONS
- Monitor the client's VS. Report abnormal findings.
- Monitor laboratory tests, e.g., complete blood count (CBC). Report abnormal findings.
- Check periodically for signs of side effects and adverse reactions to gold therapy. Side effects may include anorexia, nausea, vomiting, diarrhea, gingivitis, stomatitis, rash, itching, and decreased urine output. Most gold drugs have a long half-life; thus, a cumulative effect can result. Auranofin causes less severe adverse reactions than other gold preparations.

CLIENT TEACHING
General
- Instruct the client to perform frequent dental hygiene, including brushing the teeth with a soft toothbrush and flossing to prevent or control gingivitis and stomatitis. Use of diluted hydrogen peroxide can be helpful with mild stomatitis.
- Instruct the client to adhere to scheduled laboratory blood tests and appointments with the health care provider so any adverse reactions can be monitored.
- Inform the client that the desired therapeutic effect may take as long as 3–4 mon to occur.

Diet
- Suggest high-fiber diet and/or antidiarrheal drugs to control diarrhea. If diarrhea is continuous or severe for a prolonged time, the gold drug is usually discontinued.

Anti-inflammatory Agent: Gold

Side Effects

- Explain to the client to report early symptoms of possible gold toxicity such as a metallic taste or pruritus. A rash may occur. These symptoms should be reported to the health care provider.
- Teach the client the side effects and to report them immediately. (See list of side effects and adverse reactions.)
- Instruct the client to avoid direct sunlight because the gold drug may cause photosensitivity. Use of sunblock is necessary.
- Instruct the client to report skin conditions such as dermatitis, bruising, and petechiae. Bleeding gums and blood in the stools should be reported to the health care provider.

EVALUATION

- Evaluate the effectiveness of the gold therapy by determining if the client has less pain and inflammation.
- Evaluate the client for present or repeated side effects. The gold therapy regimen may need to be changed or discontinued.

Anti-inflammatory Drugs: Gold Preparations

Generic (Brand)	Route and Dosage	Preg Cat	Interaction	t 1/2	PB	Onset	Peak	Duration
Auranofin (Ridaura)	See Prototype Drug Chart							
Aurothioglucose (Solganal)	Increase dose weekly: A: IM: 10, 25, 50 mg (sol in oil)	C	*Increase* blood dyscrasias with immunosuppressants, cytotoxics, phenylbutazone, penicillamine	3–27 d	95%	2–3 h	4–6 h	6 mon
Gold sodium thiomalate (Myochrysine)	Increase dose weekly: A: IM: 10, 25, 50 mg (aqueous sol) until 1 g cumulative; maint: 25–50 mg q2–3wk C: Test dose: 10 mg followed by 1 mg/kg/wk × 20 wk; maint: 1 mg/kg/dose every 2–4 wk; max single dose: 50 mg	C	Same as aurothioglucose	3–27 d	95%	2–3 h	4–6 h	6 mon

KEY: For complete abbreviation key, see inside front cover.

Prototype: Antigout

Allopurinol

Allopurinol
 (Zyloprim), ❈ Alloprin, Purinol, Apo-Allopurinol
Uric acid biosynthesis inhibitor
Pregnancy Category: C
Drug Forms:
Tab 100, 300 mg

Dosage

A: PO: 200–300 mg/d (for mild gout)
 PO: 400–600 mg/d (for severe gout); max: 800 mg/d
C: PO: 10 mg/kg/d in 2–3 divided doses
 <6 y: 150 mg/d in 3 divided doses

Contraindications

Hypersensitivity, severe renal disease
Caution: Hepatic disorder

Drug-Lab-Food Interactions

Increase effect of warfarin, phenytoin, theophylline, anticancer drugs, ACE inhibitors; *increase* rash with ampicillin, amoxicillin; *increase* toxicity with thiazide diuretics
Decrease allopurinol effect with antacids
Lab: Increase AST, ALT, BUN

Pharmacokinetics

Absorption: PO: 80% absorbed
Distribution: PB: UK
Metabolism: t 1/2: Drug: 2–3 h
Metabolite: 20–24 h
Excretion: 10–20% in urine; 80–90% in feces

Pharmacodynamics

PO: Onset: 0.5–1 h
 Peak: 2–4 h
 Duration: 18–30 h

Therapeutic Effects/Uses: To treat gout and hyperuricemia; prevent urate calculi.
Mode of Action: Reduction of uric acid synthesis.

Side Effects

Anorexia, nausea, vomiting, diarrhea, stomatitis, dizziness, headache, rash, pruritus, malaise, metallic taste

Adverse Reactions

Cataracts, retinopathy
Life-threatening: Bone marrow depression, aplastic anemia, thrombocytopenia, agranulocytosis, leukopenia

KEY: For complete abbreviation key, see inside front cover.

■ NURSING PROCESS: ANTIGOUT: Allopurinol (Zyloprim)

ASSESSMENT

- Obtain a medical history from the client of any gastric, renal, cardiac, or liver disorders. Antigout drugs are excreted via kidneys, so sufficient renal function is needed. Drug dosage and drug selection might need to be changed.
- Obtain a drug history. Report possible drug-drug interactions. (See drug-lab-food interaction list.)
- Assess the serum uric acid value to be used for future comparisons.
- Assess the urine output. Use the initial urine output for future comparisons.

Antigout

- Obtain laboratory tests (BUN, serum creatinine, ALP, AST, ALT, LDH) and compare with future laboratory test results.

POTENTIAL NURSING DIAGNOSES
Impaired tissue integrity
Pain

PLANNING
- Client's "gouty pain" is absent or controlled without side effects.

NURSING INTERVENTIONS
- Report GI symptoms, gastric pain, nausea, vomiting, or diarrhea when taking antigout drugs. Take these drugs with food to alleviate gastric distress.
- Monitor the client's urine output. Because the drugs and uric acid are excreted through the urine, kidney stones might occur, so both water intake and urine output should be increased.
- Monitor laboratory tests for renal and liver function, i.e., BUN, serum creatinine, ALP, AST, and ALT.

CLIENT TEACHING
General
- Encourage the client to keep medical appointments and to have regular scheduled laboratory tests for renal, liver, and blood cell (CBC) functions. Some antigout drugs may cause blood dyscrasias; blood tests should be monitored.
- Instruct the client to increase fluid intake; it will increase drug and uric acid excretion.

Diet
- Advise the client to avoid alcohol and caffeine because they can increase uric acid levels.
- Suggest to the client not to take large doses of vitamin C while taking allopurinol; kidney stones may occur.
- Instruct the client not to ingest foods that are high in purine content, such as organ meats, salmon and sardines, gravies, and legumes. Purine foods increase the uric acid levels.
- Instruct the client to report any gastric distress. Encourage the client to take antigout drugs with food or at mealtime.

Side Effects
- Instruct the client to report side effects of antigout drugs, such as anorexia, nausea, vomiting, diarrhea, stomatitis, dizziness, rash, pruritus, or metallic taste, to the health care provider.
- Advise the client to have yearly eye examination since visual changes can result from prolonged use of allopurinol.

EVALUATION
- Evaluate the client's response to the antigout drug. If pain persists, the drug regimen may need modification.
- Determine the presence of adverse reactions. Drug therapy for gout pain may need to be changed.

Antigout Drugs

Generic (Brand)	Route and Dosage	Preg Cat	Interaction	t 1/2	PB	Onset	Peak	Duration
Anti-inflammatory Gout Drug Colchicine (Colsalide, Novocolchine)	A: PO: Initially: 0.5–1.2 mg; then 0.5–0.6 mg q1–2h for pain relief; max: 4 mg/d IV: Initially: 2 mg; then 0.5 mg q6h PRN; max: 4 mg/d	C	*Increase* effects of CNS depressants, adrenergics *Decrease* effect of vitamin B_{12} *Lab: Increase* AST, ALT	20–30 min	10–30%	20 min	0.5–2 h	9 d
Uric Acid Biosynthesis Inhibitor Allopurinol (Zyloprim)	See Prototype Drug Chart							
Uricosurics Probenecid (Benemid)	A: PO: First week: 250 mg b.i.d.; maint: 500 mg b.i.d.; max: 2 g/d C <50 kg: PO: 25–40 mg/kg/d in 4 divided doses	B	*Increase* effect of anticoagulants; *increase* toxicity of NSAIDs *Decrease* probenecid effect with aspirin, alcohol, diuretics, diazoxides, nitrofurantoin; *decrease* effect of oral hypoglycemics	4–10 h	90%	30 min	2–4 h	8 h
Sulfinpyrazone (Anturane)	A: PO: First week: 100–200 mg b.i.d.; maint: 200–400 mg b.i.d.; max: 800 mg/d	C	Similar to probenecid	3 h	90%	30 min	2–4 h	4–6 h

KEY: For complete abbreviation key, see inside front cover.

ANTI-INFECTIVE AGENTS

Antibacterials:
 Penicillins
 Cephalosporins
 Erythromycin
 Tetracyclines
 Aminoglycosides
 Quinolones
 Unclassified
 Sulfonamides
 Peptides

Antitubercular Agents

Antifungals

Antimalarials

Antivirals

Topical Anti-infectives:
 Burns
 Acne Vulgaris
 Psoriasis

Prototype: Antibacterials: Broad-Spectrum Penicillins

Amoxicillin trihydrate

Amoxicillin trihydrate (Amoxil), ♦ Apo-Amoxi
Amoxicillin-clavulanate (Augmentin), ♦ Clavulin
Broad-spectrum penicillin
Pregnancy Category: B
Drug Forms:
Cap 250, 500 mg
Tab (chewable) 125, 250 mg
Liq 62.5, 125, 250 mg/5 mL

Dosage

A: PO: 250–500 mg q8h
C: PO: 20–40 mg/kg/d in 3 divided doses

Contraindications

Allergy to penicillin, severe renal disorder
Caution: Hypersensitivity to cephalosporins

Drug-Lab-Food Interactions

Increase effect with aspirin, probenecid
Decrease effect with tetracycline, erythromycin
Lab: Increase serum AST, ALT

Pharmacokinetics

Absorption: PO: >80% (intestine)
Distribution: PB: 20%
Metabolism: t 1/2: 1–1.5 h
Excretion: Amoxicillin: 70% in urine; clavulanate: 30–40% in urine

Pharmacodynamics

PO: Onset: 0.5 h
   Peak: 1–2 h
   Duration: 6–8 h

Therapeutic Effects/Uses: To treat respiratory tract infections, urinary tract infection, otitis media, and most gram-positive and gram-negative cocci and bacilli.
Mode of Action: Inhibition of the enzyme in cell wall synthesis. Bactericidal effect.

Side Effects

Nausea, vomiting, diarrhea, rash, stomatitis, edema

Adverse Reactions

Superinfections (vaginitis)
Life-threatening: Blood dyscrasias, bone marrow depression, hemolytic anemia, respiratory distress

KEY: For complete abbreviation key, see inside front cover.

■ NURSING PROCESS: ANTIBACTERIALS: Broad-Spectrum Penicillins

ASSESSMENT

- Assess for allergy to penicillin or cephalosporins. The client who is hypersensitive to amoxicillin should not take any type of penicillin products. Severe allergic reaction could occur. A small percentage of clients who are allergic to penicillin could also be allergic to a cephalosporin product.
- Check laboratory results, especially liver enzymes. Report elevated ALP, ALT, or AST.

Antibacterials: Broad-Spectrum Penicillins

- Assess urine output. If the amount is inadequate (<30 mL/h or <600 mL/d), drug and/or drug dosage may need to be changed.

POTENTIAL NURSING DIAGNOSES
High risk for infection
High risk for impaired tissue integrity
Noncompliance with drug regimen

PLANNING
- Client's infection will be controlled and later eliminated.

NURSING INTERVENTIONS
- Send a culture of the infectious area to the laboratory to determine antibiotic susceptibility (also known as C&S) before antibiotic therapy is started.
- Check for signs and symptoms of superinfection, especially for clients taking high doses of the antibiotic for a prolonged time. Signs and symptoms include stomatitis (mouth ulcers), genital discharge (vaginitis), and anal or genital itching.
- Check the client for allergic reaction to the penicillin product, especially after the first and second doses. This may be a mild reaction, such as a rash, or a severe reaction, such as respiratory distress or anaphylaxis.
- Have epinephrine available to counteract a severe allergic reaction.
- Check the client for bleeding if high doses of penicillin are being given; a decrease in platelet aggregation (clotting) may result.
- Monitor body temperature and infectious area.
- Dilute the antibiotic for IV use in an appropriate amount of solution as indicated in the drug circular.

CLIENT TEACHING
General
- Instruct the client to take all of the prescribed penicillin product such as amoxicillin until the bottle is empty. If only a portion of the penicillin is taken, drug resistance to that antibacterial agent may develop in the future.
- Advise the client who is allergic to penicillin to wear a medical alert (Medic-Alert) bracelet or necklace and carry a card that indicates the allergy. The client should notify the health care provider during history taking of his or her allergy to penicillin.
- Keep drugs out of reach of small children. Request child safety cap bottle.
- Inform the client to report any side effects or adverse reaction that may occur while taking the drug.
- Encourage the client to increase fluid intake; it will aid in decreasing the body temperature and in excreting the drug.
- Instruct the client or child's parent that chewable tablets must be chewed or crushed before swallowing.

Diet
- Advise the client to take medication with food to decrease gastric irritation.

EVALUATION
- Evaluate the effectiveness of the antibacterial agent by determining if the infection has ceased and no side effects, including superinfection, have occurred.

Antibacterials: Penicillins

Generic (Brand)	Route and Dosage	Preg Cat	Interaction	t1/2	PB	Onset	Peak	Duration
Basic Penicillins								
Penicillin G procaine (Crysticillin, Wycillin)	A: IM: 600,000–1.2 million units/d in 1–2 divided doses C: IM: 300,000–600,000 units/d in 1–2 divided doses NB: IM: 50,000 units/kg/d	B	Same as penicillin G sodium	0.5–1 h	65%	1–2 h	1–4 h	15–18 h
Penicillin G benzathine (Bicillin)	A: IM: 1.2 million units as a single dose C: IM: >27 kg: 900,000 units/dose IM: <27 kg: 50,000 units/kg/dose or 300,000–600,000 units/dose	B	Same as penicillin G sodium	1 h	65%	Delayed	12–24 h	26 d
Penicillin G sodium/ potassium (Pentids, Pfizerpen)	A: PO: 200,000–500,000 units q6h IM: 500,000–5 million units/d in divided doses IV: 4–20 million units/d in divided doses, diluted in IV fluids C: PO: 25,000–90,000 units/d in divided doses IV: 50,000–100,000 units/kg/d in divided doses	B	*Increase* effect with aspirin, probenecid *Decrease* effect with tetracycline, erythromycin	0.5–1 h	65%	PO: 30 min IM: 15 min IV: Minutes	PO: 0.5–1 h IM: 15–30 min IV: 5–10 min	6 h

Penicillin V potassium (V-Cillin K, Veetids, Betapen VK)	A: PO: 125–500 mg q6h C: PO: 15–50 mg/kg/d in 3–4 divided doses	B	Same as penicillin G *Decrease* effect with neomycin	30 min	80%	<30 min	0.5–1 h	6 h
Broad-Spectrum Penicillins								
Amoxicillin (Amoxil) Amoxicillin-clavulanate (Augmentin)	See Prototype Drug Chart See Prototype Drug Chart							
Ampicillin (Polycillin, Omnipen)	A: PO: 250–500 mg q6h IM/IV: 2–8 g/d in divided doses C: PO: 25–100 mg/kg/d in divided doses IM/IV: 25–200 mg/kg/d in divided doses	B	*Increase* ampicillin effect with aspirin, probenecid *Decrease* effect of oral contraceptives *Decrease* ampicillin effect with tetracycline, erythromycin	1–2 h	15–28%	Rapid	PO: 1–2 h IM: 1 h IV: 5 min	6–8 h
Ampicillin-sulbactam (Unasyn)	A: IV: 1.5–3.0 g q6h	B	Same as ampicillin	1–2 h	28–38%	Immediate	5 min	UK
Bacampicillin HCl (Spectrobid)	A: PO: 400–800 mg q12h C: PO: 25–50 mg/kg/d in divided doses	B	Similar to ampicillin	1 h	17–20%	UK	0.5–1 h	5–6 h
Cyclacillin (Cyclapen)	A: PO: 250–500 mg q6h C: PO: 25–100 mg/kg/d in divided doses	B	Similar to ampicillin	0.5–1 h	20%	UK	0.5–1 h	6–8 h

continued

Antibacterials: Penicillins—Continued

Generic (Brand)	Route and Dosage	Preg Cat	Interaction	t 1/2	PB	Onset	Peak	Duration
Penicillinase-Resistant Penicillins								
Cloxacillin (Tegopen)	A: PO: 250–500 mg q6h C: PO: 50–100 mg/kg/d in 4 divided doses	B	Similar to ampicillin	0.5–1 h	90%	0.5 h	1–2 h	6 h
Dicloxacillin (Dynapen)	A: PO: 125–500 mg q6h C: PO: 12.5–25 mg/kg/d in 4 divided doses	B	Similar to ampicillin	0.5–1 h	95%	0.5 h	1–2 h	4–6 h
Methicillin (Staphcillin)	A: IM: 1 g q6h IV: 1–2 g q6h diluted in NSS C: IM/IV: 100–300 mg/kg/d in 4–6 divided doses	B	Similar to ampicillin	0.5–1 h	25–40%	IM: 20–30 min IV: Rapid	IM: 0.5–1 h IV: UK	IM: 4 h IV: 2 h
Nafcillin (Nafcin, Unipen)	A: PO: 250 mg–1 g q4–6h IM: 250–500 mg q6h IV: 500 mg–1 g q4–6h C: PO: 50–100 mg/kg/d in 4 divided doses IM: 25 mg/kg b.i.d. IV: 50–200 mg/kg/d in divided doses; max: 12 g/d	B	Similar to ampicillin	0.5–1.5 h	90%	PO: 1 h IM: <30 min	PO: 2 h IM: 0.5–1 h IV: Rapid	4–6 h

Oxacillin (Prostaphlin, Bactocill)	A: PO: 250–1 g q4–6h IM/IV: 500 mg–2 g q4h; max: IM/IV: 12 g C: PO/IM/IV: 50–100 mg/kg/d in divided doses; max: IM/IV: 300 mg/kg/d	B	Similar to ampicillin	0.5–1 h	95%	PO/IM: 0.5 h IV: Rapid	PO/IM: 0.5–2 h IV: 15 min	PO/IM/IV: 4–6 h
Anti-*Pseudomonas* Penicillins								
Carbenicillin disodium (Geocillin, Geopen)	A: PO: 1.5–3.0 g/d in divided doses IM: 1–2 g q6h or 200 mg/kg/d in 4 divided doses IV: 4–6 g q4–6h C: PO: 30–50 mg/kg/d in divided doses; max: 2–3 g/d IM: 50–200 mg/kg/d in divided doses IV: 50–500 mg/kg/d in divided doses	B	Similar to ampicillin	1–1.5 h	50%	30 min	PO: 0.5–2 h IM: 45 min–1.5 h IV: 5–10 min	UK
Mezlocillin (Mezlin)	A: IM/IV: 1.5–4 g q6h or 100–200 mg/kg/d in 4 divided doses; max: 24 g/d C: IM/IV: 50 mg/kg q4h	B	Similar to ampicillin *Lab*: May *increase* BUN, AST, ALT, ALP, bilirubin	1 h	30–40%	Rapid	IV: 5–10 min	UK

continued

Antibacterials: Penicillins—Continued

Generic (Brand)	Route and Dosage	Preg Cat	Interaction	t1/2	PB	Onset	Peak	Duration
Piperacillin (Pipracil)	A: IM/IV: 2–4 g q6h or 100–300 mg/kg/d in divided doses; max: 24 g/d C >12 y: IM/IV: 100–300 mg/kg/d in 4–6 divided doses	B	Similar to ampicillin	0.6–1.5 h	16–22%	Rapid	IM: 45 min–1 h IV: 5–10 min	UK
Piperacillin-tazobactam sodium (Zosyn) *Penicillin*	A: IV: 3.375 g q6h infused over 30 min ×7–10 d (piperacillin 3 g and tazobactam sodium 0.375 g) *Renal Insufficiency:* Cl_{cr}: 20–40 mL/min: 2.25 g q6h	B	May *increase* with probenecid *Lab:* May *increase* AST, ALT, ALP, LDH, bilirubin; may *increase* sodium and *decrease* potassium	0.7–1.2 h	30%	Immediate	Immediate	UK
Mupirocin (Bactroban)	Topical: apply 3 × d for 1–2 wk	B	Incompatible with 2% salicylic acid	NA	NA	NA	NA	NA
Ticarcillin-clavulanate (Timentin)	A: IV: 3.1 g q6h C >12 y: IV: 200–300 mg/kg/d in 4–6 divided doses	B	Similar to ampicillin	1–1.5 h	45–65%	Rapid	IM: 1–2 h	UK
Ticarcillin disodium (Ticar)	A: IM/IV: 1–2 g q6h C: IM/IV: 50–200 mg/kg/d in 4 divided doses *Systemic infections:* Dose is increased	C	Similar to ampicillin	1–1.5 h	45–65%	Rapid	IM: 1–2 h	May be present for 12 mo

KEY: For complete abbreviation key, see inside front cover.

NOTES:

Prototype: Antibacterials: Cephalosporins

Cefaclor

Cefaclor
 (Ceclor)
Second-generation cephalosporin
Pregnancy Category: B
Drug Forms:
Cap 250, 500 mg
Liq 125, 250, 325 mg/5 mL

Dosage

A: PO: 250–500 mg q8h; max: 4 g/d
C: PO: 20–40 mg/kg/d in 3 divided doses; max: 1 g/d

Contraindications

Hypersensitivity to cephalosporins
Caution: Hypersensitivity to penicillins; renal disease, lactation

Drug-Lab-Food Interactions

Increase effect with probenecid; *increase* toxicity of aminoglycosides, loop diuretics, colistin, vancomycin
Decrease effect with tetracyclines, erythromycin
Lab: May *increase* BUN, serum creatinine, AST, ALT, ALP, LDH, bilirubin

Pharmacokinetics

Absorption: PO: Well absorbed
Distribution: PB: 25%
Metabolism: t 1/2: 0.5–1 h
Excretion: 60–80% unchanged in urine

Pharmacodynamics

PO: Onset: Rapid
 Peak: 0.5–1 h
 Duration: UK

Therapeutic Effects/Uses: To treat respiratory, urinary, skin, and ear infections, or cases resistant to ampicillin/amoxicillin.
Mode of Action: Inhibition of cell wall synthesis, causing cell death; bactericidal effect.

Side Effects

Anorexia, nausea, vomiting, diarrhea, weakness, headaches, vertigo, pruritus, maculopapular rash

Adverse Reactions

Superinfection (candidiasis), proteinuria, urticaria
Life-threatening: Renal failure

KEY: For complete abbreviation key, see inside front cover.

■ NURSING PROCESS: Antibacterial: Cephalosporins

ASSESSMENT

- Assess for allergy to cephalosporins. If allergic to one type or class of cephalosporin, the client should not receive any other type of cephalosporin.
- Assess VS and urine output. Report abnormal findings, which may include an elevated temperature or a decrease in urine output.

Antibacterials: Cephalosporins

- Check laboratory results, especially those that indicate renal and liver function, such as BUN, serum creatinine, AST, ALT, ALP, and bilirubin. Report abnormal findings. Use these laboratory results for baseline values.

POTENTIAL DRUG DIAGNOSES
High risk for infection
Noncompliance with drug regimen

PLANNING
- Client's infection will be controlled and later eliminated.

NURSING INTERVENTIONS
- Culture the infectious area **before** cephalosporin therapy is started. The organism causing the infection can be determined by culture, and the antibiotics to which the organism is sensitive are determined by C&S. (Antibiotic therapy may be started before culture result is reported. The antibiotic may need to be changed after C&S test result.)
- Check for signs and symptoms of a superinfection, especially if the client is taking high doses of a cephalosporin product for a prolonged period of time. Superinfection is usually caused by the fungal organism *Candida* in the mouth (mouth ulcers) or in the genital area, such as the vagina (vaginitis).
- Refrigerate oral suspensions. For IV cephalosporins, dilute in an appropriate amount of IV fluids (50–100 mL) according to the drug circular.
- Administer IV cephalosporins over 30–45 min 2–4 times a day.
- Monitor VS, urine output, and laboratory results. Report abnormal findings.

CLIENT TEACHING
General
- Keep drugs out of reach of small children. Request child safety cap bottle.
- Instruct the client to report signs of superinfection, such as mouth ulcers or discharge from the anal or genital area.
- Advise the client to ingest buttermilk or yogurt to prevent superinfection of the intestinal flora with long-term use of a cephalosporin.
- Instruct the diabetic client not to use Clinitest tablets for urine glucose testing since false test results may occur. Tes-Tape or Clinistix may be used for urine testing, or Chemstrip bG may be used for blood glucose testing.
- Instruct the client to take the complete course of medication even when symptoms of infection have ended.

Diet
- Advise the client to take medication with food if gastric irritation occurs.

Side Effects
- Instruct the client to report any side effects from use of oral cephalosporin drug; they may include anorexia, nausea, vomiting, headache, dizziness, itching, and rash.

EVALUATION
- Evaluate the effectiveness of the cephalosporin by determining if the infection has ceased and no side effects, including superinfection, have occurred.

Antibacterials: Cephalosporins

Generic (Brand)	Route and Dosage	Preg Cat	Interaction	t1/2	PB	Onset	Peak	Duration
First Generation								
Cefadroxil (Duricef)	A: PO: 500 mg–2 g/d in 1–2 divided doses C: PO: 30 mg/kg/d in 2 divided doses	B	*Increase* nephrotoxicity with aminoglycosides, loop diuretics, colistin *Decrease* effect with tetracycline, erythromycin *Lab:* May *increase* BUN, AST, ALT, ALP	1–2 h	20%	Rapid	1 h	UK
Cefazolin sodium (Ancef, Kefzol)	A: IM/IV: 250 mg–2 g q6–8 h; max: 12 g/d C: IM/IV: 25–100 mg/kg/d in 3 divided doses; max: 6 g/d	B	Same as cefadroxil	1.5–2.5 h	75–85%	IM: Rapid IV: Immediate	IM: 0.5–2 h IV: 10–15 min	UK
Cephalexin (Keflex)	*Infection:* A: PO: 250–500 mg q6h C: PO: 25–50 mg/kg/d in 3–4 divided doses *Otitis media:* C: PO: 25–100 mg/kg/d in 4 divided doses; max: 3 g/d	B	Same as cefadroxil	0.5–1.2 h	10–15%	Rapid	1 h	UK
Cephalothin (Keflin)	A: IM/IV: 500 mg–1 g q4–6h C: IM/IV: 20–40 mg/kg q6h	B	Same as cefadroxil	30–50 min	65–80%	UK	IM: 30 min IV: 15 min	UK

Cephapirin (Cefadyl)	A: IM/IV: 500 mg–1 g q4–6h C: IM/IV: 40–80 mg/kg/d in 4 divided doses	B	Same as cefadroxil	0.5–1 h	40–50%	Rapid	IM: 30 min IV: 5–10 min	UK
Cephradine (Velosef)	A: PO: 250–500 mg q6h or 500 mg–1 g q12h IM/IV: 500 mg–1 g q6–12 h C: PO: 25–50 mg/kg/d in 4 divided doses IM/IV: 50–100 mg/kg/d in 4 divided doses	B	Same as cefadroxil	1–2 h	20%	Rapid	PO: 1 h IM: 1–2 h IV: 5–10 min	UK
Second Generation								
Cefaclor (Ceclor)	See Prototype Drug Chart							
Cefamandole (Mandol)	A: IM/IV: 500 mg–1 g q4–8h	B	Similar to cefadroxil	45 min–1 h	60–75%	IM: Rapid IV: Rapid	IM: 0.5–2 h IV: 0.5 h	UK
Cefmetazole sodium (Zefazone)	A: IV: 2 g q6–12h	B	*Increase* effect with probenecid *Decrease* effect with erythromycin, tetracyclines *Lab:* May *increase* effect of ALP, AST, ALT, LDH, BUN, creatinine	1.5–3 h	68%	IV: Rapid	End of infusion	UK
Cefonicid sodium (Monocid)	A: IM/IV: 500 mg–2 g/d single dose or b.i.d.	B	Similar to cefadroxil	4.5 h	98%	Rapid	IM: 1 h IV: 5–10 min	UK
Ceforanide (Precef)	A: IM/IV: 500 mg–1 g q12h C: IM/IV: 20–40 mg/kg/d in 2 divided doses	B	Similar to cefadroxil	3 h	80%	Rapid	IM: 1 h IV: 30 min	UK

continued

Antibacterials: Cephalosporins—*Continued*

Generic (Brand)	Route and Dosage	Preg Cat	Interaction	t1/2	PB	Onset	Peak	Duration
Cefoxitin sodium (Mefoxin)	A: IM/IV: 1–2 g q6–8h; max: 12 g/d C: IM/IV: 80–160 mg/kg/d in divided doses	B	Similar to cefadroxil	45 min–1 h	70%	Rapid	IM: 20 min–1 h IV: 5–10 min	UK
Cefpodoxime (Proxetil, Vantin)	A: PO: 100–400 mg q12h × 1–2 wk C: 6 mo–12 y: PO: 10 mg/kg/d in 2 divided doses	B	*Decrease* effect with antacids	2–3 h	20–40%	1 h	UK	UK
Cefprozil monohydrate (Cefzil)	A: PO: 250–500 mg daily or q12h C: PO: 15 mg/kg q12h × 10 d	B	*Increase* effect with probenecid; *increase* toxicity with aminoglycosides, colistin *Decrease* effect of erythromycin, tetracyclines	1–2 h	99%	UK	1–2 h	UK
Cefuroxime (Ceftin, Zinacef)	A: PO: 250–500 mg q12h IM/IV: 750 mg–1.5 g q8h C: PO: 125–250 mg q12h IM/IV: 50–100 mg/kg/d in divided doses	B	Similar to cefadroxil	1.5–2 h	50%	Rapid	PO: 2 h IM: 30 min	UK
Loracarbef (Lorabid)	A: PO: 200 mg qd × 7 d C: PO: 15 mg/kg q12h × 7 d	B	*Increase* effect with aminoglycosides, probenecid, furosemide, vancomycin	1 h	UK	30 min	45–60 min	UK

Third Generation

Cefixime (Suprax)	A: PO: 400 mg/d in 1–2 divided doses C: <12 y: PO: 8 mg/kg/d in 1–2 divided doses	B	Similar to cefadroxil	2.5–4 h	65%	Rapid	2–6 h	UK
Cefoperazone (Cefobid)	A: IM/IV: 2–4 g/d in 2 divided doses C: IV: 25–100 mg/kg q12h	B	Similar to cefadroxil	2.5 h	70–80%	IV: Rapid	IM: 1–2 h IV: 5–20 min	IM/IV: 6–8 h
Cefotaxime (Claforan)	A: IM/IV: 1–2 g q8–12h C: IM/IV: 50–180 mg/kg/d in 4–6 divided doses *Life-threatening infection:* 2 g q4h	B	Similar to cefadroxil	1–1.5 h	30–40%	UK	IM: 30 min IV: 5–10 min	UK
Cefotetan (Cefotan)	A: IM/IV: 500 mg–2 g q12h	B	Similar to cefadroxil	3–5 h	85%	Rapid	1.5–3 h	UK
Ceftazidime (Fortaz, Tazicef)	A: IM/IV: 500 mg–2 g q8–12h C: IV: 50 mg/kg q8h; max 6 g/d	B	Similar to cefadroxil	1–2 h	10–17%	Rapid	1 h	IV: End of infusion
Ceftriaxone (Rocephin)	A: IM/IV: 500 mg–2 g in single dose or q12h C: IM/IV: 50–75 mg/kg/d in 2 divided doses	B	Similar to cefadroxil	8 h	85–95%	Rapid	IM: 1–2 h IV: 10–15 min	UK
Ceftizoxime (Cefizox)	A: IM/IV: 500 mg–2 g q8–12h C: IV: 50 mg/kg q6–8h; max: 200 mg/kg/d	B	Similar to cefadroxil	2 h	30–60%	Rapid	IM: 1 h IV: 5–10 min	IV: End of infusion
Moxalactam disodium	A: IM/IV: 2–6 g/d in 2–3 divided doses C: IM/IV: 50 mg/kg q6–8h; max: 200 mg/kg/d	C	Similar to cefadroxil	2 h	25–50%	Rapid	IM: 0.5–2 h IV: 5–10 min	UK IV: End of infusion

KEY: For complete abbreviation key, see inside front cover.

Prototype: Antibacterials: Erythromycin

Erythromycin

Erythromycin
(E-Mycin, Erythrocin, Erythrocin Lactobionate [IV]), ♣ Novorythro, Erythromid, Apo-Erythro-S or base
Macrolide antibiotic
Pregnancy Category: B
Drug Forms:
Various oral preparations (cap, tab, chewables, susp)
Inj 500 mg, 1 g

Dosage

A: PO: 250–500 mg q6h
   IV: 1–4 g/d in 4 divided doses
C: PO: 30–50 mg/kg/d in 4 divided doses
   IV: 20–50 mg/kg/d in 4–6 divided doses

Contraindications

Severe hepatic disease
Caution: Hepatic dysfunction, lactation

Drug-Lab-Food Interactions

Increase effect of digoxin, carbamazepine, theophylline, cyclosporine, warfarin, triazolam
Decrease effect of penicillins, clindamycin

Pharmacokinetics

Absorption: PO: Well absorbed
Distribution: PB: 65%
Metabolism: t 1/2: PO: 1–2 h
   IV: 3–5 h
Excretion: In bile, feces, and (small amount) urine

Pharmacodynamics

PO: Onset: 1 h
    Peak: 4 h
    Duration: 6 h
IV: Onset: UK
    Peak: UK
    Duration: UK

Therapeutic Effects/Uses: To treat gram-positive and some gram-negative organisms; for clients who are allergic to penicillin.

Mode of Action: Inhibition of the steps of protein synthesis; bacteriostatic or bactericidal effect.

Side Effects

Anorexia, nausea, vomiting, diarrhea, tinnitus, abdominal cramps, pruritus, rash

Adverse Reactions

Superinfections, vaginitis, urticaria, stomatitis, hearing loss
Life-threatening: Hepatotoxicity, anaphylaxis

KEY: For complete abbreviation key, see inside front cover.

Antibacterials: Erythromycin

■ NURSING PROCESS: Antibacterials: Macrolides: Erythromycin

ASSESSMENT
- Assess VS and urine output. Report abnormal findings.
- Check laboratory tests for liver enzyme values to determine liver function. Liver enzyme tests should be periodically ordered for clients taking large doses of erythromycin for a continuous period of time.
- Obtain a history of drugs the client is currently taking. Erythromycin can increase the effects of digoxin, oral anticoagulants, theophylline, carbamazepine, and cyclosporine. Dosing for these drugs may need to be decreased.

POTENTIAL NURSING DIAGNOSES
High risk for infection
High risk for impaired tissue integrity

PLANNING
- Client's infection will be controlled and later eliminated.

NURSING INTERVENTIONS
- Obtain a culture from the infectious area and send to the laboratory for culture and (antibiotic) sensitivity (C&S) test *before* starting erythromycin therapy. Antibiotic can be initiated after culture has been obtained.
- Monitor VS, urine output, and laboratory results, especially liver enzymes: ALP, ALT, AST, and also bilirubin.
- Monitor the client for liver damage due to prolonged use and high dosage of macrolides, such as erythromycin. Signs of liver dysfunction include elevated liver enzyme levels and jaundice.
- Monitor bleeding times if the client is receiving an oral anticoagulant.
- Administer oral erythromycin 1 h before meals or 2 h after meals. Take with a full glass of water and not fruit juice. Take the drug with food if GI upset occurs. Chewable tablets should be chewed and not swallowed whole.
- For IV erythromycin, dilute in an appropriate amount of solution as indicated in the drug circular.

CLIENT TEACHING

General
- Instruct the client to take the full course of antibacterial agent as prescribed. Drug compliance is most important for all antibacterials (antibiotics).

Side Effects
- Instruct the client to report side effects, including adverse reactions. Encourage the client to report nausea, vomiting, diarrhea, abdominal cramps, and itching. Superinfection, a secondary infection due to drug therapy, such as stomatitis or vaginitis may occur.
- Instruct the client to report any symptoms of hearing impairment, such as tinnitus, vertigo, or roaring noises.

EVALUATION
- Evaluate the effectiveness of erythromycin by determining if the infection has been controlled or has ceased and no side effects, including superinfection, have occurred.

Antibacterials: Macrolides, Lincosamides, and Vancomycin

Generic (Brand)	Route and Dosage	Preg Cat	Interaction	t1/2	PB	Onset	Peak	Duration
Macrolides								
Azithromycin (Zithromax)	A: PO: Initially: 500 mg × 1 dose; maint: 250 mg/d; max: 1.5 g	C	*Increase* effects of digoxin, theophylline, methylprednisolone *Decrease* absorption with antacids; *decrease* effect of clindamycin	11–55 h	50%	2 h	4–12 h	24 h
Clarithromycin (Biaxin)	A: PO: 250–500 mg q12h × 7–14 d	C	Same as azithromycin *Lab:* May *increase* BUN and serum ALP, ALT, AST, creatinine, LDH	3–6 h	65–75%	<2 h	2–4 h	12 h
Erythromycin base (E-Mycin, Ilotycin) Erythromycin estolate (Ilosone) Erythromycin ethylsuccinate (E.E.S., E-Mycin E, Pediamycin) Erythromycin lactobionate (Erythrocin Lactobionate IV) Erythromycin stearate (Erythrocin)	See Prototype Drug Chart							

Lincosamides							
Clindamycin HCl (Cleocin)	A: PO: 150–450 mg q6–8h; max: 1,800 mg/d	B	*Decrease* effect with erythromycin, chloramphenicol *Lab*: May *increase* AST, ALT, ALP, CPK, bilirubin	2–3 h	94%	Rapid	PO: 1 h IM: 1.5 h IV: End of infusion	PO: 6 h
Clindamycin palmitate (Cleocin Pediatric)	C: PO: 25–40 mg/kg/d in 3–4 divided doses	B	Same as clindamycin HCl	2–3 h	94%	Rapid	PO: 1 h IM: 1.5 h IV: End of infusion	PO: 6 h
Clindamycin phosphate (Cleocin Phosphate)	A: IM/IV: 300–900 mg q6–8h; max: 2,700 mg/d C: IM/IV: 20–30 mg/kg/d in 3–4 divided doses	B	Same as clindamycin HCl	2–3 h	94%	Rapid	IM: 1–3 h	IM: 8–12 h
Lincomycin (Lincorex)	A: PO: 500 mg q6–8h; max: 8 g/d IM: 600 mg daily–q12h IV: 600 mg–1 g q8–12h; dilute in 100 mL of IV fluids C: PO: 30–60 mg/kg/d in 3–4 divided doses IV: 10–20 mg/kg/d in 2–3 divided doses, dilute in IV fluids	B	Similar to clindamycin HCl	4–6 h	70–75%	UK	PO: 2–4 h IM: 30 min IV: 15 min	PO: 6–8 h IM: 8–12 h IV: 10–14 h
Vancomycin							
Vancomycin HCl (Vancocin)	A: IV: 500 mg q6h or 1 g q12h C: IV: 40 mg/kg/d in 4 divided doses; dilute in IV fluids; run for 1–1.5 h	C	*Increase* nephrotoxicity effect with aminoglycosides, amphotericin B, colistin	5–11 h	10%	Rapid	30–45 min after infusion	12 h

KEY: For complete abbreviation key, see inside front cover.

Prototype: Antibacterials: Tetracyclines

Tetracycline

Tetracycline
 (Achromycin, Tetracyn, Panmycin, Sumycin), ✤ Novotetra
Pregnancy Category: D (includes child <8 y)
Drug Forms:
Tab 250, 500 mg
Cap 100, 250, 500 mg
Susp 125 mg/5 mL

Dosage

Systemic infection:
A: PO: 250–500 mg q6–12h
 IM: 250 mg/d; 300 mg/d in 2–3 divided doses
C: >8 y: PO: 25–50 mg/kg/d in 4 divided doses
 IM: 15–25 mg/kg/d in 2–3 divided doses; max: 250 mg/dose

Contraindications

Hypersensitivity, pregnancy, severe hepatic or renal disease
Caution: History of allergies, renal and hepatic dysfunction, myasthenia gravis

Drug-Lab-Food Interactions

May *increase* or *decrease* effects of anticoagulants
Decrease tetracycline absorption with antacids, iron, and zinc; *decrease* effects of oral contraceptives
Food: Dairy products (milk, cheese) *decrease* effect
Lab: Decrease serum potassium level

Pharmacokinetics

Absorption: PO: 75–80% absorbed
Distribution: PB: 20–60 h
Metabolism: t 1/2: 6–12 h
Excretion: Unchanged in the urine

Pharmacodynamics

PO: Onset: 1–2 h
 Peak: 2–4 h
 Duration: 6 h
IV: Onset: Rapid
 Peak: 0.5–1 h
 Duration: UK

Therapeutic Effects/Uses: To treat uncommon gram-positive and gram-negative organisms, skin infections or disorders, chlamydia, gonorrhea, syphilis, rickettsial infection.

Mode of Action: Inhibition of the steps of protein synthesis. Bacteriostatic or bactericidal effect.

Side Effects

Nausea, vomiting, diarrhea, rash, flatulence, abdominal discomfort, headache, photosensitivity, pruritus, epigastric distress, heartburn

Adverse Reactions

Superinfection (candidiasis)
Life-threatening: Blood dyscrasias, hepatotoxicity, nephrotoxicity, exfoliative dermatitis, intracranial hypertension

---

KEY: For complete abbreviation key, see inside front cover.

■ NURSING PROCESS: Antibacterials: Tetracyclines

ASSESSMENT

- Assess VS and urine output. Report abnormal findings.
- Check laboratory results, especially those that indicate renal and liver function, such as BUN, serum creatinine, AST, ALT, APT, and bilirubin.

Antibacterials: Tetracyclines

- Obtain a history of dietary intake and drugs the client is currently taking. Dairy products and antacids will decrease drug absorption.

POTENTIAL NURSING DIAGNOSES
High risk for infection
Noncompliance with drug regimen
High risk for impaired skin integrity

PLANNING
- Client's infection will be controlled and later eliminated.

NURSING INTERVENTIONS
- Obtain a culture from the infectious area and send to the laboratory for C&S test. Antibiotic therapy can be started after the culture has been taken.
- Administer tetracyline 1 h before meals or 2 h after meals for absorption.
- Monitor laboratory values for liver and kidney functions; these include liver enzymes, BUN, and serum creatinine.
- Monitor VS and urine output.

CLIENT TEACHING

General
- Instruct the client to store tetracycline out of the light and extreme heat. Tetracycline decomposes in light and heat, causing the drug to become toxic.
- Advise the client to check the expiration date on the bottle of tetracycline; out-of-date tetracycline can be toxic.
- Advise a woman contemplating pregnancy who has an infection to inform her health care provider and to avoid taking tetracycline because of possible teratogenic effect.
- Inform parents that children less than 8 years old should not take tetracycline because it can cause discoloration of permanent teeth.
- Instruct the client to take the complete course of tetracycline as prescribed.

Diet
- Instruct the client to avoid milk products, iron, and antacids. Tetracycline should be taken 1 h before meals or 2 h after meals with a full glass of water. If GI upset occurs, drug can be taken with food except milk products.

Side Effects
- Instruct the client to use sunblock/protective clothing during sun exposure. Photosensitivity is associated with tetracycline.
- Instruct the client to report signs of a superinfection (mouth ulcers, anal or genital discharge).
- Advise client to use additional contraceptive techniques and not to rely on oral contraceptives when taking drug because effectiveness may decrease.
- Advise the client to use effective oral hygiene several times a day to prevent or alleviate mouth ulcers (stomatitis).

EVALUATION
- Evaluate the effectiveness of tetracycline by determining if the infection has been controlled or has ceased and no side effects have occurred.

Antibacterials: Tetracyclines

Generic (Brand)	Route and Dosage	Preg Cat	Interaction	t1/2	PB	Onset	Peak	Duration
Demeclocycline HCl (Declomycin)	A: PO: 150 mg q6h or 300 mg q12h C: >8 y: PO: 6–12 mg/kg/d in 2–4 divided doses	D	May *increase* risk of digoxin toxicity *Decrease* effect with antacids, iron, calcium, magnesium, sodium bicarbonate, cimetidine Food: *Decrease* effect with dairy products	10–17 h	35–90%	1.5–3 h	3–6 h	>24 h
Doxycycline hyclate (Vibramycin)	A: PO: 100 mg q12–24 h IV: 100–200 mg/d C: >8 y: PO/IV: 2–4 mg/kg/d in 1–2 divided doses	D	Same as demeclocycline *Increase* effect of anticoagulants *Decrease* effects of penicillins, oral contraceptives	15–24 h	25–92%	1 h	1.5–4 h	UK
Minocycline HCl (Minocin)	A: PO/IV: 100 mg q12h or 50 mg q6h C: >8 y: PO/IV: 4 mg/kg/d in 2 divided doses	D	Same as doxycycline	11–20 h	55–88%	1 h	2–3 h	UK

Oxytetracycline HCl (Terramycin)	A: PO: 250–500 mg q6–12h IM: 200–300 mg/d in 2–3 divided doses IV: 250–500 mg in 2 divided doses C: >8 y: PO: 25–50 mg/kg/d in 4 divided doses IM: 15–25 mg/kg/d in 2–3 divided doses; max: 250 mg/dose IV: 10–20 mg/kg/d in 2 divided doses	D	Same as demeclocycline	6–10 h	20–40%	1–2 h	2–4 h	PO: 6 h
Tetracycline (Achromycin, Tetracyn, Sumycin, Panmycin)	See Prototype Drug Chart							

KEY: For complete abbreviation key, see inside front cover.

Prototype: Antibacterials: Aminoglycosides

Gentamicin Sulfate

Gentamicin sulfate (Garamycin)
Aminoglycoside
Pregnancy Category: C
Drug Forms:
Inj 10, 40 mg/mL
Intrathecal 2 mg/mL
Available for topical and ophthalmic use

Dosage

A: IM: 3 mg/kg/d in 3–4 divided doses
IV: 3–5 mg/kg/d in 3–4 divided doses
C: IM/IV: 2–2.5 mg/kg q8–12h
TDM: 5–10 µg/mL; peak: 10–12 µg/mL; trough: 0.5–2 µg/mL

Contraindications

Hypersensitivity, severe renal disease, pregnancy and breast feeding
Caution: Renal disease, neuromuscular disorders (myasthenia gravis, parkinsonism), heart failure, elderly, neonates

Drug-Lab-Food Interactions

Increase risk of ototoxicity with loop diuretics, methoxyflurane; *increase* risk of nephrotoxicity with amphotericin B, polymyxin, cisplatin, furosemide, vancomycin
Lab: Increase AST, ALT, LDH, bilirubin, BUN, serum creatinine
Decrease serum potassium and magnesium

Pharmacokinetics

Absorption: IM: Well absorbed
Distribution: PB: UK
Metabolism: t 1/2: 2 h
Excretion: Unchanged in urine

Pharmacodynamics

IM/IV: Onset: Rapid
Peak: 1–2 h
Duration: 6–8 h

Therapeutic Effects/Uses: To treat serious infections caused by gram-negative organisms, such as *Pseudomonas aeruginosa*, *Proteus*; to treat pelvic inflammatory disease (PID); and to treat methicillin-resistant *Staphylococcus aureus* infections.
Mode of Action: Inhibition of bacterial protein synthesis. Bactericidal effect.

Side Effects

Anorexia, nausea, vomiting, rash, numbness, tremors, tinnitus, pruritus, muscle cramps or weakness, photosensitivity

Adverse Reactions

Oliguria, deafness, urticaria, palpitation, visual disturbances, superinfection
Life-threatening: Thrombocytopenia, ototoxicity, nephrotoxicity, neuromuscular blockade, agranulocytosis, liver damage

KEY: For complete abbreviation key, see inside front cover.

■ **NURSING PROCESS: Antibacterials: Aminoglycosides**

ASSESSMENT

- Assess VS and urine output. Compare these results with future VS and urine output. An adverse reaction to most aminoglycosides is nephrotoxicity.

Antibacterials: Aminoglycosides

- Assess laboratory results to determine renal and liver functions, including BUN, serum creatinine, ALP, ALT, AST, and bilirubin. Serum electrolytes should also be checked. Aminoglycosides may decrease the serum potassium and magnesium levels.
- Obtain a medical history related to renal or hearing disorders. Large doses of aminoglycosides could cause nephrototoxicity or ototoxicity.

POTENTIAL NURSING DIAGNOSES

High risk for infection
High risk for impaired tissue integrity
High risk for altered tissue perfusion: renal

PLANNING

- Client's infection will be controlled and later eliminated.

NURSING INTERVENTIONS

- Send a culture of the infectious area to the laboratory to determine organism and antibiotic sensitivity, (C&S) before aminoglycoside is started.
- Monitor intake and output. Urine output should be at least 600 mL/d. Immediately report if urine output is decreased. Urinalysis may be ordered daily. Check results for proteinuria, casts, blood cells, or appearance.
- Check for hearing loss. Aminoglycosides can cause ototoxicity.
- Check laboratory results and compare with baseline values. Report abnormal results.
- Monitor VS. Note if body temperature has decreased.
- For IV use, dilute the aminoglycoside in 50–200 mL of NSS or D_5W solution and administer in 30–60 min.
- Check that the TDM has been ordered for peak and trough drug levels. The TDM for gentamicin is 5–10 µg/mL. Blood should be drawn 45–60 min after drug has been administered for peak levels and minutes before the next drug dosing for trough levels. Drug peak values should be 10–12 µg/mL, and trough values should be 0.5–2 µg/mL.
- Monitor for signs and symptoms of superinfection, such as stomatitis (mouth ulcers), genital discharge (vaginitis), and anal or genital itching.

CLIENT TEACHING

General

- Unless fluids are restricted, encourage the client to increase fluid intake.
- Instruct the client never to take leftover antibiotics.

Side Effects

- Instruct the client to report side effects resulting from the aminoglycosides, including nausea, vomiting, tremors, tinnitus, pruritus, and muscle cramps.
- Instruct the client to use sunblock lotion and protective clothing during sun exposure. Photosensitivity can be caused by aminoglycosides.

EVALUATION

- Evaluate the effectiveness of the aminoglycoside by determining if the infection has ceased and no side effects have occurred.

Antibacterials: Aminoglycosides

Generic (Brand)	Route and Dosage	Preg Cat	Interaction	t 1/2	PB	Onset	Peak	Duration
Amikacin SO$_4$ (Amikin)	A&C: IM/IV: 15 mg/kg/d in 2–3 divided doses; max: 1.5 g/d NB: IV: 7.5 mg/kg q12h TDM: Peak: 15–30 mg/mL; trough: 5–10 mg/mL	C	May *increase* nephrotoxicity with cephalosporins, amphotericin B, furosemide, cyclosporine *Lab:* May *increase* BUN, AST, ALT, bilirubin May *decrease* electrolyte concentrations	2–3 h	4–11%	Rapid	1–2 h	UK
Gentamicin SO$_4$ (Garamycin)	See Prototype Drug Chart							
Kanamycin SO$_4$ (Kantrex)	A: PO: 1 g q6h *Hepatic coma:* 8–12 g/d in divided doses IM/IV: 15 mg/kg/d in 2 divided doses C: IV: Same as adult	D	Similar to amikacin	2–3 h	10%	Rapid	1–2 h	UK
Neomycin SO$_4$ (Mycifradin)	A: PO: GI surgery: 1 g qh for 4 doses; then 1 g q4h for 24 h or other regimens	C	May *decrease* effects of penicillin V, digoxin	2–3 h	10%	PO: UK IM: Rapid	1–2 h 1–4 h	PO: UK IM: 6–8 h

Drug	Dose						
	Hepatic coma: 4–12 g/d in divided doses IM: 15 mg/kg/d in 4 divided doses; max: 1 g/d C: PO: 10 mg/kg in q4–6 h for 3 d						
Netilmicin (Netromycin)	A: IM/IV: 3–6 mg/kg/d in 3 divided doses C: IM/IV: 5–8 mg/kg/d in 3 divided doses TDM: Peak: 0.5–10 µg/mL; trough: <4 µg/mL	D	Similar to amikacin	2–3 h	10%	Rapid	0.5–1 h	UK
Paromomycin (Humatin)	*Intestinal amebiasis:* A&C: PO: 25–35 mg/kg/d in 3 divided doses for 5–10 d	C	*Increase* effect of oral anticoagulants *Decrease* effect of methotrexate, digoxin Lab: *Decrease* cholesterol with prolonged use	Not absorbed into systemic circulation	UK	UK	UK	UK
Streptomycin SO$_4$	*Tuberculosis:* A: IM: 1 g daily for 2–3 mo; then 1 g 3×wk *Endocarditis:* A: IM: 1 g q12h for 1 wk; dose may be decreased	C	May *increase* anticoagulant effect with warfarin	2–3 h	30%	Rapid	1–2 h	UK
Tobramycin SO$_4$ (Nebcin)	A: IM/IV: 3–5 mg/kg/d in 3 divided doses C: IM/IV: 6–7.5 mg/kg/d in 3–4 divided doses TDM: Peak: 10–12 µg/mL; trough: 0.5–2 µg/mL	D	Similar to amikacin	2–3 h	10%	Rapid	1–1.5 h	8 h

KEY: For complete abbreviation key, see inside front cover.

Prototype: Antibacterials: Quinolones

Ciprofloxacin

Ciprofloxacin
  (Cipro)
Quinolone, Fluoroquinoline
Pregnancy Category: C (X at term), breast feeding
Drug Forms:
Tab 250, 500, 750 mg
Inj 200-, 400-mg vials

Dosage

A: PO: 250–500 mg q12h
Severe infections:
A: PO: 500–750 mg q12h
  IV: 200 mg q12h
Mild to moderate infections:
A: IV: 400 mg q12h

Contraindications

Severe renal disease, hypersensitivity to other quinolones, pregnancy and breast feeding
Caution: Seizure disorders, renal disorders, children <14 y, elderly, clients receiving theophylline

Drug-Lab-Food Interactions

Increase effect with probenecid; *increase* effect of theophylline, caffeine
Decrease drug absorption with antacids, iron
Lab: Increase AST, ALT

Pharmacokinetics

Absorption: PO: 70% absorbed
Distribution: PB: 20%
Metabolism: t 1/2: 3–4 h
Excretion: 50% unchanged in urine

Pharmacodynamics

PO: Onset: 0.5–1 h
  Peak: 1–2 h
  Duration: UK

Therapeutic Effects/Uses: To treat lower respiratory, renal, bone, and joint infections.
Mode of Action: Interference with the enzyme DNA gyrase, which is needed for bacterial DNA synthesis. Bactericidal effect.

Side Effects

Nausea, vomiting, diarrhea, abdominal cramps, flatulence, headache, dizziness, fatigue, restlessness, insomnia, rash, flushing, tinnitus, photosensitivity

Adverse Reactions

Urticaria, oral candidiasis, crystalluria, hematuria, seizures

---

KEY: For complete abbreviation key, see inside front cover.

■ NURSING PROCESS: Antibacterials: Quinolones

ASSESSMENT

- Assess VS and intake and urine output. Compare these results with future VS and urine output. Fluid intake should be at least 2,000 mL/d.
- Assess laboratory results to determine renal function: BUN and serum creatinine.

Antibacterials: Quinolones

- Obtain a drug and diet history. Antacids and iron preparations decrease absorption of quinolones such as ciprofloxacin (Cipro). Ciprofloxacin can increase the effects of theophylline and caffeine.

POTENTIAL NURSING DIAGNOSES
High risk for infection
High risk for impaired tissue integrity
Noncompliance with drug regimen

PLANNING
- Client's infection will be controlled and later eliminated.

NURSING INTERVENTIONS
- Culture the infectious site and send specimen to the laboratory for C&S.
- Monitor intake and output. Urine output should be at least 750 mL/d. Client should be well hydrated, and fluid intake should be >2,000 mL/d to prevent crystalluria. Urine pH should be <6.7.
- Monitor VS. Report abnormal findings.
- Check laboratory results, especially BUN and serum creatinine. Elevated values may indicate renal dysfunction.
- Administer ciprofloxacin 1 h before or 2 h after meals or 2 h before or after antacids and iron products for absorption. Take with a full glass of water. If GI distress occurs, drug may be taken with food.
- For IV ciprofloxacin, dilute the antibiotic in an appropriate amount of solution as indicated in the drug circular. Infuse over 60 min.
- Check for signs and symptoms of superinfection such as stomatitis (mouth ulcers), furry **black** tongue, anal or genital discharge, and itching.
- Monitor serum theophylline levels. Ciprofloxacin can increase theophylline levels. Check for symptoms of CNS stimulation: nervousness, insomnia, anxiety, and tachycardia.

CLIENT TEACHING
General
- Instruct the client to drink at least 6–8 glassfuls (8 oz) of fluid daily.
- Instruct the client to avoid caffeinated products.

Side Effects
- Advise the client to avoid operating hazardous machinery or operating a motor vehicle while taking the drug or until drug stability has occurred due to possible drug-related dizziness.
- Advise the client that photosensitivity is a side effect of most quinolones. The client should use sunglasses, sunblock, and protective clothing when in the sun.
- Instruct the client to report side effects, such as dizziness, nausea, vomiting, diarrhea, flatulence, abdominal cramps, tinnitus, and rash. Older adults are more likely to develop side effects.

EVALUATION
- Evaluate the effectiveness of the quinolone by determining if the infection has ceased and the body temperature has returned within normal range.

Antibacterials: Quinolones and Unclassified

Generic (Brand)	Route and Dosage	Preg Cat	Interaction	t1/2	PB	Onset	Peak	Duration
Quinolones								
Cinoxacin (Cinobac)	A: PO: 1 g/d in 2–4 divided doses for 1–2 wk C >12 y: Same as adult	B	*Increase* effect with probenecid	1.5 h	60–80%	1–1.5 h	2–3 h	6–12 h
Ciprofloxacin HCl (Cipro)	See Prototype Drug Chart							
Enoxacin (Penetrex)	A: PO: 200–400 mg b.i.d. 7–14 d	C	*Increase* effects of probenecid; *increase* toxicity with theophylline *Decrease* enoxacin effect with antacids	3–6 h	40%	1 h	1–3 h	UK
Lomefloxacin HCl (Maxaquin)	A: PO: 200–400 mg/d × 7–14 d	C	*Increase* effects of warfarin; *increase* effect with cimetidine, probenecid *Decrease* effect with antacids, sucralfate, nitrofurantoin	6–8 h	UK	1 h	1–2 h	UK
Nalidixic acid (NegGram)	A: PO: 1 g q.i.d. for 1–2 wk; 1 g b.i.d. for long-term use C: PO: 55 mg/kg/d in 4 divided doses for 1–2 wk; 33 mg/kg/d for long-term use	B	*Increase* effects of anticoagulants	2–6 h	95%	<1 h	1–2 h	UK

Drug	Dosage						
Norfloxacin (Noroxin)	A: PO: 400 mg b.i.d., a.c. or p.c. for 1–3 wk	C	*Decrease* absorption with iron, antacids *Lab:* May *increase* AST, ALT, ALP	3–4 h	10–15%	45 min–1 h	1–2 h	UK
Ofloxacin (Floxin)	A: PO: 200–400 mg q12h × 10 d	C	Similar to lomefloxacin	5–8 h	20%	1 h	1–2 h	UK
Unclassified								
Aztreonam (Azactam)	*Urinary tract infections:* A: IM/IV: 0.5–1.0 g q8–12h *Severe infections:* A: IM/IV: 1.0–2.0 g q6–8h; max: 8 g/d	B	*Decrease* effects of cefoxitin, imipenem	1.7–2.1 h	56%	IM/IV: Rapid	IM: 1 h IV: Rapid	IM/IV: 8 h
Chloramphenicol (Chloromycetin)	A&C: PO/IV: 50 mg/kg/d in 4 divided doses (q6h) NB: 25 mg/kg/d in 4 divided doses (q6h)	C	*Increase* effects of barbiturates, oral hypoglycemics, oral anticoagulants, Cytoxan, phenytoin *Decrease* effects of penicillins, iron, folic acid	1.5–4 h	50–60% Neonate: 30%	PO: 1 h IV: Rapid	PO: 1–3 h IV: 1 h	PO: 8 h
Imipenem-cilastatin (Primaxin)	A: IM: 500–750 mg q12h IV: 250 mg–1 g q6–8h C: IV: 15–25 mg/kg q6h	C	*Decrease* effect with cephalosporins, penicillins **Not** to be mixed with other antibacterials	1 h	20%	Immediate	0.5–1 h	UK
Spectinomycin HCl (Trobicin)	A: IM: 2–4 g as single dose	B	None noted	1–3 h	10%	1 h	1–2 h	8–12 h

KEY: For complete abbreviation key, see inside front cover.

Prototype: Antibacterials: Sulfonamides (Trimethoprim-Sulfamethoxazole)

Co-Trimoxazole

Co-trimoxazole
(Bactrim, Septra)
Sulfonamide: trimethoprim (TMP)-sulfamethoxazole (SMZ)
Pregnancy Category: C
Drug Forms:
Tab 80 mg (T)/400 mg (S)
Susp 40 mg (T)/200 mg (S)/5 mL
Inj 16 mg (T)/80 mg (S)/mL

Dosage

A: PO: 160/800 mg q12h (160 mg [TMP]/800 mg [SMZ])
C: PO: 8/40 mg q12h (8 mg [TMP]/40 mg [SMZ])
Dosing is based on trimethoprim

Contraindications

Severe renal or hepatic disease, hypersensitivity to sulfonamides

Drug-Lab-Food Interactions

Increase anticoagulant effect with warfarin
Lab: Increase BUN, serum creatinine

Pharmacokinetics

Absorption: PO: Well absorbed
Distribution: PB: 50–65%; crosses placenta
Metabolism: t 1/2: 8–12 h
Excretion: In urine as metabolites

Pharmacodynamics

PO: Onset: 0.5–1 h
   Peak: 2–4 h
   Duration: UK
IV: Onset: Immediate
   Peak: 0.5–1 h
   Duration: UK

Therapeutic Effects/Uses: To treat urinary tract infection, otitis media, bronchitis, pneumonia, *Pneumocystis carinii*, rheumatic fever, burns.
Mode of Action: Inhibition of protein synthesis of nucleic acids. Bactericidal effect.

Side Effects

Anorexia, nausea, vomiting, diarrhea, rash, stomatitis, fatigue, depression, headache, vertigo, photosensitivity

Adverse Reactions

Life-threatening: Leukopenia, thrombocytopenia, increased bone marrow depression, hemolytic anemia, aplastic anemia, agranulocytosis, Stevens-Johnson syndrome, renal failure

KEY: T: trimethoprim, S: sulfamethoxazole; for complete abbreviation key, see inside front cover.

Antibacterials: Sulfonamides (Trimethoprim-Sulfamethoxazole)

■ NURSING PROCESS: Antibacterials: Sulfonamides

ASSESSMENT

- Assess the client's renal function by checking urinary output (>600 mL/d), BUN (normal, 8–25 mg/dL), and serum creatinine (normal, 0.5–1.5 mg/dL).
- Obtain a medical history from the client. Sulfonamides such as co-trimoxazole (trimethoprim-sulfamethoxazole [Bactrim, Septra]) are contraindicated for clients with severe renal or liver disease.
- Assess if the client is hypersensitive to sulfonamides. An allergic reaction can include rash, skin eruptions, and itching. A severe hypersensitivity reaction includes erythema multiforme (erythematous macular, papular, or vesicular eruption; if severe, can cover the entire body) or exfoliative dermatitis (desquamation, scaling, and itching of skin).
- Obtain a history of drugs the client is currently taking. Oral antidiabetic drugs (sulfonylureas) with sulfonamides increase the hypoglycemic effect; the use of warfarin with sulfonamides increases the anticoagulant effect.
- Assess baseline laboratory results, especially CBC. Blood dyscrasias may occur due to high doses of sulfonamides over a continuous period of time, causing life-threatening conditions.

POTENTIAL NURSING DIAGNOSES

High risk for infection
High risk for impaired tissue integrity
Altered patterns of urinary elimination

PLANNING

- Client's infection will be controlled and later alleviated.

NURSING INTERVENTIONS

- Administer sulfonamides with a full glass of water. Extra fluid intake can prevent crystalluria and kidney stone formation.
- Monitor the client's intake and output. Urine output should be at least 1,200 mL/d to decrease the risk of crystalluria. The sulfonamides sulfadiazine and sulfamethoxazole are more likely to cause crystalluria than are sulfisoxazole (Gantrisin) and combination drugs. Fluid intake should be at least 2,000 mL/d.
- Monitor VS. Note if the temperature has decreased.
- Observe the client for hematologic reaction that may lead to life-threatening anemias. Early signs are sore throat, purpura, and decreasing white blood cell and platelet counts. Check the client's CBC and compare with baseline findings.
- Check for signs and symptoms of superinfection (secondary infection caused by a different organism than the primary infection). Symptoms include stomatitis (mouth ulcers), furry **black** tongue, anal or genital discharge, and itching.

CLIENT TEACHING

General

- Instruct the client to drink several quarts of fluid daily while taking sulfonamides to avoid the complication of crystalluria.
- Advise a pregnant woman to avoid sulfonamides during the last 3 mo of pregnancy.

Antibacterials: Sulfonamides (Trimethoprim-Sulfamethoxazole)

- Instruct the client not to take antacids with sulfonamides because antacids decrease the absorption rate.
- Advise the client who has an allergy to one sulfonamide that all sulfonamide preparations should be avoided, with the health care provider's approval, due to the possibility of cross-sensitivity. Observe the client for rash or any skin eruptions.

Skill

- Instruct the client to take the sulfonamide 1 h before or 2 h after meals with a full glass of water.

Side Effects

- Instruct the client to report bruising or bleeding that could be caused from drug-induced blood disorder. Advise the client to have blood cell count monitored.
- Advise the client to avoid direct sunlight and to use sunblock and protective clothing to decrease the risk of photosensitive reactions.

EVALUATION

- Evaluate the effectiveness of the sulfonamide by determining if the infection has been alleviated and the blood cell count is within normal range.

Antibacterials: Sulfonamides

Generic (Brand)	Route and Dosage	Preg Cat	Interaction	t1/2	PB	Onset	Peak	Duration
Short Acting								
Sulfadiazine (Microsulfon)	A: PO: LD: 2–4 g; then 2–4 g/d in 4 divided doses C: PO: LD: 75 mg/kg or 2 g/m^2; then 150 mg/kg/d in 4–6 divided doses	C	*Increase* hypoglycemic effect with oral antidiabetics; *increase* anticoagulant effect with warfarin *Decrease* effect of oral contraceptives	8–12 h	20–30%	0.5–1 h	3–6 h	Short acting
Sulfamethizole (Sulfasol, Thiosulfil Forte)	A: PO: 0.5–1 g in 3–4 divided doses C: PO: 30–45 mg/kg/d in 4 divided doses	C	Same as sulfadiazine	1.5 h	90%	Rapid	2 h	Short acting
Sulfisoxazole (Gantrisin)	A: PO: LD: 2–4 g; then 4–8 g/d in 4–6 divided doses C: PO: LD: 75 mg/kg or 2 g/m^2; then 150 mg/kg/d in 4–6 divided doses	C	Same as sulfadiazine	4.5–7.5 h	85–95%	Rapid	2–4 h	Short acting

continued

Antibacterials: Sulfonamides—Continued

Generic (Brand)	Route and Dosage	Preg Cat	Interaction	t 1/2	PB	Onset	Peak	Duration
Intermediate Acting								
Sulfamethoxazole (Gantanol)	A: PO: LD: 2 g; then 2–3 g/d in 2–3 divided doses for 7–10 d C: PO: LD: 50–60 mg/kg; then 25–30 mg/kg q12h; max: 75 mg/kg/d	C	Same as sulfadiazine	7–12 h	60–70%	1 h	3–4 h	UK
Sulfasalazine (Azaline, Azulfidine, Salazoprin)	A: PO: Initially: 1 g q6–8h; maint: 2 g/d in 4 divided doses; may increase to 8 g/d C >2 y: PO: Initially: 40–60 mg/kg/d in 4–6 divided doses; maint: 20–30 mg/kg/d in 4 divided doses; max: 2 g/d	B (D, near term)	*Increase* effects of oral anticoagulants, folic acid; *increase* hypoglycemic effect with oral antidiabetics	5.5 h	99%	1 h	1.5–6 h	UK
Trimethoprim-sulfamethoxazole (Bactrim, Septra)	See Prototype Drug Chart							

KEY: For complete abbreviation key, see inside front cover.

Antibacterials: Peptides

Generic (Brand)	Route and Dosage	Preg Cat	Interaction	t1/2	PB	Onset	Peak	Duration
Bacitracin (Bactrin USP)	C <2.5 kg: IM: <900 units/kg/d in 2–3 divided doses C >2.5 kg: IM: <1000 units/kg/d in 2–3 divided doses Available in topical and ophthalmic ointment; seldom used parenterally except for children	C	Similar to polymyxin B	UK	<20%	IM: Rapid	1–2 h	6–12 h
Colistin (PO) (ColyMycin S, Polymyxin E)	A&C: PO: 5–15 mg/kg/d in 3 divided doses	C	Similar to polymyxin B *Lab:* May *increase* BUN, creatinine	2–3 h	UK	IM: UK IV: Rapid	IM: 1–2 h IV: End of infusion	IM: 8–12 h IV: UK
Colistimethate sodium (IM/IV) (Coly-Mycin M)	IM/IV: 2.5–5 mg/kg/d in divided doses		Same as colistin					
Polymyxin B SO₄ (Aerosporin)	A: IM: 25,000 units/kg/d in divided doses IV: 15,000–25,000 units/kg/d in 2 divided doses (q12h) C >2 y: Same as adult	B	May cause nephrotoxicity with aminoglycosides, amphotericin B	4.5–6 h	UK	IM: Rapid IV: Rapid	IM: 2 h IV: End of infusion	UK

KEY: For complete abbreviation key, see inside front cover.

Prototype: Antitubercular Drugs

Isoniazid

Isoniazid
  (INH, Nydrazid), ✶ Isotamine, PMS Isoniazid
Antituberculars
Pregnancy Category: C
Drug Forms:
Tab 50, 100, 300 mg
Liq 50 mg/5 mL
Inj 100 mg/mL

Dosage

A: PO/IM: 5–10 mg/kg/d in a single dose; max: 300 mg/d
Prophylaxis: 300 mg/d
C: PO/IM: 10–20 mg/kg/d in a single dose; max: 500 mg/d
Prophylaxis: 10 mg/kg/d in a single dose

Contraindications

Severe renal or hepatic disease, alcoholism, diabetic retinopathy

Drug-Lab-Food Interactions

Increase effect with alcohol, rifampin, cycloserine

Pharmacokinetics

Absorption: PO: Well absorbed
Distribution: PB: 10%
Metabolism: t 1/2: 1–4 h
Excretion: 50% unchanged in urine

Pharmacodynamics

PO: Onset: 0.5 h
    Peak: 1–2 h
    Duration: PO: 6–8 h
              IM: 6 h

Therapeutic Effects/Uses: To treat tuberculosis; prophylactic measure against tuberculosis.

Mode of Action: Inhibition of bacterial cell wall synthesis.

Side Effects

Drowsiness, tremors, rash, blurred vision, photosensitivity

Adverse Reactions

Psychotic behavior, peripheral neuropathy, vitamin B_6 deficiency
Life-threatening: Blood dyscrasias, thrombocytopenia, seizures, agranulocytosis, hepatotoxicity

KEY: For complete abbreviation key, see inside front cover.

Antitubercular Drugs

■ NURSING PROCESS: Antitubercular Drugs

ASSESSMENT
- Obtain a history from the client of any past instances of tuberculosis, last purified protein derivative (PPD) tuberculin test and reaction, last chest x-ray and result, and allergy to any of the antitubercular drugs if taken previously.
- Obtain a medical history from the client. Most antitubercular drugs are contraindicated if the client has a severe hepatic disease.
- Check laboratory tests for liver enzyme values, bilirubin, BUN, and serum creatinine. These baseline values can be compared with future laboratory test results.
- Assess the client for signs and symptoms of peripheral neuropathy, such as numbness or tingling of the extremities.
- Check the client for hearing changes if the antitubercular drug regimen includes streptomycin. Ototoxicity is an adverse reaction to streptomycin.

POTENTIAL NURSING DIAGNOSES
High risk for infection
High risk for impaired tissue integrity

PLANNING
- Client's sputum test for acid-fast bacilli will be negative in 2–3 mo after the prescribed antitubercular therapy.

NURSING INTERVENTIONS
- Administer the commonly ordered antitubercular drug isoniazid (INH) 1 h before or 2 h after meals. Food decreases absorption rate.
- Administer pyridoxine (vitamin B_6) as prescribed with isoniazid to prevent peripheral neuropathy.
- Monitor serum liver enzyme levels, especially if the client is taking isoniazid and/or rifampin. Elevated levels may indicate liver toxicity.
- Collect sputum specimens for acid-fast bacilli early in morning. Usually three consecutive morning sputum specimens are sent to the laboratory, and the routine is repeated several weeks later.
- Have eye examinations performed on clients taking isoniazid and ethambutol. Visual disturbances may result in clients taking these antitubercular drugs.
- Emphasize the importance of complying with drug regimen.

CLIENT TEACHING
General
- Instruct the client to take the antitubercular drug such as isoniazid 1 h before meals or 2 h after meals for better absorption.
- Instruct the client to take the antitubercular drugs as prescribed. Ineffective treatment of tuberculosis might occur if the drugs are taken intermittently or discontinued when symptoms are decreased or when the client is feeling better. Compliance with the drug regimen is a must.
- Instruct the client not to take antacids while taking antitubercular drug(s) because they decrease the drug absorption. The client should also avoid alcohol because it may increase the risk of hepatotoxicity.
- Advise the client to keep medical appointments and to participate in spu-

Antitubercular Drugs

tum testing. Sputum testing is important to determine the effectiveness of the drug regimen.
- Advise the woman contemplating pregnancy to first check with her health care provider about taking the antitubercular drugs ethambutol and rifampin.

Side Effects

- Instruct the client to report any numbness, tingling, or burning of the hands and feet. Peripheral neuritis is a common side effect of isoniazid. Vitamin B_6 prevents peripheral neuropathy. Neuritis may not occur if the client eats a balanced diet daily.
- Advise the client to avoid direct sunlight to decrease the risk of photosensitivity. Client should use sunblock while in the sun.
- Inform the client taking rifampin that urine, feces, saliva, sputum, sweat, and tears may be a harmless red-orange color. Soft contact lenses may be permanently stained.
- Advise the client receiving ethambutol to take daily single doses to avoid visual problems. Divided doses of ethambutol may cause visual disturbances.

EVALUATION

- Evaluate the effectiveness of the antitubercular drug(s). Sputum specimen for acid-fast bacilli should be negative after taking antitubular drugs for several weeks to months.

Antitubercular Drugs

Generic (Brand)	Route and Dosage	Preg Cat	Interaction	t 1/2	PB	Onset	Peak	Duration
Aminosalicylate sodium P.A.S. sodium	A: PO: 14–16 g/d in 2–3 divided doses C: PO: 275–420 mg/kg/d in 3–4 divided doses; take with food	C	*Decrease* effect of digoxin, vitamin B_{12}	1 h	Normal renal function: 15%	UK	1–2 h	UK
Ethambutol HCl (Myambutol)	A: PO: 15 mg/kg as a single dose *Retreatment:* A: PO: 25 mg/kg as a single dose for 2 mo; then decrease to 15 mg/kg/d C >12 y: Same as adult See Prototype Drug Chart	C	*Increase* nephrotoxicity with aminoglycosides, cisplatin	3–4 h Renal dysfunction: 8 h	10–20%	Rapid	2–4 h	UK
Isoniazid (INH, Nydrazid)								
Rifabutin (Mycobutin)	A: PO: 300 mg/d in 1 or 2 divided doses	B	Similar to rifampin	16–69 h	85%	UK	2–4 h	UK
Rifampin (Rifadin, Rimactane)	A: PO: 600 mg/d as a single dose C: PO: 10–20 mg/kg/d as a single dose; max: 600 mg/d	C	*Decrease* effect with barbiturates, corticosteroids, oral hypoglycemics, digoxin, oral contraceptives	3 h	85–90%	1–2 h	2–4 h	>24 h
Streptomycin SO_4	A: IM: 1 g daily or 7–15 mg/kg/d for 2–3 mo, then 2–3 × wk C: IM: 20–40 mg/kg/d in divided doses	C	May *increase* anticoagulant effect with warfarin	2–3 h	30%	Rapid	1–2 h	UK

KEY: For complete abbreviation key, see inside front cover.

Prototype: Antifungals

Nystatin

Nystatin
 (Mycostatin), ✤ Nadostine, Nyaderm
Antifungal
Pregnancy Category: C
Drug Forms:
Tab 500,000 U
Susp 100,000 U
Vaginal tab 100,000 U

Dosage

A: Topical use as directed
Intestinal infections:
A: PO: 500,000–1,000,000 U t.i.d. or q8h
Oral candidiasis:
A: PO: 400,000–600,000 U q6–8h
Neonate (<7 d): PO: 100,000 U q.i.d.
C: PO: 250,000–500,000 U q.i.d.

Contraindications

Hypersensitivity
Vag: Pregnancy

Drug-Lab-Food Interactions

None significant known

Pharmacokinetics

Absorption: PO: Poorly absorbed
Distribution: PB: UK
Metabolism: t 1/2: UK
Excretion: In feces unchanged

Pharmacodynamics

PO: Onset: Rapid
   Peak: UK
   Duration: 6–12 h
Vaginally: Onset: 24–72 h
   Peak: UK
   Duration: UK

Therapeutic Effects/Uses: To treat *Candida* infections.
Mode of Action: Increase permeability of the fungal cell membrane.

Side Effects

PO: Anorexia, nausea, vomiting, diarrhea (large doses), stomach cramps, rash
Vag: Rash, burning sensation

Adverse Reactions

None known

KEY: For complete abbreviation key, see inside front cover.

■ NURSING PROCESS: Antifungals

ASSESSMENT

- Obtain a medical history from the client of any serious renal or hepatic disorder. Antifungal agents such as amphotericin B, fluconazole (Diflucan), flucytosine (Ancobon), and ketoconazole (Nizoral) are contraindicated if the client has a serious renal or liver disease.
- Check laboratory tests for liver enzyme values (ALP, ALT, AST, GGT), BUN, bilirubin, and serum creatinine. Elevated levels can indicate liver or renal dysfunction. These test results may be used for future comparisons.
- Obtain baseline VS for future comparison.

Antifungals

POTENTIAL NURSING DIAGNOSES
High risk for infection
High risk for impaired tissue integrity

PLANNING
- Client's fungal infection will be resolved.

NURSING INTERVENTIONS
- Obtain a culture to determine the fungus, e.g., *Candida*.
- Monitor the client's urinary output; many of the antifungal drugs may cause nephrotoxicity.
- Monitor the laboratory results and compare with baseline findings, i.e., BUN, serum creatinine, ALP, ALT, AST, bilirubin, and electrolytes. Certain antifungals could cause hepatotoxicity as well as nephrotoxicity when taking high doses over a prolonged period of time.
- Monitor VS. Compare with baseline findings.
- Observe for side effects and adverse reactions to antifungal drugs (antimycotics), such as nausea, vomiting, headache, phlebitis, and signs and symptoms of electrolyte imbalance (hypokalemia with amphotericin B).

CLIENT TEACHING
General
- Instruct the client to take the drug as prescribed. Compliance is of utmost importance since discontinuing the drug too soon may result in a relapse.
- Advise the client to obtain laboratory testing as indicated. Serum liver enzymes, BUN, creatinine, and electrolytes should be monitored.
- Advise the client taking ketoconazole not to consume alcohol.

Skill
- Instruct the client on the administration of nystatin (Mycostatin) suspension. Place the nystatin dose, usually 1–2 teaspoons, in the mouth. Swish the solution in the mouth and swallow (swish and swallow), or after swishing, have the client expectorate the solution (check with health care provider).

Side Effects
- Advise the client to avoid operating hazardous equipment or a motor vehicle when taking amphotericin B, ketoconazole, or flucytosine because these drugs may cause visual changes, sleepiness, dizziness, or lethargy.
- Instruct the client to report side effects, such as nausea, vomiting, diarrhea, dermatitis, rash, dizziness, tinnitus, edema, and flatulence. These symptoms may occur when taking certain antifungal drugs.

EVALUATION
- Evaluate the effectiveness of the antifungal (antimycotic) drug by noting the absence of the fungal infection, e.g., decreased itching, redness, and rawness.

Antifungals

Generic (Brand)	Route and Dosage	Preg Cat	Interaction	t1/2	PB	Onset	Peak	Duration
Polyenes Amphotericin B (Fungizone)	*Test dose:* A: IV: 0.25–1.0 mg in 20 mL of D$_5$W infused over 20–30 min A: IV: 0.25–1.0 mg/kg/d in D$_5$W or 1.5 mg/kg q.o.d.; max: 1.5 mg/kg/d C: IV: Same as adult, except dilution and infuse time differ	B	May *increase* effect of digoxin, skeletal muscle relaxants; may *increase* risk of nephrotoxicity with aminoglycosides; *increase* hypokalemia with corticosteroids	Initially: 24 h Final: 15 d	90%	Rapid	1–2 h after infusion	20 h
Nystatin (Mycostatin)	See Prototype Drug Chart							
Imidazoles Fluconazole (Diflucan)	A: PO/IV: 50–400 mg/d; maint: 100–200 mg/d C: PO/IV: 3–6 mg/kg/d	C	Same as miconazole May *increase* effect of phenytoin	20–40 h	12%	PO: UK IV: Rapid	PO: 1–2 h IV: End of infusion	UK
Itraconazole (Sporanox)	A: PO: Loading dose: 200 mg q8h × 3d; maint: 200 mg/d; max: 400 mg/d in 2 divided doses	C	May *increase* effect of phenytoin *Decrease* effect of rifampin; may *decrease* effect of warfarin	21–42 h	99%	UK	1.5–5 h Steady state: 12 h	UK

Ketoconazole (Nizoral)	A: PO: 200–400 mg/d as a single dose C: PO: 3.3–6.6 mg/kg/d as single dose C <20 kg: PO: 50 mg daily	C	*Increase* effect with cyclosporine *Decrease* absorption with antacids, anticholinergics, H$_2$ blockers	Initially: 2 h Final: 8 h	95%	1 h	1–2 h	UK
Miconazole nitrate (Monistat, Micatin)	A: IV: 200–3,600 mg/d in D$_5$W in 3 divided doses; infuse IV over 30–60 min C: IV: 20–40 mg/kg/d in divided doses; max: 15 mg/kg/inf A: Supp: 100 mg vag h.s. for 7 d Available: Vaginal cream 2%; lotion	B	*Increase* effect of anticoagulants; may *increase* hypoglycemic reaction with oral hypoglycemics	Triphasic: 40 min, 2 h, 24 h	92%	Rapid	End of infusion	UK
Terbinafine HCl (Lamisil)	A&C: Topical: Cream 1%, apply 1–2× per day	B	None significant known	NA	NA	UK	UK	UK
Antimetabolites Flucytosine (Ancobon)	A: PO: 50–150 mg/kg/d in 4 divided doses C <50 kg: PO: 1.5–4.5 g/m^2/d in 4 divided doses	C	Synergistic effect with amphotericin B	3–8 h	5%	Rapid	2–6 h	UK
Antiprotozoal Atovaquone (Mepron)	A: PO: 750 mg t.i.d. with food × 21 d	C	*Increase* effect with other highly protein-bound drugs	2–3 d	99%	UK	2 peaks First: 1–8 h Second: 2–3 d	6–20 wk

KEY: For complete abbreviation key, see inside front cover.

Antimalarials

Generic (Brand)	Route and Dosage	Preg Cat	Interaction	t1/2	PB	Onset	Peak	Duration
Chloroquine HCl (Aralen HCl)	*Acute malaria:* A: PO: 600 mg base/dose; then 6 h later: 300 mg/dose; then at 24 and 48 h: 300 mg/dose IM: 200 mg/base q6h PRN C: PO: 10 mg base/kg/dose, then 6 h later: 5 mg base/kg/dose; 24–48 h later: 5 mg base/kg/dose. IM: 5 mg base/kg q12h *Prophylaxis:* 2 wk before and 6–8 wk after exposure A&C: PO: 5 mg/kg/wk; max: 300 mg base/wk	C	*Increase* effects of digoxin, anticoagulants, neuromuscular blocker *Decrease* absorption with antacids	2.5–5 d Terminal: 1–2 mo	50–65%	PO, IM: Rapid	3.5 h IV/IM: 0.5 h	Days to weeks
Hydroxychloroquine SO$_4$ (Plaquenil SO$_4$)	*Acute malaria:* A: PO: 800 mg/dose; 6 h later: 400 mg; then 400 mg daily for 2 d C: PO: 10 mg base/kg/dose; 6 h later: 5 mg base/kg; 5 mg base/kg/daily for 2 d	C	Similar to chloroquine HCl	2.5–5 d	55%	<1 h	1–2 h	UK

Drug	Dose	Preg. Cat.	Interactions	Half-life	Bioavail.	Onset	Peak	Duration
Mefloquine HCl (Lariam)	*Prophylaxis:* 1 wk before and 6–8 wk after exposure A&C: PO: 5 mg base/kg/wk; max: 300 mg base/wk	C	*Increase* ECG abnormalities with antidysrhythmics, beta blockers May *decrease* effect of valproic acid	21 d	98%	UK	7–24 h	UK
Primaquine phosphate	A: PO: Single dose: 1,250 mg; then 250 mg qwk × 4 wk	C	*Increase* toxicity of quinacrine	3.7–9.6 h	UK	UK	1–6 h	UK
Pyrimethamine (Daraprim)	*Malaria prophylaxis:* A: PO: 15 mg/d for 14 d (single doses) C: PO: 0.3 mg/kg/d for 14 d (single doses)	C	*Decrease* effect of folic acid	1.5–2 d	80%	UK	>2 h	2 wk
Quinacrine HCl (Atabrine HCl)	*Malaria prophylaxis:* A&C >10 y: PO: 25 mg/wk C <4 y: PO: 6.25 mg/wk C 4–10 y: PO: 12.5 mg/wk *Malaria suppression:* A: PO: 100 mg/d C: PO: 50 mg/d	C	*Increase* toxicity with primaquine	UK	UK	UK	8 h	4 wk
Quinine SO₄ (Quin-260, Quiphile)	*Acute malaria:* A: PO: 650 mg q8h for 3–7 d C: PO: 25 mg/kg/d in 3 divided doses (q8h) for 3–7 d	X	Similar to chloroquine HCl	6–14 h	70–95%	<1 h	1–3 h	6–8 h

KEY: For complete abbreviation key, see inside front cover.

Prototype: Antivirals

Acyclovir sodium

Acyclovir sodium
 (Zovirax)
Antiviral
Pregnancy Category: C
Drug Forms:
Cap 200 mg
Inj 500 mg/vial

Dosage

A: PO: 200 mg q4h 5×/d
  IV: 5 mg/kg q8h × 5d (diluted in D_5W)
C: IV: <12 y: 250 mg/m^2 q8h × 5 d; infuse over 1 h

Contraindications

Hypersensitivity, severe renal or hepatic disease
Caution: Electrolyte imbalance, lactation

Drug-Lab-Food Interactions

Increase nephro-neurotoxicity with aminoglycosides, probenecid, interferon
Lab: May *increase* AST, ALT, BUN

Pharmacokinetics

Absorption: PO: Slowly absorbed
Distribution: PB: 10–30%
Metabolism: t 1/2: 2–3 h
Excretion: 95% unchanged in urine

Pharmacodynamics

PO: Onset: UK
  Peak: 1.5–2 h
  Duration: 4–8 h
IV: Onset: Rapid
  Peak: 1–2 h
  Duration: 4–8 h

Therapeutic Effects/Uses: To treat herpes simplex I, genital herpes II.
Mode of Action: Interference with synthesis by the virus of DNA.

Side Effects

Nausea, vomiting, diarrhea, headache, tremors, lethargy, rash, pruritus, increased bleeding time, phlebitis at IV site

Adverse Reactions

Urticaria, anemia, gingival hyperplasia
Life-threatening: Nephrotoxicity (large doses), neuropathy, bone marrow depression, granulocytopenia, thrombocytopenia, leukopenia, seizure, acute renal failure

KEY: For complete abbreviation key, see inside front cover.

■ NURSING PROCESS: Antivirals

ASSESSMENT

- Obtain a medical history of any serious renal or hepatic disease.
- Obtain baseline VS and a complete blood count. Use these findings for comparison with future results.
- Assess baseline laboratory results, particularly BUN, serum creatinine, liver enzymes, bilirubin, and electrolytes. Use these results for future comparisons.
- Assess baseline VS and urine output. Report abnormal findings.

Antivirals

POTENTIAL NURSING DIAGNOSES
High risk of infection
High risk for impaired tissue integrity

PLANNING
- Symptoms of viral infections will be eliminated or diminished.

NURSING INTERVENTIONS
- Monitor the client's complete blood count (CBC). Report abnormal results, such as leukopenia, thrombocytopenia, and low hemoglobin and hematocrit.
- Monitor other laboratory tests, such as BUN, serum creatinine, and liver enzymes, and compare with baseline values.
- Monitor the client's urinary output. An antiviral drug such as acyclovir can affect renal function.
- Monitor VS, especially blood pressure. Acyclovir and amantadine may cause orthostatic hypotension.
- Observe for signs and symptoms of side effects. Most antiviral drugs have many side effects; see Prototype Drug Chart.
- Check for superimposed infection (superinfection) due to high dose and prolonged use of an antiviral drug such as acyclovir.
- Administer oral acyclovir as prescribed. Oral dose can be taken at mealtime.
- For IV use, dilute the antiviral drug in an appropriate amount of solution as indicated in the drug circular. Administer the IV drug over 60 min. **Never** give acyclovir as a bolus (IV push).

CLIENT TEACHING

General
- Advise the client to maintain an adequate fluid intake to ensure adequate hydration for drug therapy and to increase urine output.
- Instruct the client with genital herpes to avoid spreading the infection by sexual abstinence or the use of a condom. Advise these women to have a Pap test done every 6 mo or as indicated by the health care provider. Cervical cancer is more prevalent in women with genital herpes simplex.
- Instruct clients taking zidovudine to have blood cell count monitored.

Side Effects
- Instruct the client to perform oral hygiene several times a day. Gingival hyperplasia (red, swollen gums) can occur with prolonged use of antiviral drugs.
- Instruct the client to report adverse reactions, including decrease in urine output and CNS changes such as dizziness, anxiety, or confusion.
- Advise the client with dizziness due to orthostatic hypotension to arise slowly from a sitting to a standing position.
- Instruct the client to report any side effects associated with the antiviral drug, such as nausea, vomiting, diarrhea, increased bleeding time, rash, urticaria, or menstrual abnormalities.

EVALUATION
- Evaluate the effectiveness of the antiviral drug in eliminating the virus or in decreasing symptoms.
- Determine if side effects are absent.

Antivirals

Generic (Brand)	Route and Dosage	Preg Cat	Interaction	t1/2	PB	Onset	Peak	Duration
General								
Amantadine HCl (Symmetrel)	*Influenza A:* A: PO: 200 mg/d in 1–2 divided doses C 1–8 y: PO: 4.4–8.8 mg/kg/d in 2–3 divided doses C 9–12 y: PO: 100–200 mg/d in 1–2 divided doses	C	May *increase* anticholinergic effect; *increase* CNS action with CNS stimulants	24 h	UK	10–15 min	1–4 h	UK
Rimantadine HCl (Flumadine)	A: PO: 200 mg/d in 1 or 2 divided doses C: PO: 5–7 mg/kg/d	C	Similar to amantadine HCl	33 h	40%	UK	3–6 h	UK
Antimetabolites								
Acyclovir (Zovirax)	See Prototype Drug Chart							
Didanosine (Videx)	*HIV infections:* A >75 kg: PO: 300 mg q12h 50–75 kg: 200 mg q12h 35–50 kg: 125 mg q12h C: PO: tab: 1.1–1.4 m²: 100 mg b.i.d. 0.8–1 m²: 75 mg q12h 0.5–0.7 m²: 50 mg q12h <0.4 m²: 25 mg q12h Available in Pedi powder	B	Avoid taking with tetracyclines, ciprofloxacin	1.5 h	UK	UK	0.6–1 h	UK

Drug		Dose	Preg. cat.	Interactions					
Famciclovir (Famvir)		*Herpes zoster:* A: PO: 500 mg q8h × 7 d		*Increase* effect of digoxin	UK	UK	UK	UK	UK
Ganciclovir sodium (Cytovene)		A&C: IV: Initially: 5 mg/kg q12h × 14–21 d; maint: 5 mg/kg/d × 7 d or 6 mg/kg/d × 5 d	C	May *increase* toxicity with cytotoxic drugs May *increase* seizures with imipenem-cilastatin *Lab:* May *increase* BUN, creatinine; may *decrease* blood glucose	2.5–6 h	1–2%	3–8 d	12–14 d	>14 d
Ribavirin (Virazole)		A&C: By aerosol inhalation administration	X	May antagonize effect of zidovudine	24 h	NA	UK	1–1.5 h	UK
Vidarabine monohydrate (Vira-A)		A: IV: 10–15 mg/kg/d infused over 12–24 h	C	*Increase* CNS side effects with allopurinol	1.5–3 h	20–30%	Rapid	End of infusion	UK
Zalcitabine (Hivid)		*HIV infections:* A: PO: 0.75 mg q8h given with zidovudine 200 mg q8h	C	May cause peripheral neuropathy with aminoglycosides, amphotericin, cisplatin, INH, nitrofurantoin, phenytoin, vincristine, disulfiram	1.2–2 h	<4%	UK	1–2 h	UK
Zidovudine (Retrovir)		A: PO: 100–200 mg q4h IV: 1–2 mg/kg q4h; max: 1,200 mg/d C: PO: 90–180 mg/m^2 q6h; max: 200 mg q6h	C	May *increase* toxicity with aspirin, acetaminophen, H$_2$ blockers, lorazepam	1 h	25–38%	Rapid	0.5–1.5 h	UK

KEY: For complete abbreviation key, see inside front cover.

Prototype: Topical Anti-infectives: Burns

Mafenide acetate

Mafenide acetate
  (Sulfamylon)
Anti-infective, sulfonamide
  derivative
Pregnancy Category: C
Drug Form:
Cream: 85 mg/g as acetate

Dosage

A&C: Topical: Apply $1/16$-inch layer evenly to affected area daily/b.i.d; reapply as necessary

Contraindications

Hypersensitivity, inhalation injury

Drug-Lab-Food Interactions

None known

Pharmacokinetics

Absorption: Some absorbed
Distribution: PB: UK
Metabolism: t 1/2: UK
Excretion: In urine

Pharmacodynamics

Onset: On contact
Peak: 2–4 h
Duration: As long as applied

Therapeutic Effects/Uses: To treat second- and third-degree burns; to prevent organism invasion of burned tissue areas; to treat burn infections.

Mode of Action: Inhibits bacterial cell wall synthesis.

Side Effects

Rash, burning sensation, urticaria, pruritus, swelling

Adverse Reactions

Metabolic acidosis, respiratory alkalosis, blistering, superinfection

Life-threatening: Bone marrow suppression, fatal hemolytic anemia

KEY: For complete abbreviation key, see inside front cover.

Topical Anti-infectives: Burns

■ NURSING PROCESS: Topical Anti-infectives: Burns

ASSESSMENT
- Assess burned tissue for infection. Culture an oozing wound.
- Check client's VS. Report abnormal findings such as an elevated temperature.

POTENTIAL NURSING DIAGNOSES
High risk for infection related to loss of skin integrity
Pain related to thermal injury

PLANNING
- Aseptic technique will be enforced when caring for burned tissue, and tissue will be free from infection.

NURSING INTERVENTIONS
- Administer prescribed analgesia before application, if needed.
- Cleanse burned tissue sites using aseptic technique.
- Apply topical antibacterial drug and dressing with sterile technique.
- Monitor client's fluid balance and renal function.
- Monitor client for side effects of and adverse reactions to topical drug.
- Monitor client's VS and be alert for signs of infection. Use with caution in client with acute renal failure.
- Closely monitor client's acid-base balance, especially in the presence of pulmonary or renal dysfunction.
- Store drug in dry place at room temperature.

CLIENT TEACHING

General
- Instruct client and family about changes in respiratory status.

Skill
- Explain to client and family the care given to the burned tissue areas, using aseptic technique.
- Instruct client and family to apply topical agent and dressings to the burned areas.

EVALUATION
- Evaluate effectiveness of treatment interventions to burned tissue areas by determining if healing is proceeding and sites are free from infection.

Topical Anti-infectives: Burns, Acne Vulgaris, Psoriasis

Generic (Brand)	Route and Dosage	Preg Cat	Interaction	t1/2	PB	Action Onset	Action Peak	Action Duration
Burns								
Nitrofurazone (Furacin)	0.2% cream, ointment, sol *Adjunctive therapy:* Apply directly or to dressing daily for 2°–3° burns; q4–5d for 2° burns with scant exudate	C	None significant reported	NA	NA	UK	UK	UK
Mafenide acetate (Sulfamylon)	See Prototype Drug Chart							
Silver nitrate	0.5 sol; 10%, 25% sticks; apply only to affected area 2–3×/wk for 2–3 wk	C	Do not use with alkalis, phosphates, thimerosal, benzalkonium chloride, halogenated acids	NA	NA	UK	UK	UK
Silver sulfadiazine (Silvadene, SSD)	1% cream, apply daily–b.i.d. in 1/16-inch layer	C	May inactivate topical proteolytic enzymes concurrently applied	NA	NA	On contact	UK	As long as applied
Acne Vulgaris: Keratolytics								
Benzoyl peroxide (Bezac, Persa-Gel, Desquam)	2.5–10% daily–q.i.d. (cream, gel, or lotion)	C	*Increase* skin irritation with tretinoin	NA	NA	UK	UK	UK
Salicylic acid (Sebulex, Freezone)	*Antiacne/antiseborrheic:* 2–10% cream, gel shampoo Use as directed	C	Avoid use by aspirin-sensitive clients	NA	NA	UK	UK	UK
Resorcinol and sulfur	2% resorcinol + 5% sulfur 2% resorcin + 8% sulfur Use as directed	C	Avoid use with other acne preparations	NA	NA	UK	UK	UK

Acne Vulgaris:
Antibiotics

Tetracycline, erythromycin, clindamycin (Cleocin), and meclocycline (Meclan)	As directed	B, C	None significant known	NA	NA	UK	UK	UK
Tretinoin (Retin-A)	Cream: 0.05–0.1% Gel: 0.025–0.1% Liquid: 0.05% daily h.s.	B	*Increase* irritation with salicylic acid, resorcinol, benzoyl peroxide	NA	NA	UK	UK	UK
Isotretinoin (Accutane)	A: PO: 0.5–2 mg/kg/d in 2 divided doses for 15 wk	X	*Increase* toxicity with vitamin A	10–20 h	99%	0.5–1 h	3.2 h	4–6 h
Psoriasis Methoxsalen (8-MOP [hard gelatin], Oxsoralen-Ultra [soft gelatin]) Do *not* interchange hard and soft capsules	A&C >12 y: PO: 10–20 mg 2 h before exposure to therapeutic ultraviolet rays; dose may be increased according to weight Topical application before exposure to ultraviolet rays	C	*Increase* effects with phenothiazines, tetracyclines, thiazides, sulfonamides	2 h	80–90%	≥10 wk	UK	8 h Sensitive to sun
Etretinate (Tegison)	A: PO: 0.5–0.75 mg/kg/d in divided doses; max: 1.5 mg/kg/d	X	*Increase* absorption with milk, high-fat foods; alcohol increases triglycerides	4–8 d	99%	Weeks	Weeks–months	Years

KEY: For complete abbreviation key, see inside front cover.

URINARY AGENTS

Urinary Anti-infectives

Urinary Analgesic

Urinary Stimulant

Urinary Antispasmodics

Prototype: Urinary Anti-infectives

Nitrofurantoin

Nitrofurantoin
  (Furalan, Furan, Macrodantin),
  ♣ Apo-Nitrofurantoin
Antibacterial
Pregnancy Category: B
Drug Forms:
Cap 25, 50, 100 mg
Tab 50, 100 mg
Susp 25 mg/5 mL

Dosage

Initial/Recurrent UTI:
A: PO: 50–100 mg q.i.d. with meals and h.s.; take with food
C: PO: >1 mo: 5–7 mg/kg in 4 divided doses
Long-term Prophylaxis:
A: PO: 50–100 mg h.s.
C: PO: 1–2 mg/kg in 1–2 divided doses

Contraindications

Hypersensitivity, moderate to severe renal impairment, oliguria, anuria, Cl_{cr} <40 mL/min, infants <1 mo, term pregnancy, lactation with infant suspected of having G-6-PD deficiency

Caution: Vitamin B deficiency, electrolyte imbalance, diabetes mellitus

Drug-Lab-Food Interactions

Decrease effect with probenecid; *decrease* absorption with antacids

Pharmacokinetics

Absorption: Well absorbed from GI tract; enhanced with food
Distribution: PB: 40%; Crosses placenta and enters breast milk
Metabolism: t 1/2: 20–60 min
Excretion: In urine; small amounts in bile

Pharmacodynamics

PO: Onset: UK
  Peak: 30 min
  Duration: UK

Therapeutic Effects/Uses: To treat acute and chronic UTIs.
Mode of Action: Inhibits bacterial enzymes and metabolism.

Side Effects

Anorexia, nausea, vomiting, rust/brown discoloration of urine, diarrhea, rash, pruritus, dizziness, headache, drowsiness

Adverse Reactions

Superinfection, peripheral neuropathy, hemolytic anemia, agranulocytosis
Life-threatening: Anaphylaxis, hepatotoxicity, Stevens-Johnson syndrome

KEY: For complete abbreviation key, see inside front cover.

■ NURSING PROCESS: Nitrofurantoin

ASSESSMENT

- Obtain a history from the client of clinical problems with urinary tract infection (UTI) or other urinary tract disorders.

Urinary Anti-infectives

- Assess the client for signs and symptoms of UTI, such as pain or burning sensation on urination and frequency and urgency of urination.
- Assess CBC on clients with long-term therapy; monitor regularly.
- Assess renal and hepatic function.
- Assess urine pH; 5.5 is desired; however, alkalinization of the urine is *not* recommended.

POTENTIAL NURSING DIAGNOSES
Altered comfort; pain
High risk for infection

PLANNING
- Client will be free of signs and symptoms of UTI within 10 d.

NURSING INTERVENTIONS
- Monitor the client's output. Careful attention to output is required when administering urinary anti-infectives to clients with anuria and oliguria. Report promptly any decrease in urine output.
- Before the start of drug therapy, obtain a urine culture to determine the organism causing the UTI.
- Observe the client for side effects of and adverse reactions to urinary anti-infectives drugs. Peripheral neuropathy (tingling, numbness of extremities) may result from renal insufficiency (inability to excrete drug) or long-term use of nitrofurantoin. Peripheral neuropathy may be irreversible.
- Dilute IV nitrofurantoin in 500 mL of IV solution before administering; constitute in sterile water without preservative.

CLIENT TEACHING

General
- Advise the client not to crush tablets or open capsules.
- Advise the client to rinse mouth thoroughly after taking oral nitrofurantoin. This drug can stain the teeth.
- Avoid antacids because they interfere with drug absorption.
- Instruct client to shake suspension well before taking and protect it from freezing.
- Advise client not to drive a motor vehicle or operate dangerous machinery; drug may cause drowsiness.
- Advise the diabetic client not to use Clinitest to test for glucose because a false-positive may result.

Diet
- Instruct the client to increase fluids and take the drug with food; this minimizes GI upset.

Side Effects
- Advise the client that urine may turn a harmless brown.
- Advise the client to report any signs of secondary fungal or bacterial infection (superinfection), such as stomatitis or anogenital discharge or itching.

EVALUATION
- Evaluate the effectiveness of the urinary anti-infectives in alleviating the UTI. Client is free of side effects and adverse reactions to drug.

Urinary Anti-infectives

Generic (Brand)	Route and Dosage	Preg Cat	Interaction	t1/2	PB	Onset	Peak	Duration
Miscellaneous Anti-infectives								
Methenamine mandelate (Mandelamine)	A: PO: 1 g q.i.d. p.c. C 6–12 y: PO: 0.5 g q.i.d. p.c. C <6 y: PO: 50 mg/kg in 4 divided doses p.c.	C	May precipitate sulfonamides; may *decrease effectiveness* with urinary alkalinizers	3–6 h	UK	UK	2 h	UK
Trimethoprim (Proloprim, Trimpex)	A: PO: 100 mg q12h or 200 mg q24h; if Cl$_{cr}$ is 15–30 mL/min: 50 mg q12h; if Cl$_{cr}$ <15 mL/min: do not use	C	*Increase* risk of bone marrow depression with antineoplastics/radiation; *increase* elimination with rifampin Lab: *Increase* BUN, AST, ALT	8–11 h	44%	Rap'd	1–4 h	UK
Quinolones (Fluoroquinolones)								
Cinoxacin (Cinobac)	A: PO: 1 g/d in 2–4 doses for 1–2 wk; *Renal dysfunction:* Initially: 500 mg; if Cl$_{cr}$ is >80 mL/min: 500 mg b.i.d.; 80–50 mL/min: 250 mg t.i.d.; 50–20 mL/min: 250 mg b.i.d.; <20 mL/min: 250 mg q.d. Not recommended for infants or prepubertal children	C, although *not* recommended during pregnancy	*Decrease* effect with probenecid Lab: *Increase* AST, ALT, BUN, alkaline phosphatase, creatinine	1.5 h Impaired renal function: ≥10 h	60–80%	UK	2–4 h	6–8 h

Ciprofloxacin (Cipro)	A: PO: mild to moderate: 250 mg q12h; severe/complicated: PO: 500–750 mg q12h IV: 200–400 mg q12h (over 60 min) *Renal dysfunction:* If Cl$_{cr}$ >50 mL/min (PO), >30 mL/min (IV): Usual dose 30–50 mL/min: 250–500 mg q12h 5–29 mL/min: 250–500 mg q18h (PO); 200–400 mg q18–24h (IV) *Hemo or peritoneal dialysis:* 250–500 mg q24h after dialysis	C	*Increase* levels of drug with probenecid, theophylline *Decrease* absorption with antacids *Lab: Increase* AST, ALT, BUN	4–6 h	20–40%	PO: Rapid IV: Rapid	1–2 h End of infusion	6–8 h UK
Methenamine hippurate (Hiprex, Urex)	A: PO: 1 g b.i.d. C 6–12 y: 0.5–1 g b.i.d.	C	*Decrease* effect with urinary alkalinizers May precipitate sulfonamides	3–6 h	UK	UK	2 h	UK
Nalidixic acid (NegGram)	A: PO: 1 g q.i.d. for 1–2 wk; 1 g b.i.d. for long-term use C: PO: 55 mg/kg/d in 4 divided doses for 1–2 wk; 33 mg/kg/d for long-term use C <3 mo: *Do not use*	B	*Increase* effects of oral contraceptives *Decrease* effects of antacids	1–2 h Elderly: 12 h	93%	1–2 h	1–2 h	UK

continued

Urinary Anti-infectives —Continued

Generic (Brand)	Route and Dosage	Preg Cat	Interaction	t1/2	PB	Onset	Peak	Duration
Norfloxacin (Noroxin)	A: PO: 400 mg b.i.d. for 1–2 wk on empty stomach *Uncomplicated cystitis due to E. coli, K. pneumoniae, P. mirabilis:* 400 mg b.i.d. ×3 d *Uncomplicated due to any other organism:* 400 mg b.i.d. ×7–10 d *Complicated:* 400 mg b.i.d. ×10–21 d *Renal impairment (Cl$_{cr}$ <30 mL/min):* 400 mg q.d.	C	*Increase* toxicity with theophylline *Decrease* absorption with sucralfate iron, antacids; decrease effects with nitrofurantoin *Lab: Increase* AST, ALT, BUN, alkaline phosphatase	3–4 h	10–15%	UK	1–3 h	UK
Other								
Aztreonam (Azactam)	A: IM/IV: 500 mg–1 g q8–12h C: 30 mg/kg q6–8h	B	*Increase* effects with furosemide, probenecid, cefoxitin, imipenem	1.5–2 h	56–60%	IM: Rapid IV: Fapid	1 h End of infusion	UK UK
Co-trimoxazole or sulfamethoxazole-trimethoprim (Bactrim, Septra)	See Anti-infectives: Sulfonamides							

Enoxacin (Penetrex)	*Uncomplicated UTI:* A: PO: 200 mg q12h for 7 d *Complicated or severe UTI:* A: PO: 400 mg q12h for 14 d If Cl$_{cr}$ <30 mL/min, reduce dose by 50%	C Pregnant, X	*Increase* effects of oral anticoagulants, probenecid, theophylline *Decrease* absorption with antacids, oral iron, sucralfate	3–6 h	UK	UK	1–2 h	UK
Imipenem/cilastatin sodium (Primaxin)	A: IV: 250 mg – 1 g q6–8h; max: 4 g/d or 50 mg/kg/d, whichever is the lesser amount IM: 500—750 mg q12h C: Safety and efficacy not established Dosing adjustment with renal impairment	C	*Increase* risk of seizures with ganciclovir *Decrease* effects with cephalosporins, penicillins, aztreonam	1 h	I: 20% C: 40%	UK UK	I: 2 h C: 1 h	UK UK
Methylene blue (Urolene Blue)	*Cystitis, urethritis:* A: PO: 60–125 mg b.i.d./t.i.d. p.c. with glass of water	C	None significant	UK	UK	UK	UK	UK
Nitrofurantoin (Furalan, Macrodantin)	See Prototype Drug Chart							
Polymyxin B SO$_4$ (Aerosporin)	A&C: IV: 15,000–25,000 U/kg/d in divided doses q12h	B	*Increase* nephrotoxicity with vancomycin, aminoglycosides, amphotericin B; *increase* effects of neuromuscular blockers	4–6 h	UK	Rapid	2 h	UK

KEY: For complete abbreviation key, see inside front cover.

Prototype: Urinary Analgesic

Phenazopyridine

Phenazopyridine
  (Pyridium, Urodine), 🍁 Phenazo, Pyronium
Antipruritic, local anesthetic
Pregnancy Category: B
Drug Forms:
Tab 100, 200 mg

Dosage

A: PO: 100–200 mg t.i.d. p.c. × 2 d
C: PO: 12 mg/kg in 3 divided doses

Contraindications

Severe liver or renal disease, pregnancy or breast feeding

Drug-Lab-Food Interactions

May interfere with urinalysis color reactions, urinary glucose, ketones, proteins, steroids

Pharmacokinetics

Absorption: PO: Well absorbed
Distribution: PB: UK
Metabolism: t 1/2: UK
Excretion: In urine

Pharmacodynamics

PO: Onset: UK
  Peak: 5–6 h
  Duration: 6–8 h

Therapeutic Effects/Uses: For relief of UTI from infection, trauma, and surgery (use with urinary antiseptic).

Mode of Action: Produces analgesia/local anesthesia on urinary tract mucosa. Exact mechanism of action unknown.

Side Effects

Anorexia, nausea, vomiting, diarrhea, heartburn, red-orange discoloration of urine, rash, pruritus, headache, vertigo

Adverse Reactions

Life-threatening: Agranulocytosis, hepatotoxicity, nephrotoxicity, thrombocytopenia, leukopenia, hemolytic anemia

KEY: For complete abbreviation key, see inside front cover.

Urinary Analgesic

■ NURSING PROCESS: Urinary Analgesic: Phenazopyridine (Pyridium)

ASSESSMENT
- Obtain a history from the client of clinical problems with the urinary tract.
- Obtain a drug history; report probable drug-drug interactions.
- Assess the client for signs and symptoms of UTI such as pain or burning sensation on urination and frequency and urgency of urination.
- Assess hepatic function studies, especially serum liver enzymes, with long-term therapy.

POTENTIAL NURSING DIAGNOSES
Altered patterns of urinary elimination
Pain due to renal problem

PLANNING
- The client will be free of urinary tract pain within 3 d.

NURSING INTERVENTIONS
- Administer drug with food or milk to decrease gastric distress. Chewable tablets should be chewed.
- Observe client for side effects of and adverse reaction to urinary analgesic.

CLIENT TEACHING
General
- Instruct client to take medication exactly as ordered; not to exceed recommended dosage. Advise to take with food or milk.

Side Effects
- Advise the client that urine will be harmless reddish orange but does permanently stain clothing and contact lens.
- Instruct client to report signs of hepatotoxicity, including yellowing of skin or sclera, clay-colored stools, abdominal pain, diarrhea, dark urine, or fever.

EVALUATION
- Evaluate the effectiveness of the drug in alleviating the urinary tract pain. Client is free of side effects and adverse reactions to drug.

Urinary Analgesic, Stimulant, and Antispasmodics

Generic (Brand)	Route and Dosage	Preg Cat	Interaction	t 1/2	PB	Onset	Peak	Duration
Urinary Analgesic Phenazopyridine HCl (Pyridium, Urodine)	See Prototype Drug Chart							
Urinary Stimulant Bethanechol Cl (Urecholine, Duvoid, Urabeth)	A: PO: 10–50 mg t.i.d./q.i.d. 1 h a.c. or 2 h p.c. SC: 2.5–10 mg t.i.d./q.i.d. PRN C: PO: 0.6 mg/kg/d in 3–4 divided doses	C	*Increased* effect with cholinergics *Decrease* action with procainamide, quinidine Hypotension with ganglionic blockers	UK	UK	PO: 30–90 min SC: 5–15 min	1 h 15–30 min	6 h 2 h

Urinary Antispasmodics

Dimethyl sulfoxide (DMSO, Rimso-50)	*Bladder instillation:* 50 mL of 50% sol retained for 15 min; repeat q2wk until relief	C	None significant	UK	UK	UK	4–8 h	UK
Flavoxate HCl (Urispas)	A: PO: 100–200 mg t.i.d. or q.i.d.	B	None significant	UK	UK	1 h	UK	UK
Oxybutynin Cl (Ditropan)	A: PO: 5 mg b.i.d. or t.i.d. C >5 y: PO: 5 mg b.i.d. C 1–5 y: PO: 0.2 mg/kg b.i.d./q.i.d.	B	None significant	1–3 h	UK	PO: 30–60 min	3–6 h	7–10 h
Propantheline bromide (Pro-Banthīne)	A: PO: 15 mg t.i.d. 30 min a.c and 30 mg h.s.; max: 120 mg/d Elderly: 7.5 mg t.i.d./q.i.d. C: PO: 2–3 mg/kg/d in divided doses	C	*Increase* chance of extrapyramidal reactions *Decrease* absorption of ketoconazole	1.5 h	UK	30–45 min	2–6 h	6 h

KEY: For complete abbreviation key, see inside front cover.

ANTINEOPLASTIC AGENTS

Alkylating Drugs

Antimetabolites

Miscellaneous Anticancer Drugs

Biologic Response Modifiers:
  Epoetin Alfa
  Granulocyte Colony–Stimulating Factor
  Granulocyte Macrophage Colony–Stimulating Factor
  Interferons

Prototype: Antineoplastic: Alkylating Drug

Cyclophosphamide

Cyclophosphamide
 (Cytoxan), ❦ Procytox
Alkylating drug
Pregnancy Category: D
Drug Forms:
Inj IV (powder) 100, 200, 500 mg;
 1, 2 g
Tab 25, 50 mg

Dosage

A: PO: Initially: 1–5 mg/kg over
 2–5 d; maint: 1–5 mg/kg/d
IV: Initially: 40–50 mg/kg in
 divided doses over 2–5 d
C: PO/IV: Initially: 2–8 mg/kg in
 divided doses for 6 d; maint:
 2–5 mg/kg
If bone marrow depression occurs,
 dosage adjustment is necessary

Contraindications

Hypersensitivity, severe bone
 marrow depression
Caution: Pregnancy, liver or kidney
 disease

Drug-Lab-Food Interactions

Thiazides, anticoagulants, digoxin,
 phenobarbital, rifampin

Lab: Uric acid, Pap test, purified
 protein derivative (PPD), mumps,
 candida

Pharmacokinetics

Absorption: PO: Well absorbed
Distribution: PB: 50%
Metabolism: t 1/2: 3–12 h
Excretion: 25–40% in urine
 unchanged; 5–20% in feces

Pharmacodynamics

Effects on blood count:
PO/IV: Onset: 7 d
 Peak: 10–14 d
 Duration: 21 d

Therapeutic Effects/Uses: To treat breast, lung, ovarian cancers; Hodgkin's disease; leukemias; and lymphomas; an immunosuppressant agent.

Mode of Action: Inhibition of protein synthesis through interference with DNA replication by alkylation of DNA.

Side Effects

Nausea, vomiting, diarrhea, weight
 loss, hematuria, alopecia,
 impotence, sterility, ovarian
 fibrosis, headache, dizziness,
 dermatitis

Adverse Reactions

Hemorrhagic cystitis, secondary
 neoplasm
Life-threatening: Leukopenia,
 thrombocytopenia, cardiotoxicity
 (very high doses), hepatotoxicity
 (long term)

KEY: For complete abbreviation key, see inside front cover.

■ NURSING PROCESS: Cyclophosphamide

ASSESSMENT

- Assess CBC, differential, and platelet count weekly. Withhold drug if platelets < 75,000 cells/mm^3 or WBC < 4,000 cells/mm^3; notify health care provider.
- Assess results of pulmonary function tests, chest x-rays, and renal and liver function studies during therapy.
- Assess temperature; fever may be early sign of infection.

Antineoplastic: Alkylating Drugs

POTENTIAL NURSING DIAGNOSES
High risk for infection
Body image disturbance

PLANNING
- Client will experience improved blood count status indicative of improvement/remission of the specific cancer growth.

NURSING INTERVENTIONS
- Hydrate client with IV and/or oral fluids before chemotherapy starts.
- Administer antacid before oral drug.
- Administer antiemetic 30–60 min before giving drug.
- Monitor IV site frequently for irritation and phlebitis.
- Increase fluids to 2–3 L/d to reduce risk of hemorrhagic cystitis, urate deposition, or calculus formation.
- Store drug in airtight container at room temperature.

CLIENT TEACHING

General
- Advise women who are contemplating pregnancy while taking antineoplastics to first seek medical advice. There may be teratogenic effects to the fetus. Pregnancy should be avoided for 3–4 mo after completing antineoplastic therapy in most situations. Some sources recommend that both men and women avoid conception for 2 y after completing treatment.
- Remind client to consult health care provider before administration of any vaccination.

Diet
- Advise client to follow diet low in purines (organ meats, beans, and peas) to alkalize urine.
- Advise client to avoid citric acid.

Side Effects
- Instruct client about good oral hygiene with soft toothbrush for stomatitis; do not use toothbrush when platelet count is <50,000 cells/mm^3.
- Emphasize with client protective isolation precautions. Advise the client not to visit anyone with any type of respiratory infection. A decreased WBC puts the client at high risk for acquiring an infection.
- Instruct client to report promptly signs of infection (fever, sore throat), bleeding (bleeding gums, petechiae, bruises, hematuria, blood in the stool), and anemia (increased fatigue, dyspnea, orthostatic hypotension).
- Remind client that she may experience amenorrhea, menstrual irregularities, or sterility and that he may experience impotence.
- Advise client of possible hair loss; recommend consideration of wig or hairpiece.

EVALUATION
- Client will be free of cancer as indicated by improved blood counts and free of side effects of drug.

Antineoplastics: Alkylating Drugs

Generic (Brand)	Route and Dosage*	Preg Cat	Interaction	t 1/2	PB	Onset	Peak	Duration
Nitrogen Mustards								
Chlorambucil (Leukeran)	A: PO: 0.1–0.2 mg/kg/d	D	*Increase* toxicity with other antineoplastics and radiation	1.5 h	99%	WBC: 7–14 d	7–14 d	12–28 d
Cyclophosphamide (Cytoxan)	See Prototype Drug Chart							
Estramustine phosphate sodium (Emcyt)	*Palliation prostate cancer:* A: PO: 10–16 mg/kg/d in 3–4 divided doses for 28–90 d; determine if response occurred	C	*Increase* toxicity with hepatotoxic agents, smoking, virus vaccines, *Decrease* absorption with calcium-rich foods and supplements, milk	20 h	UK	Effect tumor spread 30–90 d	2–3 h	Hemotologic effects: 6 wk
Ifosfamide (Ifex)	A: IV: 1.2 g/m²/d for 5 d q21–28 d	D	*Increase* toxicity with antineoplastics, radiation, live virus vaccines, phenobarbital, phenytoin, chloral hydrate	High dose: 12–15 h Low dose: 4–8 h	UK	UK	UK	UK
Mechlorethamine HCl (Mustargen)	A: IV: 0.4 mg/kg/dose or 6–10 mg/m² as single dose or in divided doses	D	Similar to chlorambucil	<1 min	UK	24 h	7–12 d	10–21 d
Melphalan (Alkeran)	A: PO: 6 mg/d	D	Similar to chlorambucil	1.5 h	≤30%	4–5 d	2–3 wk	5–6 wk
Uracil mustard	*Palliation chronic lymphocytic leukemia, non-Hodgkin's lymphoma:* A: PO: 0.15 mg/kg/wk for 4 wk C: PO: 0.30 mg/kg/wk for 4 wk	X	*Increase* toxicity with antineoplastics, radiation, virus vaccines; dosage adjustment of antigout agents *Lab: Increase* blood uric acid	UK	UK	UK	UK	2 h

Nitrosoureas							
Carmustine (BiCNU)	A: IV: 75–100 mg/m² /d for 2 d or 200 mg/m² q6 wk as single dose or divided into 2 doses on successive days; next course is dependent on blood count	D	*Increase* bone marrow toxicity with cimetidine; hepatic dysfunction with etoposide	15–30 min	UK	Platelets: 3–5 d	3–5 wk	6 wk
Lomustine (CeeNu)	A: PO: 130 mg/m² as single dose	D	Similar to ifosfamide	1–2 d	50%	UK	4–6 wk	1–2 wk
Streptozocin (Zanosar)	A: IV: 500 mg/m²/d for 5 or 1 g/m²/wk	C	*Increase* toxicity with antineoplastics and radiation	35–45 min	UK	Tumor response: 15 d	35 d	UK
Alkyl Sulfonates							
Busulfan (Myleran)	A: PO: 4–8 mg/d; max: 12 mg/d C: PO: 0.06–0.12 mg/kg/d	D	Similar to streptozocin	UK	UK	10–14 d	3 wk	<1 mo
Alkylating-like							
Altretamine (Hexalen)	A: PO: 4–12 mg/kg/d in 3–4 divided doses for 28–90 d *Solid tumors:* C: IV: 560 mg/m² once q4 wk	D	*Increase* toxicity with MAOIs; may cause severe orthostatic hypotension *Decrease* effect with phenobarbital	13 h	6%	Effect on blood counts: UK	3–4 wk	6 wk
Carboplatin (Paraplatin)	A: IV: 360 mg/m² q4 wk	D	*Increase* bone marrow depression with nephrotoxic agents	2–6 h	0%	UK	21 d	28 d
Cisplatin (Platinol)	A: IV: 20 mg/m²/d for 5 d; then 50–70 mg/m² q3 wk or 100 mg/m² q4 wk	D	Similar to streptozocin *Increase* toxicity with aminoglycosides, loop diuretics, phenytoin	alpha: 30–60 min beta: 60–72 h	>90%	Effect on blood count: UK	18–21 d	35–40 d

continued

Antineoplastics: Alkylating Drugs—Continued

Generic (Brand)	Route and Dosage*	Preg Cat	Interaction	t1/2	PB	Onset	Peak	Duration
Dacarbazine (DTIC)	*Hodgkin's disease:* A: IV: 150 mg/m² daily for 5 d; repeat course q28d or 375 mg/m² on day 1 of combination therapy: repeat course q15d *Metastatic malignant melanoma:* A: IV: 2–4.5 mg/kg daily for 10 d; repeat q28d	C	*Increase* toxicity with antineoplastics, radiation, virus vaccines, phenobarbital, phenytoin	5 h	5–10%	WBC: 18–24 d Platelets: UK	21–25 d 14–16 d	3–5 d 3–5 d
Pipobroman (Vercyte)	*Chronic myelocytic leukemia:* A: PO: Initially: 1.5–2.5 mg/kg/d for 30 d; maint: 10–175 mg/d	D	Similar to cyclophosphamide	UK	UK	UK	UK	UK
Procarbazine HCl (Matulane)	A: PO: Initially: 2–4 mg/kg/d in divided doses for 7 d; then increase to 4–6 mg/kg/d until desired leukocyte/platelet counts	D	*Increase* CNS depression with phenothiazines, narcotics, barbiturates; *increase* toxicity with tyramine-rich foods	10 min	UK	14 d	2–8 wk	4–6 wk
Triethylenethio-phosphoramide (thiotepa)	A: IV: 0.2 mg/kg/d for 4–5 d; then 0.3–0.4 mg/kg at 2- to 4- wk intervals	D	Similar to carboplatin; *increase* toxicity with antineoplastics or radiation, neuromuscular blocking agents (e.g., succinylcholine)	1.5–2 h	UK	10 d	14 d	20 d

KEY: For complete abbreviation key, see inside front cover.
*Refer to individual protocol.

NOTES:

Prototype: Antineoplastic: Antimetabolite

Fluorouracil

Fluorouracil
  (Adrucil, 5-FU)
Pregnancy Category: D
Antimetabolite
Drug Forms:
Inj IV 50 mg/mL
Sol/cream 2%, 5%

Dosage

A: IV: 12 mg/kg/d ×4d; max: 800 mg/d; repeat with 6 mg/kg on day 6, 8, 10, and 12
Maint: 10–15 mg/kg/wk as single dose; max: 1 g/wk
Topical: 1–2% sol/cream b.i.d. to head/neck lesions; 5% to other body areas
Refer to specific protocol.

Contraindications

Hypersensitivity, pregnancy, severe infection, myelosuppression, marginal nutritional status

Drug-Lab-Food Interactions

Bone marrow depressants, live virus vaccines, cimetidine, calcium
Lab: Liver function studies, albumin, AST, ALT

Pharmacokinetics

Absorption: Topical: 5–10%
Distribution: PB: UK
Metabolism: t 1/2: 10–20 min
Excretion: In urine and expired carbon dioxide

Pharmacodynamics

Effects on blood count:
IV: Onset: 1–9 d
  Peak: 9–21 d
  Duration: 30 d
Topical: Onset: 2–3 d
  Peak: 2–6 wk
  Duration: 4–8 wk

Therapeutic Effects/Uses: To treat cancer of breast, cervix, colon, liver, ovary, pancreas, stomach, and rectum. In combination with levamisole after surgical resection in clients with Duke's Stage C colon cancer.

Mode of Action: Prevention of thymidine production, thereby inhibiting DNA and RNA synthesis. Not phase specific.

Side Effects

Nausea, vomiting, diarrhea, stomatitis, alopecia, rash

Adverse Reactions

Anemia
Life-threatening: Thrombocytopenia, myelosuppression, hemorrhage, renal failure

---

KEY: For complete abbreviation key, see inside front cover.

■ NURSING PROCESS: Fluorouracil

ASSESSMENT

- Assess the client's VS and use for future comparison.
- Assess CBC and platelet count weekly. Notify health care provider and withhold drug if WBC is <3,500/mm^3 or platelet count is <100,000 cells/mm^3.
- Assess renal function studies before and during drug therapy.
- Assess temperature every 4–6 h; fever may be early sign of infection.

Antineoplastic: Antimetabolite

POTENTIAL NURSING DIAGNOSES
High risk for infection
Altered nutrition; less than body requirements
Body image disturbance

PLANNING
- Client will have blood tests with values in the desired range.
- Client will be free of adverse reactions to drug therapy.
- Client's neoplasm will decrease in size.

NURSING INTERVENTIONS
- Handle drug with care during preparation; avoid direct skin contact with anticancer drugs. (Follow protocols.) Solution is colorless to light yellow.
- Administer IV dose over 1–2 min. Apply firm prolonged pressure to injection site if thrombocytopenia is present.
- Monitor IV site frequently. Extravasation produces severe pain. If this occurs, apply ice pack and notify health care provider.
- Administer antiemetic 30–60 min before drug to prevent vomiting.
- Offer the client food and fluids that may decrease nausea, such as cola, crackers, or ginger ale.
- Administer antibiotics prophylactically for infection, analgesics for pain, and antispasmodics for diarrhea, as ordered.
- Maintain strict medical asepsis.
- Encourage fluid intake of 2–3 L/d, unless contraindicated, to prevent dehydration.
- Support good oral hygiene; brush teeth with soft toothbrush and use waxed dental floss.
- Monitor fluid intake and output and nutritional intake. GI effects are common on the fourth day of treatment.

CLIENT TEACHING
General
- Emphasize protective precautions, as necessary.
- Teach the client to examine mouth daily and report stomatitis (ulceration in mouth). Good oral hygiene several times a day is essential. If stomatitis occurs, rinse mouth with baking soda or saline. Do not use a toothbrush when the platelet count is <50,000/mm^3.
- Advise women who are contemplating pregnancy while taking antineoplastics to first seek medical advice. Teratogenic effects to the fetus can occur from antineoplastics. Pregnancy should be avoided for 3–4 mo after completing antineoplastic therapy in most situations. Some sources recommend that both men and women avoid conception for 2 y after completion of treatment.
- Advise the client not to visit anyone with any type of respiratory infection. A decreased WBC count puts the client at high risk for acquiring an infection.

Side Effects
- Advise the client to promptly report signs of bleeding, anemia, and infection to the health care provider.

EVALUATION
- The client's tumor size will be decreased.
- Evaluate the client's blood tests results.
- Evaluate for side effects or adverse reactions to drug therapy.

Antineoplastics: Antimetabolites

Generic (Brand)	Route and Dosage*	Preg Cat	Interaction	t 1/2	PB	Onset	Peak	Duration
Folic Acid Antagonist Methotrexate (Mexate)	A: PO/IM: 3.3 mg/m²/d for 4–6 wk; maint: 30 mg/m²/wk in divided doses (2 wk)	D	*Increase* toxicity of drug with NSAIDs, 5-FU, sulfonamides, live virus vaccines	8–16 h	50%	5–7 d	7–14 d	21 d
Pyrimidine Analogs Cytarabine HCl (Cytosar-U, ara-C)	A: IV: 100–200 mg/m²/d or 3 mg/kg/d as continuous 12- or 24-h infusion	D	*Decrease* absorption of po digoxin	1–3 h	15%	24 h	7–10 d	12 d
Floxuridine (FUDR)	A: Intra-arterial: 0.1–0.6 mg/kg/d for 14 d IV: 0.5–1 mg/kg/d for 7–15 d	D	*Increase* bone marrow depression with radiation or antineoplastics	20 h	UK	1–10 d	10–21 d	30 d
5-Fluorouracil (Adrucil, 5-FU)	See Prototype Drug Chart							
Purine Analogs Cladribine (Leustatin)	*Hairy cell leukemia:* A: IV: 0.09 mg/kg/d for 7 d	D	*Increase* bone marrow depression with radiation or other antineoplastics	5.5 h	20%	UK	UK	UK

Fludarabine (Fludara)	A: IV: 25 mg/m² over 30 min daily for 5 consecutive d; repeat course q28d C: IV: 10 mg/m² bolus over 15 min; then 30 mg/m²/d over 5 d	D	*Increase* toxicity with myelosuppressive agents *Lab: Increase* uric acid	9 h	UK	Blood counts: UK	14–16 d	UK
6-Mercaptopurine (Purinethol)	A&C: PO: 1.5–2.5 mg/kg/d; max: 5 mg/kg/d	D	Allopurinol *increases* bone marrow depression	A: 45 min C: 20 min	19%	5–10 d	14 d	21 d
Thioguanine	A&C: PO: 2–3 mg/kg/d	D	Similar to 5-fluorouracil hepatotoxicity with busulfan	2–11 h	UK	Effect on blood count 7–10 d	14 d	21 d
Ribonucleotide Reductase Inhibitor								
Hydroxyurea (Hydrea)	*Palliation:* A: PO: 20–30 mg/kg/d or 80 mg/kg q3d C: No dosage regimens established	D	*Increase* toxicity with cytotoxic agents, radiation; *increase* neurotoxicity with fluorouracil *Lab: Increase* uric acid, BUN, creatinine	3–4 h	UK	Blood counts: 7 d	10 d	21 d

KEY: For complete abbreviation key, see inside front cover.
*Refer to specific protocol.

Antineoplastic: Miscellaneous

Generic (Brand)	Route and Dosage*	Preg Cat	Interaction	t1/2	PB	Onset	Peak	Duration
Antimicrotubule Paclitaxel (Taxol)	*Ovarian cancer:* A: IV: 135 mg/m² for 24 h q3wk; shortened infusions approved for refractory breast cancer	D	*Decrease* metabolism of drug with ketoconazole	5–17 h	80–90%	UK	11 d	3 wk
Enzyme Inhibitor Pentostatin (Nipent)	*Hairy cell leukemia:* A: IV: 4 mg/m² every other wk	D	*Increase* toxicity with fludarabine	6 h	UK	5 mo	UK	>8 mo
Podophyllotoxin Derivative Etoposide (VePesid, VP-16)	A: IV: 50–100 mg/m²/d on days 1–5, q3–4 wk for 3–4 treatment therapy	D	*Increase* bone marrow depression with radiation or other antineoplastics, sodium salicylate, tolbutamide	4–11 h	97%	7 d	14 d	20 d
Antitumor Antibiotics Bleomycin SO₄ (Blenoxane)	A: IM/IV: 10–20 units/m²/wk or 0.25–0.5 units/kg/wk Reduce dose with renal impairment	D	*Increase* toxicity with other antineoplastics *Decrease* effects of digoxin, phenytoin	2 h	1%	7 d	14 d	21 d

Dactinomycin (Actinomycin D, Cosmegen)	A: IV: 500 µg/m²/d for 5 d; may repeat at 2–4 wk; max: 15 µg/kg/d or 400–600 µg/m²/d for 5 d C: IV: 10–15 µg/kg/d for 5 d	C	*Increase* effects of radiation therapy; may interfere with antibacterial drug levels; not compatible with heparin	36 h	80–90%	7 d	14 d	21 d
Daunorubicin HCl (Cerubidine)	*Leukemias:* A: IV: 30–60 mg/m²/d for 2–3 d; repeat dose in 3–4 wk Reduce dose with hepatic/renal impairment	D	Severe local tissue necrosis with extravasation	19 h	80%	7–10 d	14 d	21 d
Doxorubicin (Adriamycin)	*Solid tumors:* A: IV: 60–75 mg/m²; repeat q21d Reduce dose with hepatic impairment	D	*Increase* effects of barbiturates, digoxin, radiation	3–22 h	80–90%	7–10 d	14 d	21 d
Idarubicin (Idamycin)	*Solid tumor:* A: IV: 12–15 mg/m²/d for 3 d *Leukemia:* A: IV: 10–12 mg/m²/d for 3–4 d; repeat q3 wk Reduce dose with hepatic/renal impairment	D	Similar to daunorubicin	22 h	97%	UK	UK	UK
Mitomycin (Mutamycin)	A: IV: 10–20 mg/m² q6–8wk Reduce dose with renal impairment	D	*Increase* toxicity with vinca alkaloids; cardiotoxicity with doxorubicin	17 min	UK	4 wk	8 wk	10 wk

continued

Antineoplastic: Miscellaneous—Continued

Generic (Brand)	Route and Dosage*	Preg Cat	Interaction	t1/2	PB	Onset	Peak	Duration
Plicamycin (Mithracin, mithramycin)	*Testicular tumor:* A: IV: 25–30 µg/kg/d for 8–10 d *Hypercalcemia:* A: IV: 15–25 µg/kg/d for 3–4 d Reduce dose with renal impairment	X	*Increase* toxicity with aspirin, glucogen, calcium products, etidronate	2–8 h	0%	Calcium decrease 24 h	48–72 h	5–15 d
Vinca Alkaloids								
Teniposide (Vumon, VM 26)	*Leukemia:* A: IV over ≥30–60 min: 165 mg/m² and cytarabine 300 mg/m² 2×/wk for 8–9 doses	D	*Increase* toxicity with tolbutamide, sodium salicylate, sulfamethizole	10–38 h	>99%	UK	16–18 d	15 d
Vinblastine SO₄ (Velban)	A: IV: 0.1 mg/kg/wk or 3.7 mg/m²/wk or q2 wk; max: 0.5 mg/kg or 18.5 mg/m²	D	*Increase* toxicity with mitomycin-C *Decrease* effect of phenytoin	1–25 h	75%	5 d	10 d	14 d
Vincristine SO₄ (Oncovin)	A: IV: 0.4–1.4 mg/m²/wk; max: 2 mg/dose C: IV: 1–2 mg/m²/wk; max: 2 mg/dose	D	*Increase* toxicity with digoxin, L-asparaginase *Decrease* effect of phenytoin	19–155 h	75%	7 d	14 d	21 d
Vinorelbine (Navelbine)	A: IV: 30 mg/m² weekly; combination with cisplatin 120 mg/m²	D	Similar to vinblastine	UK	UK	UK	UK	UK

Androgens						
Testolactone (Teslac) CSS III	*Palliation breast carcinoma:* A: PO (females): 250 mg q.i.d.	C	*Increase* effects of oral anticoagulants *Lab: Increase* calcium, creatinine	UK	Clinical effects: 6–12 wk	UK	UK
Trimetrexate glucuronate (Neutrexin)	A: IV: 45 mg/m^2/d by infusion over 1–1.5 h with Leucovorin 20 mg/m^2 q6h (PO or IV) Administer drugs through separate lines	D	Alter P-450 enzyme system with erythromycin, rifampin, ketoconazole	13.6 h	86–94%	UK	UK
Other						
Aldesleukin (Interleukin-2)	*Metastatic renal cell carcinoma:* A: IV: 0.037 mg/kg/d q8h (15 min IV); treatment: two 5-d cycles with 9-d rest between; max: 28 doses per course	C	*Increase* toxicity with analgesics, antiemetics, sedatives, narcotics, tranquilizers; nephrotoxic, hepatotoxic, and myelotoxic agents; *increase* hypotension with beta blockers	20–120 mo	UK	UK	UK
Aminoglutethimide (Cytadren)	A: PO: 250 mg q6h; increased q2 wk to 2 g/d in 2–3 divided doses to decrease nausea and vomiting	D	*Decrease* effect of digitoxin, warfarin, dexamethasone, theophylline *Lab: Decrease* thyroxine	7–15 h	20–25%	*Adrenal* suppression: 3–5 d	UK	36–72 h; 1 yr after long term

continued

Antineoplastic: Miscellaneous — Continued

Generic (Brand)	Route and Dosage*	Preg Cat	Interaction	t1/2	PB	Onset	Peak	Duration
Other								
Asparaginase (Elspar)	Start with intradermal skin test A: IV/IM: 6,000 units/m^2 q.o.d. for 3–4 wk or 1,000–20,000 units/m^2 for 10–20 d	C	*Increase* toxicity with vincristine, prednisone *Decrease* effect of methotrexate	8–30 h	30%	Immediate	IM: 14–24 h IV: UK	24–36 d
Flutamide (Eulexin)	A: PO: 250 mg q8h *Note:* Give simultaneously with LHRH analog therapy, e.g., leuprolide acetate, 7.5 mg IM/mo	D	None known	5–6 h Elderly: 10 h	94–96%	UK	UK	UK
Goserelin acetate (Zoladex)	*Palliation prostate cancer:* A: SC: 3.6 mg into upper abdomen q28d	X	None known *Lab: Decrease* after initial increase in follicle-stimulating hormone, testosterone, luteinizing hormone	4–6 h	UK	UK	12–15 d	29 d
Mitotane (Lysodren)	*Palliation adrenal cortical carcinoma:* A: PO: 1–6 g/d in divided doses; increasing to 8–10 g/d in 3–4 divided doses; max: 18 g/d	C	*Increase* toxicity with CNS depressants *Decrease* effect of phenytoin, warfarin, barbiturates	20–160 d	UK	*Decrease* adrenocortical function 2–3 d	TR: 6 wk	UK

Megestrol acetate	*Breast cancer:* A: PO: 40 mg q.i.d. *Endometrial cancer:* A: PO: 40–320 mg/d in divided doses; max: 800 mg/d	X	*Decrease* effects with bromocriptine *Lab:* Altered liver function and thyroid tests	15–20 h	UK	response 6–8 wk	1–3 h	3–12 mo
Mitoxantrone (Novantrone)	*Solid tumor:* A: IV: 12 mg/m^2/d × 3; dilute with 50 mL NSS or D$_5$W over 15–30 min	D	Similar to daunorubicin	6 d	78%	7–10 d	14 d	21 d
Polyestradiol PO$_4$ (Estradurin)	*Palliation prostate cancer:* A: IM: 40 mg q2–4 wk; max: 80 mg	X	Unknown	UK	UK	UK	UK	UK
Progesterone (Gesterol 50, Progestaject, Progestasert)	*Endometrial and breast carcinoma:* A: IM: 5–10 mg/d for 6–8 d	X	*Lab:* Altered thyroid, liver function, coagulation tests	5 min	UK	UK	UK	24 h
Tamoxifen citrate (Nolvadex)	*Palliation/adjunctive treatment of breast carcinoma:* A: PO: 10–20 mg b.i.d	D	*Increase* toxicity of warfarin, cyclosporine, allopurinol *Lab: Increase* T$_4$	7 d	UK	Tumor response: 4–10 wk	3–6 mo	UK

KEY: For complete abbreviation key, see inside front cover.
*Refer to specific protocol.

Prototype: Biologic Response Modifiers

Epoetin Alfa (Erythropoietin [EPO])

Epoetin Alfa (Erythropoietin [EPO]) (Epogen, Procrit)
Pregnancy Category: C
Drug Forms:
Inj 2,000, 4,000 U/mL

Dosage

A: 50–100 U/kg 3 × wk
  IV: Dialysis clients
IV/SC: Nondialysis, CRF clients
IV/SC: 100 U/kg 3 × wk for 8 wk in AZT-treated HIV-infected clients
Initial dose to those with EPO levels <500 mU/mL and receiving <4,200 mg of AZT/wk. Clients with EPO level >500 mU/mL are unlikely to respond to EPO therapy.

Contraindications

Uncontrolled hypertension, hypersensitivity to mammalian cell–derived products or human albumin
Caution: Pregnancy, lactation, porphyria; safety in children not known

Drug-Lab-Food Interactions

Drug: None known
Lab: Increase hematocrit, decreased plasma volume

Pharmacokinetics

Absorption: UK
Distribution: PB: UK
Metabolism: t 1/2: 4–13 h in clients with CRF; 20% less in those with normal renal function
Excretion: In urine

Pharmacodynamics

IV: Onset: 1 wk to 10 d
  Peak: 2–4 wk
  Duration: UK
SC: Onset: 1 wk to 10 d
  Peak: 5–24 h
  Duration: UK

Therapeutic Effects/Uses: To treat anemia secondary to CRF or AZT (zidovudine) treatment of HIV infections. Use in clients with anemia secondary to cancer or its treatment is under investigation.

Mode of Action: Increased production of RBCs, triggered by hypoxia or anemia.

Side Effects

Sense of well-being, hypertension, arthralgias, nausea, edema, fatigue, injection site reaction, rash, diarrhea, shortness of breath

Adverse Reactions

Seizures, hyperkalemia
Life-threatening: Cerebral vascular accident, MI

KEY: For complete abbreviation key, see inside front cover.

Biologic Response Modifiers

■ NURSING PROCESS: Biologic Response Modifiers

ASSESSMENT
- Obtain baseline information about the client's physical status, including height, weight, VS, laboratory values (CBC, uric acid, electrolytes, BUN, creatinine, and liver function tests), cardiopulmonary assessment, intake and output, skin assessment, daily activities status (ability to perform activities of daily living, sleep-rest cycle), nutritional status, presence or absence of underlying symptoms of disease, and the use of current or past medication and treatment.
- Assess CBC and platelet count (with **filgrastim** and **sargramostim**) before therapy and biweekly throughout therapy to avoid leukocytosis. Assess renal and hepatic function tests in clients with dysfunction (liver enzymes, BUN, serum creatinine). With **erythropoietin**, assess blood pressure before start and especially early in therapy. Most clients will need supplemental iron. Desired levels are >100 ng/mL for serum ferritin and >20% for serum iron transferrin saturation.
- Obtain baseline data regarding the client's psychosocial status, including educational level, ability and desire to learn, support systems, past coping strategies, presence or absence of emotional difficulties, and self-care abilities.
- Assess the client for signs and symptoms of biologic response modifiers (BRM), such as fatigue, chills, diarrhea, and weakness. With **filgrastim**, be alert to changes in clients with preexisting cardiac conditions.
- Assess the client's and family's ability to administer subcutaneous BRM.
- Determine the client's and family's understanding of BRM and related side effects.

POTENTIAL NURSING DIAGNOSES
Altered nutrition; less than body requirements
High risk for infection
High risk for fluid volume deficit
Altered oral mucous membrane
Fatigue
Body image disturbance
Anxiety
Fear
High risk for caregiver role strain

PLANNING
- Client and family will verbalize an understanding of the importance of reporting BRM-related side effects.
- Client and family will demonstrate correct and safe BRM administration.
- Client and family will identify strategies to deal with BRM-related side effects.
- Client will remain free of infection (**filgrastim** and **sargramostim**).

NURSING INTERVENTIONS
- Monitor the client's temperature at the onset of chills.
- Administer prescribed meperidine 25–50 mg IV to decrease rigors.
- Premedicate the client with acetaminophen to reduce chills and fever and with diphenhydramine to reduce nausea.
- Cover the client with blankets to promote warmth during chills.

(text continues on page 235)

Prototype: Granulocyte Colony–Stimulating Factor

Filgrastim

Filgrastim
  (Neupogen)
Granulocyte colony–stimulating factor (G-CSF)
Pregnancy Category: C
Drug Forms:
Vial 300 µg/mL; 480 µg/1.6 mL

Dosage

A: IV inf/SC: 5 µg/kg/d
C: 5–10 µg/kg/d
Refer to specific protocols.

Contraindications

Hypersensitivity to *E. coli*–derived proteins; 24 h before or after cytotoxic chemotherapy
Caution: Pregnancy, lactation; safety in children not known

Drug-Lab-Food Interactions

Drug: None known
Lab: Increase lactic acid, LDH, alkaline phosphatase; transient *increase* in neutrophils

Pharmacokinetics

Absorption: SC: Well absorbed
Distribution: PB: UK
Metabolism: t 1/2: 2–3.5 h
Excretion: Probably in urine

Pharmacodynamics

IV/SC: Onset: 24 h
  Peak: 3–5 d
  Duration: 4–7 d

Therapeutic Effects/Uses: To decrease incidence of infection in clients receiving myelosuppressive chemotherapeutic agents; adjunct to chemotherapy for both solid tumor and hematologic malignancies.

Mode of Action: Increases production of neutrophils and enhances their phagocytosis.

Side Effects

Nausea, vomiting, skeletal pain, alopecia, diarrhea, fever, skin rash, anorexia, headache, cough, chest pain, sore throat, constipation

Adverse Reactions

Neutropenia, dyspnea, splenomegaly, psoriasis, hematuria
Life-threatening: Thrombocytopenia, myocardial infarction, adult respiratory distress syndrome in clients with sepsis

KEY: For complete abbreviation key, see inside front cover.
See page 233 for Nursing Process.

Biologic Response Modifiers *(Continued)*

- Encourage the client to rest when tired and to notify health care provider if profound fatigue or anorexia occurs.
- Encourage the client to drink at least 2 L of fluid a day to promote excretion of cellular breakdown products.
- Administer antiemetic as necessary. Premedicate the client with antiemetic and administer antiemetic around the clock for 24 h after BRM administration to further delay nausea or vomiting.
- Consult the dietitian, social worker, and physical or occupational therapist as necessary.
- Provide the client and family the opportunity to discuss the effect of BRM therapy on the quality of life.
- Refer the client and family to a financial counselor if reimbursement of BRM therapy is problematic.
- Administer BRM at bedtime to decrease the consequences of fatigue.
- Continue with the same brand of BRM, and notify the health care provider if you are considering changing the brand.
- Remember, with **sargramostim**, use only one dose per vial; be alert for expiration date. Avoid shaking vial. Reconstituted solutions are clear; use within 6 h and discard unused portion. Recall that albumin may be added, depending on drug concentration, to prevent adsorption of drug to components of the drug delivery system.
- Remember, with **filgrastim**, drug vials are for one-time use; any vial left at room temperature for more than 6 h should be discarded. Drug vials are preservative free. Store in refrigerator at 2–8°C. Avoid shaking vials.

CLIENT AND FAMILY TEACHING

General

- Explain to the client and family the rationale for BRM therapy.
- Explain the frequency and rationale for studies and procedures during BRM therapy.
- Inform the client and family that most BRM side effects disappear within 72–96 h after discontinuation of therapy.
- Instruct clients of childbearing age to use contraceptives during BRM therapy and for 2 y after completion of therapy.
- Provide the client with information regarding the effect on sexuality of BRM-related fatigue.

Side Effects

- Advise the client to report episodes of difficulty in concentration, confusion, or somnolence.
- Report weight loss.
- Report dyspnea, palpitations, and signs of infection or bleeding.

Skill

- Demonstrate correct drug administration techniques.
- Provide the client and family with written or video instructions regarding BRM self-administration.

EVALUATION

- Evaluate the client's and family's education strategies by asking them to discuss the potential effect of BRM therapy on the quality of life.
- Evaluate the client's and family's BRM self-administration technique.

(text continues on page 237)

Prototype: Granulocyte Macrophage Colony–Stimulating Factor

Sargramostim

Sargramostim
  (Leukine, Prokine)
Granulocyte macrophage colony–stimulating factor (GM-CSF)
Pregnancy Category: C
Drug Forms:
Powder in vial 250 µg (Leukine only) and 500 µg of sargramostim

Dosage

A: IV: 250 µg/m^2/d as a 2-h inf for 21 d after autologous BMT; a maximum tolerated dose has not been determined
Some protocols use SC administration.

Contraindications

Within 24 h of chemotherapy administration or within 12 h after last dose of radiation therapy, excessive leukemia myeloid blast cells in bone marrow, hypersensitivity to GM-CSF, yeast-derived products

Caution: Pregnancy, lactation, congestive heart failure; safety in children not established; not FDA approved for children

Drug-Lab-Food Interactions

Lithium and steroids may *increase* effect
Lab: Increase in WBC and platelet counts

Pharmacokinetics

Absorption: IV: Essentially complete
Distribution: PB: UK
Metabolism: t 1/2: 2 h
Excretion: Probably in urine

Pharmacodynamics

IV: Onset: 7–14 d
  Peak: UK
  Duration: Baseline WBC by 1 wk after administration

Therapeutic Effects/Uses: To accelerate growth and development of bone marrow and circulating blood cell activity in autologous BMT.

Mode of Action: Increased production and functional activity of eosinophils, macrophages, monocytes, and neutrophils.

Side Effects

Generally well tolerated; diarrhea, fatigue, chills, weakness, local irritation at injection site, peripheral edema, rash

Adverse Reactions

Pleural/pericardial effusion, rigors, GI hemorrhage, dyspnea

KEY: For complete abbreviation key, see inside front cover.
See pages 233, 235, 237 for Nursing Process.

Biologic Response Modifiers *(Continued)*

- Evaluate periodically the client's and family's management of BRM-related side effects.
- There will be a decreased incidence of infection in clients after autologous bone marrow transplant.

Biologic Response Modifiers: Interferons

Generic (Brand)	Route and Dosage	Preg Cat	Interaction	t1/2	PB	Onset	Peak	Duration
Interferon alfa-2a (Roferon-A)	*Hairy cell leukemia, condylomata acuminata:* A: SC/IM: 3 million IU daily for 16–24 wk	C	*Increase* toxicity with vinblastine; *increase* effects of theophylline, cimetidine	IM/IV: 2–3 h SC: 3 h	UK	Myelosuppression: 7–10 d	6–8 h Nadir: 14 d	Recovery: 21 d
Interferon alfa-2b (Intron-A)	A: SC: 2 million IU/m² 3×wk *Kaposi sarcoma:* A: IM/SC/IV: Initially: 36 million IU daily for 10–12 wk; maint: 36 million IU 3×wk	C	*Increase* toxicity effect with vinblastine, cimetidine	IM/IV: 2 h SC: 3 h	UK	7–10 d	14 d	21 d
Interferon gamma-1b (Actimmune)	*Body surface area >0.5 m²:* A: SC: 50 µg/m² 3×wk *Body surface area <0.5 m²:* A&C <1 y: SC: 1.5 µg/kg 3×wk	C	*Increase* bone marrow depression with other antineoplastics or radiation therapy	SC: 6 h IM: 3 h IV: 0.5 h	UK	UK	SC: 7 h IM: 4 h IV: UK	UK
Interferon alfa-N3 (Alferon N)	*Condylomata acuminata:* A: Inject into wart: 250,000 U (0.05 mL) twice weekly; max: 8 wk Do *not* repeat for >3 mo after end of therapy	C	Similar to interferon alfa-2a	UK	UK	7–10 d	14 d	21 d
Interferon beta-1b (Betaseron)	*Reduce number of clinical exacerbations of multiple sclerosis:* A >18 y: SC: 8 million U q.o.d. C: Not recommended	C	Not fully evaluated; none significant known	0.5–4 h	UK	UK	1–8 h	UK

KEY: *For complete abbreviation key, see inside front cover.*

238

NOTES:

RESPIRATORY AGENTS

Antihistamines

Antitussives and Expectorants

Decongestants

Bronchodilators:
 Adrenergic
 Methylxanthine

Prototype: Antihistamine

Diphenhydramine HCl

Diphenhydramine HCl (Benadryl), ✽ Allerdryl
Antihistamine
Pregnancy Category: B
Drug Forms:
Cap 25, 50 mg
Tab 50 mg
Elix, syrup 12.5 mg/5 mL
Inj 10, 50 mg/mL
Topical 1–2% cream, lotion

Dosage

A: PO: 25–50 mg q6–8h
A: IM/IV: 10–50 mg as single dose q4–6h; max: 400 mg/d
C: PO/IM/IV 5 mg/kg/d in 4 divided doses; max: 300 mg/d

Contraindications

Acute asthmatic attack, severe liver disease, lower respiratory disease, neonate, MAOIs

Caution: Narrow-angle glaucoma, benign prostatic hypertrophy, pregnancy, newborn or premature infant, breast feeding; urinary retention

Drug-Lab-Food Interactions

Increase CNS depression with alcohol, narcotics, hypnotics, barbiturates; avoid use of MAOIs

Pharmacokinetics

Absorption: PO: Well absorbed
Distribution: PB: 82%
Metabolism: t 1/2: 2–7 h
Excretion: In urine as metabolites

Pharmacodynamics

PO: Onset: 15–45 min
    Peak: 1–4 h
    Duration: 4–8 h
IM: Onset: 15–30 min
    Peak: 1–4 h
    Duration: 4–7 h
IV: Onset: Immediate
    Peak: 0.5–1 h
    Duration: 4–7 h

Therapeutic Effects/Uses: To treat allergic rhinitis, itching; to prevent motion sickness; sleep aid; antitussive.

Mode of Action: Blocks histamine, thereby decreasing allergic response. Affects respiratory system, blood vessels, and GI system.

Side Effects

Drowsiness, dizziness, fatigue, nausea, vomiting, urinary retention, constipation, blurred vision, dry mouth and throat, reduced secretions, hypotension, epigastric distress, vision and hearing disturbances; excitation in children, photosensitivity

Adverse Reactions

Life-threatening: Agranulocytosis, hemolytic anemia, thrombocytopenia

KEY: For complete abbreviation key, see inside front cover.

Antihistamine

■ NURSING PROCESS: Diphenhydramine

ASSESSMENT
- Obtain baseline VS.
- Obtain drug history; report if drug-drug interaction is probable.
- Assess for signs and symptoms of urinary dysfunction, including retention, dysuria, and frequency.
- Assess CBC during drug therapy.
- Assess cardiac and respiratory status.
- If allergic reaction, obtain history of environmental exposures, drugs, recent foods, and stress.

POTENTIAL NURSING DIAGNOSES
Fluid volume deficit, potential
Sleep pattern disturbance

PLANNING
- Client will have improvement of histamine-associated (allergy) effects.
- Client will have improved sleep, if used as a sleep aid.

NURSING INTERVENTIONS
- Give with food to decrease gastric distress.
- Administer IM in large muscle. Avoid SC injection.

CLIENT TEACHING
General
- Instruct client to avoid driving a motor vehicle and other dangerous activities if drowsiness occurs or until stabilized on drug.
- Avoid alcohol and other CNS depressants.
- Instruct client to take drug as prescribed. Notify health care provider if confusion or hypotension occurs.
- For prophylaxis of motion sickness, take drug 30 min before offending event and then before meals and h.s. during the event.

EVALUATION
- Evaluate effectiveness of drug in relieving allergic symptoms or as a sleep aid.

Antihistamines for Treatment of Allergic Rhinitis

Generic (Brand)	Route and Dosage	Preg Cat	Interaction	t1/2	PB	Onset	Peak	Duration
Antihistamines Chlorpheniramine maleate (Chlor-Trimeton, Kloromin, Phenetron, Telachlor, Teldrin)	A: PO: 2–4 mg q4–6h; max: 24 mg/24 h SR: 8–12 mg q8–12 h C: 6–12 y: PO: 2 mg q4–6h	C	*Increase* effect of drug with MAOIs; *increase* CNS depression *Decrease* effects of oral anticoagulants, heparin	20–24 h	72%	20–60 min	6 h	8–12 h
Diphenhydramine (Benadryl)	See Prototype Drug Chart							
Phenothiazines (Antihistamine Action) Promethazine HCl (Phenergan, Prometh, Prorex, V-Gan)	A: PO/IM: 12.5–25 mg q4–6h PRN a.c. & h.s.; max: 150 mg/d C: PO/IM: 0.5 mg/kg q4–6h; max: 18.75 mg/d Tab & suppository not recommended <2 y	C	Similar to chlorpheniramine	UK	UK	PO: 20 min IM: 3–5 min	UK	4–6 h
Trimeprazine tartrate (Temaril)	A: PO: 2.5 mg q.i.d. C 3–12 y: PO: 2.5 mg t.i.d. C 0.5–3 y: 1.25 mg t.i.d. SR: A: PO: 5 mg q12h C >6 y: PO: 5 mg/d	C	Similar to chlorpheniramine	5 h	UK	15–60 min	4 h	UK
Piperazine Derivative Hydroxyzine HCl (Atarax, Vistaril)	A: PO: 25–100 mg t.i.d./q.i.d. C >6 y: 50–100 mg/d in divided doses For pruritus: C: <6 y: PO: 50 mg/d in divided doses	C	*Increase* CNS depression with alcohol, analgesics, barbiturates, narcotics *Decrease* effects of epinephrine	3 h	UK	15–30 min	<2 h	4–6 h

Butyrophenone Derivative Terfenadine (Seldane)	A: PO: 60 mg b.i.d. C >6 y: PO: 30 mg b.i.d. C 3–6 y: PO: 15 mg b.i.d.	C	Cardiotoxic effects with erythromycin, ketoconazole *Increase* effects with pseudoephedrine	20 h	97%	60–90 min	3–4 h	>12 h
Ethanolamine Derivative Carbinoxamine and pseudoephedrine (Carbiset, Carbodec, Rondec)	A: PO: 5 mL q.i.d. or 1 tab q.i.d. C <18 mo: PO: 0.25–1 mL q.i.d. C 1.5–6 y: PO: 2.5 mL t.i.d./q.i.d. C >6 y: PO: 5 mL b.i.d./q.i.d.	C	*Increase* toxicity of tricyclic antidepressants, barbiturates; *increase* toxicity with MAOIs	10–20 h	UK	15–60 min	UK	UK
Clemastine fumarate (Tavist)	A: PO: 1.34–2.68 mg b.i.d./t.i.d.; max: 8 mg/d C <12 y: PO: 0.67–1.34 mg b.i.d.	C	*Increase* toxicity with tricyclic antidepressants, CNS depressants, MAOIs, phenothiazines	UK	UK	15–60 min	5–7 h	12 h
Ethylenediamine Derivative Tripelennamine HCl (Pelamine)	A: PO: 25–50 mg q4–6h or SR: 100 mg q8–12h; max: 600 mg/d C: PO: 5 mg/kg/d in 4–6 divided doses; max: 300 mg/d (Note: 5 mL of tripelennamine citrate elix = 25 mg HCl)	B	*Increase* CNS depression with alcohol, CNS depressants; *increase* anticholinergic effects with MAOIs	UK	UK	15–30 min	2–3 h	4–6 h SR: 8 h

continued

Antihistamines for Treatment of Allergic Rhinitis —Continued

Generic (Brand)	Route and Dosage	Preg Cat	Interaction	t1/2	PB	Onset	Peak	Duration
Piperidine Derivatives								
Azatadine maleate (Optimine)	A: PO: 1–2 mg b.i.d./t.i.d. C <12 y: PO: not recommended	B	Increase effect/toxicity with CNS depressants, alcohol, tricyclic antidepressants, procarbazine	9–12 h	UK	Rapid	4 h	12 h
Cyproheptadine HCl (Periactin)	A: PO: 4–20 mg/d divided q8h; max: 0.5 mg/kg/d C >6 y: PO: 4 mg q8–12h; max: 16 mg/d C 2–6 y: PO: 2 mg q8–12h	B	Increase toxicity with MAOIs	UK	UK	15–60 min	UK	8 h
Propylamine Derivatives								
Brompheniramine maleate (Bromphen, Dimetane, Histaject, Nasahist B, Oraminic II)	A: PO: 4 mg q4–6h or SR: 8 mg q8–12h; max: 12 mg/d IM/IV/SC: 10 mg q6–12h; max: 40 mg/d C 6–12 y: PO: 2 mg q4–6h; max: 12–16 mg/d	C	Increase toxicity with MAOIs, tricyclic antidepressants, CNS depressants	25–36 h	UK	15–60 min	3–9 h	4–25 h
Dexchlorpheniramine maleate (Dexchlor, Poladex, Polaramine)	A: PO: 2 mg q4–6h or SR: 4–6 mg q8–10h or h.s. C >6 y: PO: 1 mg q4–6h or SR: 4 mg h.s.	B	Increase toxicity with MAOIs, tricyclic antidepressants, CNS depressants, phenothiazines, guanabenz	UK	UK	15–60 min	3 h	3–6 h
Triprolidine and pseudoephedrine (Actifed)	A: PO: 1 tab q4–6h; max: 4 tab/d C >6 y: PO: 1/2 tab q6–8h; max: 2 tab/d	B	Increase effect with MAOIs	3 h	UK	15–60 min	2–3 h	4–8 h

Triprolidine HCl (Alleract, Myidyl)	A: PO: 2.5 mg q6–8h; max: 10 mg/d C 6–12 y: PO: 1.25 mg q6–8h; max: 5 mg/d C 2–5 y: PO: 0.6 mg t.i.d./q.i.d.; max: 2.5 mg/d C 4 mo–2 y: PO: 0.3 mg t.i.d./q.i.d.; max: 1.25 mg/d	C	*Increase* effects with alcohol, CNS depressants, MAOIs	3 h	UK	Rapid	3–5 h	8 h
Other								
Cromolyn sodium (Intal)	*Prophylaxis bronchial asthma:* A&C >5 y: Inhal: 2 metered sprays or PO: 20 mg ≦1 h before exercise *Allergic rhinitis:* A&C >5 y: 1 spray per nostril t.i.d./q.i.d.; max: 6 per day	B	None significant reported *Not* used for acute asthma attacks	90 min	UK	PO: UK Inhal: <1 wk Spray: <1 wk	2–3 wk 2–4 wk 2–4 wk	UK UK UK
Miscellaneous								
Astemizole (Hismanal)	A: PO: 30 mg on day 1; 20 mg on day 2, 10 mg on day 3 and thereafter; take on empty stomach C 6–12 y: PO: 5 mg/d C <6 y: PO: 0.2 mg/kg/d	C	*Increase* toxicity with CNS depressants; cardiotoxicity with triazole antifungals, macrolide antibiotics	2.5 d	96%	2–3 d	9–12 d	Weeks after discontinuing drug
Cetirizine (Zyrtec)	A: PO: 5–10 mg/d	C	Caution with erythromycin, ketoconazole	8 h	93%	15–60 min	1 h	UK
Loratadine (Claritin)	A: PO: 10 mg daily	B	None significant reported	8–11 h	UK	30 min	4–6 h	>24 h
Methdilazine HCl (Tacaryl)	A: PO: 8 mg b.i.d./q.i.d. C >3 y: PO: 4 mg b.i.d./q.i.d.	C	*Increase* toxicity with CNS depressants	UK	UK	15–60 min	UK	6–12 h

KEY: For complete abbreviation key, see inside front cover.

Prototype: Antitussive

Dextromethorphan hydrobromide

Dextromethorphan hydrobromide (Robitussin DM, Romilar, Sucrets Cough Control, PediCare 1, ✥ Balminil DM, Nao-DM, Ornex DM Benylin DM, and others)
OTC preparation
Antitussive

Pregnancy Category: C

Drug Forms:
Lozenge 5 mg
Sol 5, 7.5, 10, 15 mg/mL

Dosage

A: PO: 10–30 mg q4–8h; max: 120 mg/24 h
C 6–12 y: PO: 5–10 mg q4–6h; max: 60 mg/d
C 2–5 y: PO: 2.5–7.5 mg q4–8h; max: 30 mg/d

Sustained Action Liquid (Delsym):
A: 60 mg q12h
C 6–12 y: 30 mg q12h
C 2–5 y: 15 mg q12h

Contraindications

Chronic obstructive pulmonary disease, chronic productive cough, hypersensitivity, clients taking MAOIs

Drug-Lab-Food Interactions

Increase effect/toxicity with MAOIs, narcotics, sedative-hypnotics, barbiturates, antidepressants, alcohol

Pharmacokinetics

Absorption: PO: Rapidly absorbed
Distribution: PB: UK
Metabolism: t 1/2: UK
Excretion: In urine, UK

Pharmacodynamics

PO: Onset: 15–30 min
Peak: UK
Duration: 3–6 h

Therapeutic Effects/Uses: To provide temporary suppression of a nonproductive cough; to reduce viscosity of tenacious secretions.

Mode of Action: Inhibition of the cough center in the medulla.

Side Effects

Nausea, dizziness, drowsiness, sedation

Adverse Reactions

Hallucinations at high doses
Life-threatening: None known

KEY: For complete abbreviation key, see inside front cover.

Antitussive

■ NURSING PROCESS: Dextromethorphan Hydrobromide

ASSESSMENT
- Obtain baseline VS. Report and document abnormal findings.

POTENTIAL NURSING DIAGNOSES
Fatigue
Sleep deprivation due to chronic coughing
High risk for infection

PLANNING
- Client will be free of nonproductive cough. A secondary bacterial infection does not occur.

NURSING INTERVENTIONS
- Monitor VS.
- Observe color of secretions.

CLIENT TEACHING
General
- Instruct the client to maintain adequate fluid intake.
- Advise the client not to drive a motor vehicle or operate dangerous machinery.
- Instruct the client to avoid environmental pollutants, smoking, and dust.
- Instruct the client to get adequate rest.
- Instruct the client not to take a cold remedy near or at bedtime. Insomnia may occur if it contains a decongestant.
- Instruct the client/parents to have child perform three effective coughs before bedtime to promote uninterrupted sleep.
- Instruct the client/parents to keep the drug stored out of reach of small children; request child safety caps.
- Advise the client to contact the health care provider if cough persists for >1 wk or is combined with chest pain, fever, or headache.

Skill
- Instruct the client to cough effectively, to take deep breaths before coughing and be in the upright position.

EVALUATION
- Evaluate the effectiveness of the drug therapy. Determine that the client is free of a nonproductive cough, has adequate fluid intake and rest, and is afebrile.

Antitussives and Expectorants

Generic (Brand)	Route and Dosage	Preg Cat	Interaction	t 1/2	PB	Onset	Peak	Duration
Narcotic Antitussives								
Codeine CSS II	A: PO: 10–20 mg q4–6h; max: 120 mg/d C 6–12 y: 5–10 mg q4–6h; max: 60 mg/d C 2–5 y: 2.5–4.5 mg q4–6h; max: 18 mg/d	C	*Increase* CNS depression with alcohol, narcotics, barbiturates, antipsychotics, muscle relaxants	2–4 h	7%	15–30 min	1–2 h	4–6 h
Guaifenesin and codeine (Cheracol, Robitussin A-C) CSS V	*Temporary relief of cough due to minor irritation:* A: PO: 5–10 mL q6–8h C 2–6 y: PO: 2.5 mL q6–8h PRN	C	*Increase* sedation with CNS depressants	UK	UK	15–30 min	UK	UK
Hydrocodone bitartrate (Hycodan) CSS III	A: PO: 5–10 mg q4–6h; max: 15 mg/d C: PO: 0.6 mg/kg/d in 3–4 divided doses, not to exceed 10 mg/single dose	C	*Increase* CNS depression with alcohol barbiturates, antipsychotics, general anesthesia, tricyclic antidepressants	3–4 h	UK	30–60 min	UK	3–6 h
Nonnarcotic Antitussives								
Benzonatate (Tessalon)	*Relief of nonproductive cough:* A: PO: 100 mg t.i.d. or q4h; max: 600 mg/d C <10 y: 8 mg/kg/d in 3–6 divided doses	C	*Increase* sedation with CNS depressants	UK	UK	15–30 min	UK	3–8 h

Dextromethorphan hydrobromide (Benylin, Sucrets cough control, and others)	See Prototype Drug Chart					
Diphenhydramine HCl (Benadryl)	See Prototype Drug Chart					
Promethazine with dextromethorphan	A: PO: 5 mL q4–6h; max: 30 mL/d C 6–12 y: PO: 2.5–5 mL q4–6h; max: 20 mL/d C 2–6 y: PO: 1.25–5 mL q4–6h	C	*Increase* sedation with CNS depressants	UK	15–30 min	UK	6–12 h
Expectorants						
Guaifenesin (Robitussin, Anti-Tuss, Glycotuss)	A: PO: 200–400 mg q4h; max: 2.4 g/d C 6–12 y: PO: 100–200 mg q4h; max: 1.2 g/d C 2–5 y: PO: 50–100 mg q4h; max: 600 mg/d	C	None significant	UK	30 min	UK	4–6 h
Iodinated glycerol (Iophen)	A: PO: 60 mg q.i.d.; sol: 20 gtt q.i.d.; elix: 5 mL q.i.d. C: PO: Up to half adult dose according to weight	X	*Increase* toxicity with MAOIs, lithium, CNS depressants	UK	UK	UK	UK
Potassium iodide (SSKI)	A: PO: 300–650 mg t.i.d/q.i.d. C: PO: 60–250 mg q6–8h	D	*Increase* toxicity with lithium	UK	UK	UK	UK
Antitussive/ Expectorant						
Guaifenesin and dextromethorphan (Robitussin-DM)	A: PO: 10 mL q6–8h C 6–12 y: 5 mL q6–8h C 2–5 y: 2.5 mL q6–8h	C	*Increase* toxicity with MAOIs	UK	15–30 min	UK	4–6 h

KEY: For complete abbreviation key, see inside front cover.

Systemic and Nasal Decongestants (Sympathomimetic Amines)

Generic (Brand)	Route and Dosage	Preg Cat	Interaction	t1/2	PB	Onset	Peak	Duration
Ephedrine SO$_4$ (Ectasule, Vatronol)	A: PO: 25–50 mg t.i.d/q.i.d. PRN SC/IM/IV: 10–50 mg; may repeat q10min; max: 150 mg/24 h	C	May cause hypertensive crises with MAOIs *Increase* adverse reactions to theophylline	3–6 h	UK	PO: 15–60 min IM: 30–60 min	UK	3–5 h 12 h
Flunisolide (Nasalide)	A: Initially: 2 sprays q nostril b.i.d.; max: 8 sprays q nostril/d C 6–14 y: Initially: 1 spray q nostril t.i.d.; max: 4 sprays q nostril/d	C	None significant known	1.8 h	UK	UK	UK	UK
Naphazoline HCl (Allerest, Albalon)	A&C >12 y: 2 gtt or 0.05% spray in each nostril; q3–6h ≤ 5 d C 6–12 y: 0.025%, 1–2 gtt q nostril	C	Similar to phenylephrine	UK	UK	<10 min	UK	2–6 h
Oxymetazoline HCl (Afrin)	A&C >6 y: 0.05% 2–3 gtt or 1–2 sprays q nostril b.i.d. C 2–5 y (0.025% gtt only): 2–3 gtt q10–12h	C	Similar to phenylephrine	UK	UK	5–10 min	UK	5–6 h
Phenylephrine HCl (Neo-Synephrine, Sinex)	A: Sol (0.25–1%): 2–3 gtt or 1–2 sprays in each nostril q4h C 6–12 y: Sol (0.25%): 2–3 gtt or sprays in each nostril q4h C 6 mo–5 y: Sol (0.125–0.16%): 1–2 gtt in each nostril q4h	C	*Increase* pressor effects with MAOIs, beta blockers	2.5 h	UK	15–30 min	UK	1–4 h

Phenylpropanolamine HCl (Allerest)	A: PO: 25–50 mg t.i.d./q.i.d.; max: 150 mg/d C 6–12 y: 12.5 mg q4h; max: 75 mg/d C 2–5 y: 6.25 mg q4h; max: 37.5 mg/d	B	Similar to phenylephrine	3–4 h	UK	PO: 15–30 min SR: 60 min	UK	3 h 12–14 h
Pseudoephedrine (Actifed, Novafed, Sudafed, Efidac)	A: PO: 60 mg q4–6h; 120 mg SR q12h; max: 240 mg/d C 6–12 y: 30 mg q4–6h; max: 120 mg/d C 2–5 y: 15 mg q4–6h; max: 60 mg/d	C	Similar to phenylephrine	9–15 h	UK	PO: 15–30 min SR: 60 min	UK	4–6 h 12 h
Tetrahydrozoline HCl (Tyzine)	A&C >6 y: 2–4 gtt (0.1%) or spray q4–6h PRN C 2–6 y: 2–3 gtt (0.05%) q4–6h PRN Direct medical supervision for use >3–4 d	C	Hypotension with reserpine, methyldopa; may cause hypertensive crises with MAOIs	UK	UK	UK	UK	4–8 h
Xylometazoline HCl (Otrivin)	A&C >12 y: 2–3 gtt (0.1%) or spray q8–10h; max: t.i.d. C <12 y: 2–3 gtt (0.5%) or spray q8–10h; max: t.i.d.	C	Similar to tetrahydrozoline	UK	UK	<5–10 min	UK	5–10 h

KEY: For complete abbreviation key, see inside front cover.

Prototype: Bronchodilator: Adrenergic

Metaproterenol SO$_4$

Metaproterenol SO$_4$
(Alupent, Metaprel)
Adrenergic bronchodilator
Pregnancy Category: C
Drug Forms:
Tab 10, 20 mg
Syrup 10 mg/mL
Sol neb 0.6%, 5%
Aerosol 0.65 mg/dose

Dosage

A&C >9 y and >27 kg: PO: 20 mg q6–8h
C: 6–9 y or <27 kg: PO: 10 mg q6–8h
A&C >12 y: MDI: 2–3 inhalations as single dose; wait 2 min before second dose, if necessary; use only q3–4h to maximum of 12 inhalations/d

Contraindications

Hypersensitivity, cardiac dysrhythmias
Caution: Narrow-angle glaucoma, cardiac disease, hypertension

Drug-Lab-Food Interactions

Increase action of both with sympathomimetics
Decrease with beta blockers
Lab: Decreased serum potassium

Pharmacokinetics

Absorption: PO: Well absorbed
Distribution: PB: UK
Metabolism: t 1/2: UK
Excretion: In urine as metabolites

Pharmacodynamics

PO: Onset: 15–30 min
    Peak: 1 h
    Duration: 4 h
MDI: Onset: 1–5 min
    Peak: 1 h
    Duration: 3–4 h

Therapeutic Effects/Uses: To treat bronchospasm, asthma; to promote bronchodilation.

Mode of Action: Relaxation of smooth muscle of bronchi.

Side Effects

Nervousness, tremors, restlessness, insomnia, headache, nausea, vomiting, hyperglycemia, muscle cramping in extremities

Adverse Reactions

Tachycardia, palpitations, hypertension
Life-threatening: Cardiac dysrhythmias, cardiac arrest, paradoxical bronchoconstriction

KEY: For complete abbreviation key, see inside front cover.

■ NURSING PROCESS: Bronchodilator: Adrenergic

ASSESSMENT

- Obtain a medical and drug history; report probable drug-drug interactions.
- Obtain baseline VS for abnormalities and for future comparisons.
- Assess for wheezing, decreased breath sounds, cough, and sputum production.
- Assess sensorium levels for confusion and restlessness due to hypoxia and hypercapnia.
- Assess hydration; diuresis may result in dehydration in the elderly and children.

Bronchodilator: Adrenergic

POTENTIAL NURSING DIAGNOSES
Airway clearance, ineffective
Noncompliance with drug therapy

PLANNING
- Client will be free of wheezing and lung fields will be clear within 2–5 d.
- Client is taking oral drug(s) and using inhaler as prescribed.

NURSING INTERVENTIONS
- Monitor VS. Blood pressure and heart rate can increase greatly. Check for cardiac dysrhythmias.
- Provide adequate hydration. Fluids aid in loosening secretions. Monitor drug therapy. Observe for side effects.
- Administer medication after meals to decrease GI distress.

CLIENT TEACHING
Skill
- Instruct to correctly use the inhaler or nebulizer. Caution against overuse since side effects and tolerance may result.

Correct use of metered-dose inhaler to deliver beta$_2$ agonist:
1. Insert the medication canister into the plastic holder.
2. Shake the inhaler well *before* using. Remove cap from mouthpiece.
3. Breathe *out* through the mouth. Open mouth wide and hold mouthpiece 1–2 inches from mouth. *Do not* put mouthpiece in mouth unless using a spacer. Discuss technique with health provider.
4. With mouth open, take *slow deep* breath through mouth and at same time push the top of the medication canister once.
5. Hold breath for a few seconds; then exhale slowly through pursed lips.
6. If a second dose is required, wait 2 min and repeat the procedure by first shaking the canister in the plastic holder with the cap on.
7. If the inhaler has not been used recently or when it is first used, "test spray" before administering the metered dose.
8. If a glucocorticoid inhalant is to be used with a bronchodilator, wait 5 min before using the inhaler containing the steroid for the bronchodilator effect.

- Teach client to monitor pulse rate.
- Teach client to monitor amount of medication remaining in the canister.
- Advise client not to take OTC preparations without first checking with the health care provider. Some OTC products may have an additive effect.
- Instruct the client to avoid smoking. Smoking increases drug elimination.
- Discuss ways to alleviate anxiety such as relaxation techniques and music.
- Advise client having asthma attacks to wear an ID bracelet or tags.

EVALUATION
- Evaluate the effectiveness of the bronchodilator. The client is breathing without wheezing and without side effects of the drug.

Sympathomimetics: Adrenergic Bronchodilators

Generic (Brand)	Route and Dosage	Preg Cat	Interaction	t1/2	PB	Action Onset	Action Peak	Action Duration
Alpha- and Beta-adrenergic								
Ephedrine SO₄ Alpha₁, beta₁, beta₂	A: PO: 25–50 mg q3–4h; max: 150 mg/d PRN; SC/IM/IV: 12.5–25 mg PRN C >2 y: PO: 2–3 mg/kg/d in 4–6 divided doses C 6–12 y: PO: 6.25–12.5 mg q4h; max: 75 mg	C	*Increase* effects with tricyclic antidepressants, MAOIs, guanethidine, furazolidine	3–6 h	UK	15–60 min	15–60 min	2–4 h
Epinephrine (Adrenalin, Primatene Mist, Bronkaid Mist) Alpha₁, beta₁, beta₂	A: SC: 0.1–0.5 mg or mL of 1:1,000 sol; may repeat q10–15 min C: SC: 0.01 mg or mL of 1:1,000 sol; may repeat q20min–4h Inhal: 1–2 puffs of 1:100 q15 min × 2 dose, then q3h	C	Hypertension with MAOIs; additive effect with other sympathomimetics	UK	UK	Inhal: 1 min SC: 3–5 min	20 min 20 min	1–3 h 20 min
Beta-Adrenergic								
Albuterol (Proventil, Ventolin) Beta₂	A&C >6 y: Inhal: 1–2 puffs q4–6h or 2 puffs 15 min before exercise A: PO: 2–4 mg t.i.d. or q.i.d.; max: 8 mg q.i.d. SR: 4–8 mg q12h C 6–12 y: PO: 2 mg t.i.d./q.i.d. C 2–6 y: PO: 0.1 mg/kg t.i.d.	C	Similar to isoetharine	PO: 4–5 h Inhal: 2–3 h	UK	Inhal: 5–15 min PO: 30 min PO/SR: 30 min	30–90 min 2–3 h 2–3 h	4–6 h 4–6 h 8–12 h

Bitolterol mesylate (Tornalate) Beta$_1$ (some), beta$_2$	A: Inhal: 2 (1–3 min apart) q4–6 h; max: 12 inhal/d	C	Similar to isoproterenol	3 h	UK	3–5 min	0.5–2 h	5–8 h
Isoetharine HCl (Bronkosol) Beta$_1$ (some), beta$_2$	Inhal: 1–2 puffs A: IPPB: 0.5–1.0 mL of 5% sol or 0.5 mL of 1% sol diluted in 3 mL of NSS	C	Similar to isoproterenol; hypertensive crisis with MAOIs	UK	UK	Inhal: Immediate	5–15 min	1–4 h
Isoproterenol sulfate (Isuprel) Beta$_1$ and beta$_2$	A&C: Inhal: 1–2 puffs q4–6h A: SL: 10–20 mg q6–8h C: SL: 5–10 mg q6–8h	C	*Increase* effects with other sympathomimetics *Decrease* action with beta blockers	2–5 min	UK	Inhal: Immediate SL: 15–30 min	UK 1–2 h	1 h 2 h
Metaproterenol sulfate (Alupent, Metaprel) Beta$_1$ (some) and beta$_2$	See Prototype Drug Chart							
Pirbuterol acetate (Maxair) Beta$_2$	*Prevention:* A&C >12 y: Inhal: 2 puffs q4–6h *Bronchospasm:* A&C >12 y: Inhal: 2 puffs (1–3 min apart) followed by 1 puff; max: 12 inhal/d	C	*Increase* toxicity with MAOIs, tricyclic antidepressants, beta agonists	2–3 h	UK	<5 min	2–3 h	5 h
Salmeterol (Serevent) Beta$_2$	*Maintenance bronchodilation:* A&C >12 y: Inhal: 2 puffs q12h *Prevention exercise-induced bronchospasm:* A&C >12 y: Inhal: 2 ≥30–60 min before exercise	C	*Increase* effects of MAOIs, tricyclic antidepressants	5.5 h	94–98%	10–20 min	3 h	12 h

continued

Sympathomimetics: Adrenergic Bronchodilators—Continued

Generic (Brand)	Route and Dosage	Preg Cat	Interaction	t 1/2	PB	Onset	Peak	Duration
Terbutaline SO$_4$ (Brethine, Bricanyl) Beta$_2$	Inhal: 1–2 puffs q4–6h A: PO: 2.5–5 mg t.i.d. SC: 0.25–0.5 mg q8h IV: 10 µg/min, gradually increase; max: 80 µg/min C >12 y: PO: 2.5 mg t.i.d.	B	Similar to isoetharine	3–11 h	25%	Inhal: 5–30 min PO: 30 min SC: 6–15 min	1–2 h 1–2 h 30–60 min	3–6 h 4–8 h 1.5–4 h
Ethylnorepinephrine HCl (Bronkephrine)	Asthma-related bronchospasm: A: SC/IM: 0.5–1 mL C: SC/IM: 0.1–0.5 mL	C	Increased CNS stimulation with CNS stimulants, xanthine derivatives; *increase* risk of dysrhythmias with digitalis, levodopa; *decrease* effects of nitrates	UK	UK	6–12 min	UK	1–2 h
Anticholinergics Ipratropium bromide (Atrovent)	COPD: A: Inhal: 2 t.i.d./q.i.d. >4 h intervals; max: 12 inhal/d nasal spray	B	Avoid use with anticholinergics Forms precipitate with cromolyn sodium	1.5–2 h	UK	5–15 min	1.5–2 h	4–6 h

KEY: For complete abbreviation key, see inside front cover.

NOTES:

Prototype: Bronchodilator: Methylxanthine

Theophylline

Theophylline
(Theo-Dur, Theophyllin KI, Elixophyllin-KI, Somophyllin, Slo-phyllin, Slo-bid, Quibron), ♣ PMS Theophylline, Pulmophylline)
Methylxanthine, respiratory smooth muscle relaxant

Pregnancy Category: C

Drug Forms:
Cap 50, 100, 200, 250 mg
Cap SR 50, 65, 100, 125, 130, 200, 250, 260, 300, 400, 500 mg
Tab 100, 125, 200, 225, 250, 300 mg
Tab SR 100, 200, 250, 300, 400, 500 mg
Susp 300 mg/15 mL
Elix 80, 11.25 mg/15 mL
Liq 80, 150, 160 mg/15 mL
Sol 80 mg/15 mL, with/without alcohol

Dosage

Bronchospasm, Bronchial Asthma:
A: PO: 250–500 mg q8–12h
C: PO: 50–100 mg q6h; max: 12 mg/kg/d
Dosing is highly individualized and is based on therapeutic serum levels between 10 and 20 μg/mL. Monitor levels and client response.

Contraindications

Severe cardiac dysrhythmias, hyperthyroidism, hypersensitivity to xanthines, peptic ulcer disease, uncontrolled seizure disorder

Caution: With young children and elderly

Drug-Lab-Food Interactions

Increase effect with allopurinol, oral contraceptives, ciprofloxacin, cimetidine, ranitidine, calcium blockers, and erythromycin
Decrease effects of neuromuscular blockers, phenytoin, lithium; *decrease* effect with smoking, rifampin, phenobarbital, corticosteroids, and others
Food: Increase metabolism with low-carbohydrate, high-protein diet
Decrease elimination with high-carbohydrate diet (*increase* t 1/2)
Lab: Interaction with laboratory result is not common; however, check with each laboratory

Pharmacokinetics

Absorption: PO: Well absorbed; SR: slowly absorbed
Distribution: PB: Approx 60%
Metabolism: t 1/2: 7–9 h nonsmokers; 4–5 h smokers
Excretion: In urine

Pharmacodynamics

PO: Onset: 30 min
    Peak: 1–2 h
    Duration: 6 h
PO/SR: Onset: 1–3 h
    Peak: 4–8 h
    Duration: 8–24 h
IV: Onset: Rapid
    Peak: UK
    Duration: 6–8 h

Bronchodilator: Methylxanthine

> *Therapeutic Effects/Uses:* To promote bronchodilation; to treat asthma and chronic obstructive pulmonary disease.
>
> *Mode of Action:* Increased cyclic AMP results in bronchodilation, diuresis; cardiac, CNS, and gastric acid stimulation.

Side Effects	Adverse Reactions
Anorexia, nausea, vomiting, restlessness, dizziness, insomnia, flushing, rash, headache	Irritability, tremors, tachycardia, palpitations, urticaria *Life-threatening:* Seizures, cardiac dysrhythmias, convulsions

KEY: For complete abbreviation key, see inside front cover.

■ NURSING PROCESS: Bronchodilator

ASSESSMENT

- Obtain a medical and drug history; report probable drug-drug interaction.
- Obtain baseline VS for identifying abnormalities and for future comparisons.
- Assess for wheezing, decreased breath sounds, cough, and sputum production.
- Assess sensorium levels for confusion and restlessness due to hypoxia and hypercapnia.
- Assess theophylline blood levels. Toxicity occurs at a higher frequency with levels of >20 μg/mL.
- Assess hydration; diuresis may result in dehydration in the elderly and children.

POTENTIAL NURSING DIAGNOSES

Airway clearance, ineffective
Activity intolerance
Knowledge deficit related to OTC drugs

PLANNING

- Client will be free of wheezing or significantly improved and lung fields will be clear within 2–5 d.
- Client is taking oral drug(s) and using inhaler as prescribed.

NURSING INTERVENTIONS

- Monitor VS. Blood pressure may decrease and heart rate may increase. Check for cardiac dysrhythmias.
- Provide adequate hydration. Fluids aid in loosening secretions. Monitor drug therapy. Observe for side effects.
- Check serum and plasma theophylline levels (normal level is 10–20 μg/mL).
- Administer medication at regular intervals around the clock to have a sustained therapeutic level.
- Administer medication after meals to decrease GI distress.
- Do *not* crush enteric-coated or SR tablets or capsules.

Bronchodilator: Methylxanthine

CLIENT TEACHING
General
- Advise the client that if allergic reaction occurs (rash, urticaria), drug should be discontinued and health care provider notified.
- Advise the client not to take OTC preparations without first checking with the health care provider. Some OTC products may have an additive effect.
- Encourage the client to stop smoking under medical supervision. Avoid changing smoking amounts acutely since levels are titrated to 10–20 μg/mL. Smoking increases drug elimination.
- Discuss ways to alleviate anxiety such as relaxation techniques and music.
- Advise the client having frequent or severe asthma attacks to wear an ID bracelet or tags.
- Encourage the client contemplating pregnancy to seek medical advice before taking a theophylline preparation.
- Advise the client to keep drug stored out of reach of small children; request child safety caps.

Skill
- Instruct the client to correctly use the nebulizer in conjunction with theophylline.
- Teach the client to monitor pulse rate and report any irregularities in comparison to baseline to health care provider.

Diet
- Advise the client that a high-protein, low-carbohydrate diet increases theophylline elimination. Conversely, a low-protein, high-carbohydrate diet prolongs the half-life; dosage may need adjustment.

EVALUATION
- Evaluate the effectiveness of the bronchodilators. The client is breathing without wheezing and without side effects of the drug.
- Evaluate serum theophylline levels to make sure they are within the accepted range.
- Evaluate tolerance to activity.

Theophylline Preparations

Generic (Brand)	Route and Dosage	Preg Cat	Interaction	t 1/2	PB	Onset	Peak	Duration
Aminophylline (theophylline ethylenediamine, Somophyllin)	A: LD 500 mg; then 250–500 mg q6–8h IV: LD 6 mg/kg over 30 min; then 0.2–0.9 mg/kg/h C: PO: LD: 7.5 mg/kg; then 3–6 mg/kg q6–8h; IV: LD 5.6 mg/kg then 1 mg/kg/h *Caution:* Need to stress that individual titration is based on serum theophylline levels	C	Similar to prototype theophylline	A: 9 h Smokers: 4 h C: 4–16 h	UK	PO: 15–60 min PO SR: UK IV: Rapid Rect: Rapid	1–2 h 4–7 h End of infusion 1–2 h	6–8 h 8–12 h 6–8 h 6–8 h
Dyphylline (dihydroxypropyl theophylline) (Dyline, Dilor, Lufyllin)	A: PO: 200–800 mg q.i.d. or q6h A: IM: 250–500 mg q6h C >6 y: PO: 4–7 mg/kg/d in 4 divided doses Therapeutic serum theophylline range is 10–20 μg/mL	C	Not hepatically metabolized, thus theophylline-like interactions do not apply. Caution with probenicid *Lab:* Use specific assay for drug; theophylline assay will give zero concentration	2 h	UK	UK	1 h	6 h
Oxtriphylline (choline theophyllinate) (Choledyl)	A: PO: 200 mg q.i.d. or q6h C: 2–12 y: PO: 4 mg/kg q6h Therapeutic serum theophylline range is 10–20 μg/mL	C	Similar to prototype theophylline	3–13 h	UK	PO: Liq: UK PO: Tab: 15–60 min PO SR: UK	1 h 5 h 4–7 h	UK 6–8 h 12 h
Theophylline	See Prototype Drug Chart							

KEY: For complete abbreviation key, see inside front cover.

CARDIOVASCULAR AGENTS

Cardiac Glycosides

Antianginals

Antidysrhythmics

Diuretics
Thiazides
Loop (High Ceiling), Osmotic, and Carbonic Anhydrase Inhibitors
Potassium Sparing

Antihypertensives
Beta Blockers and Central Alpha$_2$ Agonist

Adrenergic Blockers (Sympatholytics):
Alpha Blockers, Alpha-Beta Blockers, Peripherally Acting Blockers, and Direct-Acting Vasodilators
Angiotensin Antagonists and Calcium Blockers

Anticoagulants, Antiplatelets, and Anticoagulant Antagonists

Thrombolytics

Antilipemics

Vasodilators (Peripheral)

Prototype: Cardiac Glycosides (Cardiotonics)

Digoxin

Digoxin (Lanoxin); ❦ *novo-digoxin*
Cardiac glycoside

Pregnancy Category: C

Drug Forms:
Tab 0.125, 0.25, 0.5 mg
Cap 0.1, 0.2 mg
Elix 0.05 mg/mL (50 µg/mL)
Inj 0.1, 0.25 mg/mL

Dosage

A: PO: 0.5–1 mg initially in 2 divided doses (digitalization); maint: 0.125–0.5 mg/d; elderly: 0.125 mg/d
IV: Same as PO dose given over 5 min
C: PO: 1 mo–2 y: 0.01–0.02 mg/kg in 3 divided doses
2–10 y: 0.012–0.04 mg/kg in divided doses; maint: 0.012 mg/kg/d in 2 divided doses (pediatric elixir form)
IV: Dosage varies

Contraindications

Ventricular dysrhythmias, 2nd- or 3rd-degree heart block
Caution: AMI, renal disease, hypothyroidism, hypokalemia

Drug-Lab-Food Interactions

Increase digoxin serum level with quinidine, flecainide, verapamil
Decrease digoxin absorption with antacids, colestipol
Increase risk for digoxin toxicity with thiazide diuretics, loop diuretics
Lab: hypokalemia, hypomagnesemia, hypercalcemia

Pharmacokinetics

Absorption: PO: 60–76%; liq PO: 90%
Distribution: PB: 25%
Metabolism: t 1/2: 30–45 h
Excretion: 70% in urine; 30% by liver metabolism

Pharmacodynamics

PO: Onset: 1–5 h
Peak: 6–8 h
Duration: 2–4 d
IV: Onset: 5–30 min
Peak: 1–5 h
Duration: 2–4 d

Therapeutic Effects/Uses: To treat CHF, atrial tachycardia, flutter, or fibrillation.

Mode of Action: It inhibits the sodium-potassium ATPase, thus promoting increased forced of cardiac contraction, cardiac output, and tissue perfusion; decreases ventricular rate.

Side Effects

Anorexia, nausea, vomiting, headache, blurred vision (yellow-green halos), diplopia, photophobia, drowsiness, fatigue, confusion

Adverse Reactions

Bradycardia, visual disturbances
Life-threatening: Atrioventricular block, cardiac dysrhythmias

---

KEY: For complete abbreviation key, see inside front cover.

■ NURSING PROCESS: Cardiac Glycosides

ASSESSMENT

- Obtain a drug history. Report if a drug-drug interaction is probable. If the client is taking digoxin and a potassium-wasting diuretic or cortisone drug, hypokalemia might result, causing digitalis toxicity. A low serum potassium level enhances the action of digoxin. A client taking a thiazide and/or cortisone along with digoxin should be taking a potassium supplement.

Cardiac Glycosides (Cardiotonics)

- Obtain a baseline pulse rate for future comparisons. Apical pulse should be taken for a full minute and should be >60 bpm.
- Assess for signs and symptoms of digitalis toxicity. Common symptoms include anorexia, nausea, vomiting, bradycardia, cardiac dysrhythmias, and visual disturbances. Report symptoms immediately to the health care provider.

POTENTIAL NURSING DIAGNOSES

Decreased cardiac output
Altered tissue perfusion (cardiopulmonary, cerebral)
Anxiety related to cardiac problem

PLANNING

- Client checks pulse rate daily before taking digoxin. Client will report pulse rate of <60 bpm or a marked decline in pulse rate.
- Client eats foods rich in potassium to maintain a desired serum potassium level (see Client Teaching, Diet).

NURSING INTERVENTIONS

- Do *not* confuse **digoxin** with **digitoxin**. Read the drug labels carefully. Digoxin has a long half-life but has a shorter half-life than digitoxin.
- Check the apical pulse rate before administering digoxin. Do *not* administer if pulse rate is <60 bpm.
- Check for signs of peripheral and pulmonary edema, which indicate CHF.
- Check the serum digoxin level. The normal therapeutic drug range for digoxin is 0.5–2.0 ng/mL. A serum digoxin level of >2.0 ng/mL is indicative of digitalis toxicity. Check serum potassium level (normal range, 3.5–5.3 mEq/L) and report if hypokalemia (<3.5 mEq/L) is present.

CLIENT TEACHING

General

- Explain to the client the importance of compliance with the drug therapy. A visiting nurse may ensure that the medications are properly taken.
- Advise the client not to take OTC drugs without first consulting the health care provider to avoid adverse drug interactions.
- Keep drugs out of reach of small children. Request child safety cap bottle.

Skill

- Instruct the client how to check the pulse rate before taking digoxin and to call the health care provider for pulse rate <60 bpm or irregular pulse.

Diet

- Advise the client to eat foods rich in potassium such as fresh and dried fruits, fruit juices, and vegetables, including potatoes.

Side Effects

- Instruct the client to report side effects such as a pulse rate of <60 bpm, nausea, vomiting, headache, and visual disturbances, including diplopia.

EVALUATION

- Evaluate the effectiveness of digoxin by noting the client's response to the drug and the absence of side effects. Continue monitoring the pulse rate.

Cardiac Glycosides

Generic (Brand)	Route and Dosage	Preg Cat	Interaction	t 1/2	PB	Onset	Peak	Duration
Rapid-Acting Digitalis Digoxin (Lanoxin)	See Prototype Drug Chart							
Long-Acting Digitalis Digitoxin (Crystodigin)	A: PO/IV: LD: 0.8–1.2 mg; maint: PO: 0.05–3 mg/d	C	Decrease effects with barbiturate, phenytoin, cholestyramine, colestipol; decrease digitoxin level with thyroid drugs	1–3 wk	97%	0.5–2 h	4–12 h	2–3 wk
Positive Inotropic Bipyridines Amrinone lactate (Inocor)	A: IV: LD: 0.75 mg/kg within 2–3 min; maint: 5–10 µg/kg/min; max: 10 mg/kg/d	C	*Increase* hypotensive effect with disopyramide *Lab:* May *increase* serum liver enzyme	3.6–7 h	10–50%	2–5 min	10 min	0.5–2 h
Milrinone lactate (Primacor)	A: IV: Initially: 50 µg/kg/over 10 min *Continuous infusion:* 0.375–0.75 µg/kg/min with 0.45–0.9% saline	C	Do *not* mix with furosemide	1.5–2.5 h	70%	UK	2 min	3–6 h

Key: For complete abbreviation key, see inside front cover.

NOTES:

Prototype: Antianginals

Nitroglycerin

Nitroglycerin
(Nitrostat, Nitro-Bid, Transderm-Nitro patch, NTG); ♣ Nitrol, Nitrogard SR
Nitrate
Pregnancy Category: C
Drug Forms:
Tab SL 0.15, 0.3, 0.4, 0.6 mg
Cap SR 2.5, 6.5, 9 mg
Oint 2% topical
Patch transderm 2.5, 5.0, 7.5, 10, 15 mg
Inj 0.5, 0.8, 5 mg/mL

Dosage

A: PO/SL: 0.3, 0.4, 0.6 mg; repeat q5min ×3 as needed.
SR: 2.5 mg q8–12 h
IV: Initially: 5 μg/min; dose may be increased
Oint 2%: 1–2 in
Patch: 2.5–15 mg/d

Contraindications

Marked hypotension, AMI, increased intracranial pressure (ICP), severe anemia
Caution: Severe renal or hepatic disease, early MI

Drug-Lab-Food Interactions

Increase effect with alcohol, beta blockers, calcium blockers, antihypertensives
Decrease effect of heparin

Pharmacokinetics

Absorption: SL: >75% absorbed; oint and patch: slow absorption
Distribution: PB: 60%
Metabolism: t 1/2: 1–4 min
Excretion: Liver and urine

Pharmacodynamics

SL: Onset: 1–3 min
　　Peak: 4 min
　　Duration: 20–30 min
SR: Cap: Onset: 20–45 min
　　Duration: 3–8 h
Oint: Onset: 20–60 min
　　Peak: 1–2 h
　　Duration: 3–8 h
Patch: Onset: 30–60 min
　　Peak: 1–2 h
　　Duration: 20–24 h
IV: Onset: 1–3 min
　　Duration: 0.5–2 h

Therapeutic Effects/Uses: To control anginal pectoris (pain).
Mode of Action: Decrease myocardial demand for oxygen; decrease preload by dilating veins, thus indirectly decreasing afterload.

Side Effects

Nausea, vomiting, headache, dizziness, syncope, weakness, flushing, confusion, pallor, rash, dry mouth

Adverse Reactions

Hypotension, reflex tachycardia, paradoxical bradycardia
Life-threatening: Circulatory collapse

KEY: For complete abbreviation key, see inside front cover.

Antianginals

■ NURSING PROCESS: Antianginals: Nitroglycerin (Nitrostat, NTG)

ASSESSMENT
- Obtain baseline VS for future comparisons.
- Obtain medical and drug histories. Nitroglycerin is contraindicated for marked hypotension or AMI.

POTENTIAL NURSING DIAGNOSES
Decreased cardiac output
Anxiety related to cardiac problem(s)

PLANNING
- Client takes nitroglycerin or other antianginals and angina pain is controlled.

NURSING INTERVENTIONS
- Monitor VS. Hypotension is associated with most antianginal drugs.
- Have the client sit or lie down when taking a nitrate for the first time. After administration, check the VS while the client is lying down and then sitting up. Have the client rise slowly to a standing position.
- Offer sips of water before giving SL nitrates; dryness may inhibit drug absorption.
- Monitor effects of IV nitroglycerin. Report angina that persists.
- Apply Nitro-Bid ointment to the designated mark on paper. Do *not* use fingers because the drug can be absorbed; use a tongue blade or gloves. For the Transderm-Nitro patch, do not touch the medication portion.
- Do *not* apply the Nitro-Bid ointment or the Transderm-Nitro patch in any area on the chest in the vicinity of defibrillator-cardioverter paddle placement. Explosion and skin burns may result.

CLIENT TEACHING
General
- A nitroglycerin SL tablet is used if chest pain occurs. Repeat in 5 min if the pain has not subsided and again in another 5 min if it persists. Do *not* give more than 3 tablets. If the chest pain persists >15 min, immediate medical help is necessary.
- Instruct the client not to ingest alcohol while taking nitroglycerin to avoid hypotension, weakness, and faintness.
- Tolerance to nitroglycerin can occur. If the client's chest pain is not completely alleviated, the client should notify the physician.

Skill
- Instruct the client about SL nitroglycerin tablets. The tablet is placed under the tongue for quick absorption. A stinging or biting sensation may indicate the tablet is fresh. With the newer SL nitroglycerin, the biting sensation may not be present. The bottle is stored away from light and kept dry.
- Instruct the client about the Transderm-Nitro patch. Apply once a day, usually in the morning. Rotation of skin sites is necessary. Usually the patch is applied to the chest wall; however, the thighs and arms are used. Avoid hairy areas.

Side Effects
- Headaches commonly occur when first taking nitroglycerin products and last about 30 min. Acetaminophen is suggested for relief.
- If hypotension results from SL nitroglycerin, place the client in supine position with legs elevated.

EVALUATION
- Evaluate the nitrate product for relieving anginal pain. Note headache, dizziness, or faintness.

Antianginals

Generic (Brand)	Route and Dosage	Preg Cat	Interaction	t 1/2	PB	Onset	Peak	Duration
Nitrates								
Amyl nitrite	A: Inhal: 0.18–0.3 mL amp PRN	C	*Increase* hypotensive effect with alcohol antihypertensives, beta blockers *Decrease* effects of epinephrine	1–4 min	UK	30 sec	UK	3–5 min
Isosorbide dinitrate (Isordil, Sorbitrate)	A: SL: 2.5–10 mg q.i.d. Chewable: 5–10 mg PRN PO: 2.5–30 mg q.i.d. a.c. and h.s. SR: 40 mg, q6–12h	C	*Increase* hypotensive effect with alcohol, phenothiazides, antihypertensives including beta blockers	1–4 h	UK	SL: 3–30 min Chewable tab: 3–20 min PO: 1 h	SL: 15 min–1 h Chewable tab: 15 min–1 h PO: 1–2 h	SL: 1–4 h Chewable tab: 1–3 h PO: 4–6 h
Isosorbide mononitrate (Imdur)	A: PO: SR: 30–60 mg q morning; max: 240 mg/d	C	Same as isosorbide	6.6 h	5%	1 h	3–4 h	12 h
Nitroglycerin (Nitrostat, Nitro-Bid, Transderm-Nitro)	See Prototype Drug Chart							
Pentaerythritol tetranitrate (Peritrate)	A: PO: 10–40 mg t.i.d./q.i.d. SR: 20–80 mg q12h	C	Same as isosorbide	10 min	UK	PO: 20–60 min SR: 0.5 h	PO: UK SR: UK	PO: 4–5 h SR: 8–12 h

Beta-Adrenergic Blockers							
Atenolol (Tenormin)	A: PO: 50–100 mg/d; max: 200 mg/d	C	*Increase* hypotensive effects with diuretics, antihypertensives; *increase* absorption with anticholinergics; Lab: may *increase* lidocaine levels	6–7 h	5–15%	1 h	2–4 h	24 h
Metoprolol tartrate (Lopressor)	A: PO: Initially: 50–100 mg/d in 1–2 divided doses; maint: 100–400 mg/d SR: 100 mg/d; max: 400 mg/d	C	*Increase* bradycardia with digoxin; *increase* hypotensive effects with alcohol, antihypertensives, anesthetics	3–7 h	12%	15 min–1 h	1.5–4 h	6–12 h
Propranolol HCl (Inderal)	A: PO: Initially: 10–20 mg t.i.d./q.i.d.; maint: 20–60 mg t.i.d./q.i.d.; max: 320 mg/d SR: 80–160 mg/d IV: See Antidysrhythmics	C	Same as atenolol	3–6 h	90%	0.5–1 h	1–1.5 h SR: 6 h	12 h
Calcium Channel Blockers								
Amlodipine (Norvasc)	A: PO: Initially: 10 mg; maint: 2.5–10 mg/d	C	May *increase* hypotension with beta blockers, anesthetics *Decrease* effect with NSAIDs, adrenergics	30–50 h	95%	UK	6–12 h	24 h

continued

Antianginals —Continued

Generic (Brand)	Route and Dosage	Preg Cat	Interaction	t 1/2	PB	Onset	Peak	Duration
Bepridal HCl (Vascor)	A: PO: Initially: 200 mg/d × 10 d; maint: 300 mg/d; max: 400 mg/d	C	*Increase* hypotensive effect with anesthesia; may *increase* effect of beta blockers *Lab:* May *increase* ALP, AST, ALT, CPK, LDH, liver enzymes	2–24 h	99%	1 h	2–3 h	UK
Diltiazem HCl (Cardizem)	A: PO: 30–60 mg q.i.d.; may increase to 360 mg/d in 4 divided doses SR: 60 mg q12h; max: 360 mg/d CD: 120–180 mg/d; max: 360 mg/d	C	Similar to nifedipine	3.5–9 h	70–85%	PO: 30 min SR: UK	PO: 2–3 h SR: 6–11 h	PO: 6–8 h SR: 12–24 h
Isradipine (DynaCirc)	A: PO: 2.5–7.5 mg t.i.d.	C	*Increase* effect of digoxin; *increase* effect with cimetidine, carbamazepine	5–11 h	99%	1–2 h	2–3 h	12 h

Nicardipine HCl (Cardene, Cardene SR)	A: PO: 20 mg t.i.d.; maint: 20–40 mg t.i.d. SR: 30 mg b.i.d.; maint: 30–60 mg b.i.d.	C	*Increase* effect with cimetidine, propranolol, theophylline *Decrease* effect with barbiturates, phenytoin *Lab: Increase* ALP, AST, ALT, creatine phosphokinase, LDH	5 h	95%	20 min	1–2 h	PO: 6–8 h
Nifedipine (Procardia, Adalat)	A: PO: 10–30 mg q6–8h; max: 180 mg/d	C	*Increase* effect with cimetidine; *increase* effects of theophylline, beta blockers, antihypertensives	2–5 h	92–98 h	PO: 20 min SR: UK	PO: 1–4 h SR: UK	PO: 6–8 h SR: 24 h
Verapamil HCl (Calan, Isoptin, Verelan)	A: PO: 40–120 mg t.i.d.; max: 480 mg/d IV: 5–10 mg over 2 min	C	*Increase* effect with cimetidine; *increase* effects of theophylline, beta blockers, antihypertensives *Decrease* effect of lithium	3–8 h	90%	PO: 1–2 h SR: UK	PO: 0.5–1.5 h SR: 4–8 h	PO: 3–7 h SR: 24 h

KEY: For complete abbreviation key, see inside front cover.

Prototype: Antidysrhythmics

Procainamide HCl

Procainamide HCl
(Procan, Pronestyl)
Fast channel (sodium) blocker (type I)
Pregnancy Category: C
Drug Forms:
Tab and Cap 250, 375, 500 mg

Dosage

A: PO: 250–500 mg q3–4h
SR: 250 mg–1 g q6h or
50 mg/kg/d in 4 divided doses
IV: 20–30 mg/min; maint:
1–4 mg/min; max: 17 mg/kg
C: PO: 40–60 mg/kg/d in 4 divided doses
IV: 3–6 mg/kg q10–30 min; max: 100 mg/dose
TDM: 4–8 µg/mL

Contraindications

Hypersensitivity to procaine, blood dyscrasias, heart block, cardiogenic shock, myasthenia gravis
Caution: Hypotension, CHF, MI, renal or hepatic insufficiency

Drug-Lab-Food Interactions

Increase effects with histamine$_2$ blockers; *increase* hypotensive effects with antihypertensives, nitrates
Decrease effects with barbiturates
Lab: May *increase* ALP, AST, LDH, bilirubin

Pharmacokinetics

Absorption: PO: 75–95%
Distribution: PB: 20%
Metabolism: t 1/2: 3–4 h
Excretion: 60% unchanged in urine (half as an active metabolite)

Pharmacodynamics

PO: Onset: 30 min
Peak: 1–1.5 h
Duration: 3–4 h (SR: 8 h)
IV: Onset: Minutes
Peak: 25–60 min
Duration: 3–4 h

Therapeutic Effects/Uses: To control cardiac dysrhythmias (premature ventricular contractions [PVCs], ventricular tachycardia)

Mode of Action: Depression of myocardial excitability by slowing conduction of cardiac tissue through the atrium, bundle of His, and ventricle to decrease cardiac dysrhythmias.

Side Effects

Anorexia, nausea, vomiting, diarrhea, headache, dizziness, weakness, flushing, rash, pruritus, lupus-like syndrome with rash

Adverse Reactions

Life-threatening: Atrioventricular block, pleural effusion, ventricular tachycardia/fibrillation, thrombocytopenia, agranulocytosis, cardiovascular collapse, torsade des pointes

KEY: For complete abbreviation key, see inside front cover.

Antidysrhythmics

■ NURSING PROCESS: Antidysrhythmics

ASSESSMENT
- Obtain health and drug histories. The history may include heart palpitations, coughing, chest pain (type, duration, and severity), previous angina or cardiac dysrhythmias, and drugs that the client is currently taking.
- Obtain baseline VS and ECG for future comparisons.
- Check early cardiac enzyme results (AST, LDH, CPK) to compare with future laboratory results.

POTENTIAL NURSING DIAGNOSES
Decreased cardiac output
Anxiety related to irregular heartbeat
High risk for activity intolerance

PLANNING
- Client will no longer experience abnormal sinus rhythm.
- Client will comply with the antidysrhythmic drug regimen.

NURSING INTERVENTIONS
- Monitor VS. Hypotension can occur.
- When the drug is ordered IV push or bolus, administer it over a period of 2–3 min or as prescribed.
- Monitor ECG for abnormal patterns and report findings, such as PVCs, increased PR and QT intervals, and/or widening of the QRS complex. Increased QT interval is a risk factor for torsade des pointes.

CLIENT TEACHING

General
- Instruct the client to take the prescribed drug as ordered. Drug compliance is essential.
- Provide specific instructions for each drug, such as photosensitivity for amiodarone.

Side Effects
- Instruct the client to report side effects and adverse reactions to the health care provider. These can include dizziness, faintness, nausea, and vomiting.
- Advise the client to avoid alcohol, caffeine, and cigarettes. Alcohol can intensify the hypotensive reaction; caffeine increases the catecholamine level; and cigarette smoking promotes vasoconstriction.

EVALUATION
- Evaluate the effectiveness of the prescribed antidysrhythmic by comparing heart rates with the baseline heart rate and assessing the client's response to the drug. Report side effects and adverse reactions. The drug regimen may need to be adjusted. A proarrhythmic effect may occur, which may require discontinuation of the drug.

Antidysrhythmics

Generic (Brand)	Route and Dosage	Preg Cat	Interaction	t1/2	PB	Onset	Peak	Duration
Fast (Sodium) Channel Blockers I								
Disopyramide phosphate (Norpace, Napamide)	A: PO: 100–200 mg q6h CR: 300 mg q12h C 4–12 y: PO: 10–15 mg/kg/d in divided doses 13–18 y: PO: 6–15 mg/kg/d in divided doses	C	*Increase* effect with other antidysrhythmics, beta blockers, lidocaine *Decrease* effect with phenytoin, rifampin *Lab:* May *increase* serum liver enzymes	4–10 h	50–65%	0.5–3.5 h	1–2 h	1.5–8 h
Procainamide (Pronestyl, Procan)	See Prototype Drug Chart							
Quinidine sulfate, polygalactorate, gluconate (Quinidex, Duraquin)	A: PO: 200–400 mg t.i.d./q.i.d. C: PO: 30 mg/kg or 900 mg/m² in 5 divided doses	C	*Increase* effect with beta blockers, thiazides, histamine₂ blockers, verapamil, sodium bicarbonate; *increase* effects of digoxin, warfarin *Decrease* effect with barbiturates, nifedipine, phenytoin, rifampin	6–7 h	80%	1–3 h	1–2 h	6–8 h
Fast (Sodium) Channel Blockers II								
Flecainide (Tambocor)	A: PO: Initially: 50–100 mg q12h; maint: 150 mg q12h; max: 300 mg/d	C	Similar to tocainide HCl	12–27 h	UK	1 h	2–3 h	UK

Encainide HCl **Available for compassionate use only**	A: PO: 25 mg q8h; may increase to 50–75 mg q8h	B	*Increase* effect with histamine$_2$ blockers	3–12 h	75–85%	1–3 h	UK	8–12 h
Lidocaine (Xylocaine)	A: IV: 50–100 mg bolus in 2–3 min; may repeat; then 20–50 µg/kg/min, inf.	B	*Increase* effect with beta blockers, histamine$_2$ blockers, other antihypertensives	1.5–2 h	60–80%	1–2 min	1–2 min	10–12 min
Mexiletine HCl (Mexitil)	A: PO: 200–400 mg q8h	C	*Increase* effect with H$_2$ blockers *Decrease* effect with barbiturates, phenytoin, antitubercular drugs, smoking	10–12 h	50–60%	0.5–2 h	2–3 h	8–12 h
Phenytoin (Dilantin)	A: IV: 100 mg q5–10 min until dysrhythmia ceases; max: 1000 mg	D	*Decrease* effects of steroids, oral contraceptives; decrease effect with barbiturate, theophylline, folic acid, antacids, CNS depressants *Food: Decrease* with calcium, vitamin D, folic acid	22 h	95%	UK	1.5–3 h	5 h
Tocainide HCl (Tonocard)	A: PO: LD: 600 mg PO: 400 mg q8h; max: 2.4 g/d	C	*Increase* effect with beta blockers, quinidine, other antihypertensives	10–17 h	70–80%	0.5–1 h	1–2 h	8–12 h

continued

Antidysrhythmics—Continued

Generic (Brand)	Route and Dosage	Preg Cat	Interaction	t 1/2	PB	Onset	Peak	Duration
Beta-Adrenergic Blockers *(Type II)*								
Acebutolol HCl (Sectral)	A: PO: 200 mg b.i.d.; may increase dose	B	*Increase* hypotensive effect with diuretics, other antihypertensives	3–13 h	26%	1 h	4–6 h	10 h
Propranolol HCl (Inderal)	A: PO: 10–30 mg t.i.d./q.i.d. A: IV bolus: 0.5–3 mg at 1 mg/min	C	Same as acebutolol	3–6 h	90%	0.5–1 h	1.5–4 h	UK
Sotalol HCl (Betapace)	A: PO: 80 mg b.i.d.; max: 240–320 mg/d Increase dose interval with renal dysfunction	B	May *increase* bradycardia with amiodarone; may *increase* hypoglycemic effect with oral antidiabetics *Food: Decrease* effect with milk and milk products	12 h	0%	UK	2–3 h	24 h
Calcium Channel Blockers *(Type IV)*								
Verapamil HCl (Calan)	A: PO: 240–480 mg/d in 3–4 divided doses IV: 5–10 mg IV push	C	*Increase* effect with cimetidine; *increase* effects of theophylline, beta blockers, antihypertensives *Decrease* effect of lithium	3–8 h	90%	PO: 0.5–1.5 h	PO: 1–2 h	PO: 3–7 h

Prolong Repolarization
(Type III)

Adenosine (Adenocard)	A: IV: 6 mg (bolus; 1–2 sec); repeat if necessary, 12 mg bolus	C	May *increase* effect with dipyridamole *Decrease* effect with theophylline	<10 s	UK	<10 s	20–30 s	UK
Amiodarone HCl (Cordarone)	A: PO: LD: 400–1,600 mg/d in divided doses; maint: 200–600 mg/d	C	*Increase* effects of digoxin, other antidysrhythmics, phenytoin *Lab:* May *increase* liver enzymes AST, ALT, ALP	5–100 d	1–3 wk	2–3 d	UK	Weeks, months
Bretylium tosylate (Bretylol)	A: IM: 5–10 mg/kg q6–8h; IV: 5–10 mg/kg; repeat in 15–30 min, IV drip or IV bolus	C	May *increase* hypotensive effect with beta blockers, other antidysrhythmics	4–17 h	UK	IM: 1–6 h IV: 5 min	IM: 6–9 h IV: End of infusion	IM/IV: 6–24 h
Propafenone HCl (Rythmol)	A: PO: 150–300 mg q8h; max: 900 mg/d	C	*Increase* digoxin effect May *prolong* clotting; Warfarin *Increase* effect with: cimetidine *Increase* effect of: Metoprolol, propranolol	5–8 h	97%	UK	1–3.5 h	UK

Key: For complete abbreviation key, see inside front cover.

Prototype: Diuretic: Thiazides

Hydrochlorothiazide

Hydrochlorothiazide
 (HydroDIURIL, HCTZ, Esidrix,
 Oretic); ♣ Apo-Hydro, Urozide
Thiazide diuretic

Pregnancy Category: B

Drug Forms:
Tab 25, 50, 100 mg
Oral sol 10, 100 mg/mL

Dosage

A: PO: Hypertension: 12.5–100 mg/d
 Edema: Initially: 25–200 mg in
 divided doses: maint:
 25–100 mg/d
C: PO: 1–2 mg/kg/d in divided
 doses
C: <6 mo: PO: 1–3 mg/kg/d in
 divided doses

Contraindications

Renal failure with anuria, electrolyte depletion

Caution: Hepatic cirrhosis, renal dysfunction, diabetes mellitus, gout, systemic lupus erythematosus (SLE)

Drug-Lab-Food Interactions

Increase digitalis toxicity with digitalis and hypokalemia; *increase* potassium loss with steroids; potassium loss

Decrease antidiabetic effect; decrease thiazide effect with cholestyramine and colestipol

Lab: Increase serum calcium, glucose, uric acid

Decrease serum potassium, sodium, magnesium

Pharmacokinetics

Absorption: Readily absorbed from the GI tract
Distribution: PB: 65%
Metabolism: t 1/2: 6–15 h
Excretion: In urine

Pharmacodynamics

PO: Onset: 2 h
 Peak: 3–6 h
 Duration: 6–12 h

Therapeutic Effects/Uses: To increase urine output. To treat hypertension, edema from CHF, hepatic cirrhosis, renal dysfunction.

Mode of Action: Action is on the renal distal tubules by promoting sodium, potassium, and water excretion. Acts on arterioles, causing vasodilation, thus decreasing blood pressure.

Side Effects

Dizziness, vertigo, weakness, nausea, vomiting, diarrhea, hyperglycemia, constipation, rash, photosensitivity

Adverse Reactions

Severe dehydration, hypotension
Life-threatening: Severe potassium depletion, marked hypotension, uremia, aplastic anemia, hemolytic anemia, thrombocytopenia, agranulocytosis

KEY: For complete abbreviation key, see inside front cover.

Diuretic: Thiazides

■ NURSING PROCESS: Diuretics: Thiazides

ASSESSMENT
- Assess VS, weight, urine output, and serum chemistry values (electrolytes, glucose, uric acid) for baseline levels.
- Check peripheral extremities for presence of edema. Note pitting edema.
- Obtain a history of drugs that are taken daily. Review for drugs that may cause drug interaction, including digoxin, corticosteroids, antidiabetics.

POTENTIAL NURSING DIAGNOSIS
High risk for fluid volume deficit

PLANNING
- Client's blood pressure will be decreased and/or return to normal value.
- Client's edema will be decreased.
- Client's serum chemistry levels remain within normal ranges.

NURSING INTERVENTIONS
- Monitor VS and serum electrolytes, especially potassium and glucose levels. Report changes. If client is taking digoxin and hypokalemia occurs, digitalis toxicity frequently results.
- Observe for signs and symptoms of hypokalemia, such as muscle weakness, leg cramps, and cardiac dysrhythmias.
- Check the client's weight daily at a specified time. A weight gain of 2.2–2.5 lb is equivalent to an excess liter of body fluids.
- Monitor urine output to determine fluid loss or retention.

CLIENT TEACHING

General
- Suggest that the client take hydrochlorothiazide in early morning to avoid sleep disturbance due to nocturia.
- Keep drugs out of reach of small children. Request child safety cap bottle.

Skill
- Instruct the client or family member how to take and record his or her blood pressure. Record daily results.

Diet
- Instruct the client to eat foods rich in potassium, such as fruits, fruit juices, and vegetables. Potassium supplements may be ordered.
- Advise the client to take drugs with food to avoid GI upset.

Side Effects
- Instruct the client to change positions from lying to standing slowly because dizziness may occur due to orthostatic (postural) hypotension.
- Advise the client who may be prediabetic to have blood sugar checked periodically because large doses of hydrochlorothiazide increase blood glucose levels.
- Advise the client to use sunscreen when in direct sunlight.

EVALUATION
- Evaluate the effectiveness of drug therapy. Client's blood pressure and edema will be reduced and blood chemistry will remain within normal range.
- Determine the absence of side effects and adverse reactions to therapy.

Diuretics: Thiazides

Generic (Brand)	Route and Dosage	Preg Cat	Interaction	t 1/2	PB	Onset	Peak	Duration
Short Acting								
Chlorothiazide (Diuril, Diachlor)	*Hypertension:* A: PO: 250–500 mg q.d. or b.i.d. *Edema:* A: PO: 500–2,000 mg q.d. or b.i.d. C >1 y: PO: 20 mg/kg/d C <6 mon: PO: 10–30 mg/kg/d in divided doses	D	May *increase* potassium and magnesium loss with digitalis, corticosteroids; *increase* toxicity with lithium *Decrease* effects of antidiabetics; *decrease* chlorothiazide absorption with colestipol	1–2 h	20–80%	1–2 h	4 h	6–12 h
Hydrochlorothiazide	See Prototype Drug Chart							
Intermediate Acting								
Bendroflumethiazide (Naturetin)	A: PO: 2.5–20 mg/d C: PO: maint: 0.05–0.1 mg/kg/d or 1.5–3 mg/m^2/d	UK	Same as chlorothiazide	3–4 h	94%	1–2 h	6–12 h	18–24 h
Benzthiazide (Aquatag, Hydrex)	*Hypertension:* A: PO: 25–100 mg/q.d. or 25–100 mg in divided doses *Edema:* A: PO: 25–200 mg q.d. C: PO: 1–4 mg/kg/d in 3 divided doses	D	Same as chlorothiazide	UK	UK	2 h	4–6 h	12–18 h
Hydroflumethiazide (Saluron, Diucardin)	*Hypertension:* A: PO: 50–100 mg/d *Edema:* A: PO: 25–200 mg/d C: PO: 1 mg/kg/d	C	Same as chlorothiazide	17 h	74%	1–2 h	3–4 h	18–24 h

Long Acting							
Methyclothiazide (Aquatensen, Enduron)	*Hypertension/edema:* A: PO: 2.5–10 mg/d C: PO: 0.05–0.1 mg/kg/d	C	*Increase* hypokalemic effect with digitalis, glucocorticosteroids; *increase* hypoglycemic effect with antidiabetics (oral and insulin); *increase* toxicity with lithium; may *increase* risk of renal failure with NSAIDs	UK	UK	2 h	6 h	>24 h
Polythiazide (Renese-R)	*Hypertension:* A: PO: 2–4 mg/d *Edema:* A: PO: 1–4 mg/d C: PO: 0.02–0.08 mg/kg/d	D	Similar to methyclothiazide	25 h	84%	2 h	6 h	24–48 h
Trichlormethiazide (Metahydrin, Naqual)	*Hypertension:* A: PO: 2–4 mg *Edema:* A: PO: 1–4 mg q.d. or b.i.d. C: PO: 0.075 mg/kg/d in divided doses	B	Similar to methyclothiazide	2.5–7 h	UK	2 h	6 h	24 h
Thiazide-Like Diuretics								
Chlorthalidone (Hygroton)	*Hypertension:* A: PO: 12.5–50 mg/d *Edema:* A: PO: 25–100 mg/d C: PO: 2 mg/kg 3×wk	C	Similar to methyclothiazide	40–54 h	75%	2 h	3–6 h	24–72 h
Indapamide (Lozol)	*Hypertension and edema:* A: PO: 2.5 mg/d; may increase to 5 mg/d	B	Similar to methyclothiazide	14–18 h	75%	1–2 h	<2 h	24–36 h
Metolazone (Zaroxolyn)	*Hypertension:* A: PO: 2.5–5.0 mg/d *Edema:* A: PO: 5–20 mg/d	D	Similar to methyclothiazide	8–14 h	33%	1 h	2–8 h	12–24 h
Quinethazone (Hydromox)	A: PO: 50–100 mg/d; max: 200 mg/d in divided doses	D	Similar to methyclothiazide	UK	UK	2 h	6 h	18–24 h

KEY: For complete abbreviation key, see inside front cover.

Prototype: Diuretic: Loop (High Ceiling)

Furosemide

Furosemide
(Lasix); ❀ Fumide, Furomide
High ceiling (loop) diuretic
Pregnancy Category: C
Drug Forms:
Tab 20, 40, 80 mg
Oral sol 10 mg/mL, 40 mg/5 mL
Inj 10 mg/mL

Dosage

A: PO: 20–80 mg single dose; repeat in 6–8 h max: 600 mg/d
IM/IV: 20–100 mg single dose; over 1–2 min IV; repeat 20 mg in 2 h
C: PO: 2 mg/kg single dose; repeat in 6–8 h; max: 6 mg/kg/d
IM/IV: 1 mg/kg single dose; repeat 1 mg/kg in 2 h

Contraindications

Presence of severe electrolyte imbalances, hypovolemia, anuria, hypersensitivity to sulfonamides, hepatic coma

Drug-Lab-Food Interactions

Increase orthostatic hypotension with alcohol; *increase* ototoxicity with aminoglycosides; *increase* bleeding with anticoagulants; *increase* potassium loss with steroids; *increase* digitalis toxicity and cardiac dysrhythmias with digitalis and hypokalemia
Lab: Increase BUN, blood/urine glucose, serum uric acid, ammonia
Decrease potassium, sodium, calcium, magnesium, chloride serum levels

Pharmacokinetics

Absorption: Readily absorbed from the GI tract
Distribution: PB: 95%
Metabolism: t 1/2: 30–50 min
Excretion: In urine, some in feces; crosses placenta

Pharmacodynamics

PO: Onset: <60 min
   Peak: 1–2 h
   Duration: 6–8 h
IV: Onset: 5 min
   Peak: 20–30 min
   Duration: 2 h

Therapeutic Effects/Uses: To treat fluid retention/fluid overload due to CHF, renal dysfunction, cirrhosis; hypertension; acute pulmonary edema.

Mode of Action: Inhibition of sodium and water reabsorption from the loop of Henle and distal renal tubules. Potassium, magnesium, and calcium also may be excreted.

Side Effects

Nausea, diarrhea, electrolyte imbalances, vertigo, cramping, rash, headache, weakness, ECG changes, blurred vision, photosensitivity

Adverse Reactions

Severe dehydration; marked hypotension
Life-threatening: Renal failure, thrombocytopenia, agranulocytosis

KEY: For complete abbreviation key, see inside front cover.

Diuretic: Loop (High Ceiling)

■ NURSING PROCESS: Diuretics: Loop (High Ceiling)

ASSESSMENT
- Obtain a history of drugs that are taken daily. Note if client is taking a drug(s) that may cause an interaction, such as alcohol, aminoglycosides, anticoagulants, corticosteroids, or digitalis. Recognize that furosemide is highly protein-bound and can displace other protein-bound drugs such as Coumadin.
- Assess VS, serum electrolytes, weight, and urine output for baseline levels.
- Compare client's drug dose with recommended dose and report discrepancy.

POTENTIAL NURSING DIAGNOSIS
High risk for fluid volume deficit

PLANNING
- Client's edema and/or hypertension will be decreased.
- Client's serum chemistry levels will remain within normal ranges.

NURSING INTERVENTIONS
- Check the half-life of furosemide. With a short half-life, the drug can be repeated or given more than once a day.
- Check onset of action for furosemide, orally and intravenously. If the drug is given intravenously, the urine output should increase in 5–20 min. If urine output does not increase, notify the health care provider. Severe renal disorder may be present.
- Monitor urinary output to determine body fluid gain or loss. Urinary output should be at least 25 mL/h or 600 mL/24 h.
- Check the client's weight to determine fluid loss or gain. A loss of 2.2–2.5 lb is equivalent to a fluid loss of 1 liter.
- Monitor VS. Be alert for marked decrease in blood pressure.
- Administer IV furosemide slowly; hearing loss may occur if rapidly injected.
- Observe for signs and symptoms of hypokalemia (<3.5 mEq/L), such as muscle weakness, abdominal distention, and/or cardiac dysrhythmias.
- Check serum potassium levels, especially when a client is taking digoxin. Hypokalemia enhances the action of digitalis, causing digitalis toxicity.

CLIENT TEACHING
General
- Instruct the client to take furosemide early in the morning and *not* in the evening, to prevent sleep disturbance and nocturia.

Diet
- Suggest taking furosemide at mealtime or with food to avoid nausea.

Side Effects
- Instruct the client to arise slowly to prevent dizziness due to fluid loss.

EVALUATION
- Evaluate the effectiveness of drug action: decreased fluid retention or fluid overload, decreased respiratory distress, and increased cardiac output.
- Check for side effects and increase in urine output.

Diuretics: Loop (High Ceiling), Osmotics, Carbonic Anhydrase Inhibitors

Generic (Brand)	Route and Dosage	Preg Cat	Interaction	t1/2	PB	Onset	Peak	Duration
Loop (High Ceiling)								
Bumetanide (Bumex)	A: PO: 0.5–2.0 mg/d; max: 10 mg/d IV: 0.5–1.0 mg/dose; repeat in 2–4 h C: PO: 0.015 mg/kg/d	C	*Increase* risk of ototoxicity with aminoglycosides, vancomycin, cisplatin; *increase* risk of toxicity with digoxin, lithium; *increase* drug effect with antihypertensives *Decrease* effects of antidiabetics (oral and insulin)	1–1.5 h	95%	PO: 0.5–1 h IV: 5–10 min	1–2 h 15–45 min	4–6 h 3–4 h
Ethacrynic acid (Edecrin)	A: PO: 50–200 mg/d IV: 0.5–1.0 mg/kg/dose C: PO: 25 mg/d	B	Similar to bumetanide	1–1.5 h	95%	PO: 30 min IV: 5–10 min	1–2 h 15–30 min	6–8 h 2–3 h
Furosemide	See Prototype Drug Chart							
Torsemide (Demadox)	*Hypertension* A: PO/IV: Initially: 5 mg/d; maint: PO: 5–10 mg/d IV: In 2 min *CHF*: A: PO/IV: 10–20 mg/d	C	Similar to furosemide	2–4 h	97–99%	30–60 min	1–4 h	6 h

Osmotics Mannitol	*ICP, IOP:* A: IV: 1.5–2.0 g/kg; 15–25% sol infused over 30–60 min *Edema and ascites:* A: IV: 100 g; 10–20% sol infused over 2–6 h	C	*Incompatible* with whole blood *Decrease* effect of lithium	1.5 h	UK	IV: 1–3 h	UK	4–6 h
Urea (Ureaphil)	A: IV: 1.0–1.5 g/kg of 30% sol C >2 y: IV: 0.5–1.5 g/kg of 30% sol	C	Same as Mannitol	1.5 h	UK	<1 h	1–2 h	3–10 h
Carbonic Anhydrase Inhibitors								
Acetazolamide (Diamox)	A: PO/IV: 250 mg q12h; dose may vary C: PO: 10–15 mg/kg/d in divided doses C: IV: 5–10 mg/kg q6h		*Increase* effects of amphetamines, antidysrhythmics, tricyclic antidepressants; *increase* toxicity with salicylates; *increase* hypokalemia with other diuretics, corticosteroids, amphotericin B	2.5–5.5 h	90%	PO: 1–1.5 h PO/SR: 2 h IV: 2 min	2–4 h 8–12 h 15 min	6–12 h 18–24 h 4–5 h
Dichlorphenamide (Daranide, Oratrol)	A: PO: 100 mg q12h; maint: 25–50 mg q.d./t.i.d.	C	Similar to acetazolamide *Decrease* effect of dichlorphenamide	UK	UK	PO: 0.5–1 h	2–4 h	6–12 h
Methazolamide (Neptazane)	A: PO: 50–100 mg b.i.d./t.i.d.	C	Same as dichlorphenamide	14 h	50–60%	2–4 h	6–8 h	10–18 h

KEY: For complete abbreviation key, see inside front cover.

Prototype: Diuretic: Potassium Sparing

Triamterene

Triamterene
  (Dyrenium)
Potassium-sparing diuretic
Pregnancy Category: B
Drug Forms:
Cap 50, 100 mg

Dosage

A: PO: Edema: 100 mg q.d., b.i.d.; not to exceed 300 mg/d
C: PO: 2–4 mg/kg/d in divided doses

Contraindications

Severe kidney or hepatic disease, severe hyperkalemia
Caution: Renal or hepatic dysfunction, diabetes mellitus

Drug-Lab-Food Interactions

Increase serum potassium level with potassium supplements; *increase* effects of antihypertensives and lithium
Lab: Increase serum potassium level; may *increase* BUN, AST, alkaline phosphatase levels
Decrease serum sodium, chloride

Pharmacokinetics

Absorption: Rapidly absorbed from GI tract
Distribution: PB: 67%
Metabolism: t 1/2: 1.5–2.5 h
Excretion: In urine, mostly as metabolites and bile

Pharmacodynamics

PO: Onset: 2–4 h
  Peak: 6–8 h
  Duration: 12–16 h

Therapeutic Effects/Uses: To increase urine output; to treat fluid retention/overload associated with CHF, hepatic cirrhosis, or nephrotic syndrome.

Mode of Action: Action on the distal renal tubules to promote sodium and water excretion and potassium retention.

Side Effects

Nausea, vomiting, diarrhea, rash, dizziness, headache, weakness, dry mouth, photosensitivity

Adverse Reactions

Life-threatening: Severe hyperkalemia, thrombocytopenia, megaloblastic anemia

KEY: For complete abbreviation key, see inside front cover.

Diuretic: Potassium Sparing

■ NURSING PROCESS: Diuretic: Potassium Sparing

ASSESSMENT
- Obtain a history of drugs that are taken daily. Note if the client is taking a potassium supplement or using a salt substitute.
- Assess VS, serum electrolytes, weight, and urinary output for baseline levels.
- Compare the client's drug dose with the recommended dose and report any discrepancy.

POTENTIAL NURSING DIAGNOSIS
High risk for fluid volume deficit

PLANNING
- Client's fluid retention and blood pressure will be decreased.
- Client's serum electrolytes remain within their normal values.

NURSING INTERVENTIONS
- Check the half-life of triamterene. With a long half-life, drug dose is usually administered once a day and sometimes twice a day.
- Monitor urinary output. Urine output should increase. Report if urine output is <30 mL/h, or 600 mL/day.
- Monitor VS. Report abnormal changes.
- Observe for signs and symptoms of hyperkalemia (increased serum potassium level: >5.3 mEq/L), such as nausea, diarrhea, abdominal cramps, tachycardia and later bradycardia, peaked narrow T wave (ECG), or oliguria.
- Administer triamterene in the early morning and not in the evening, to avoid nocturia.

CLIENT TEACHING
General
- Instruct the client to take triamterene with or after meals to avoid nausea.

Diet
- Advise clients with high average serum potassium levels to avoid foods rich in potassium when taking potassium-sparing diuretics.

Side Effects
- Instruct the client to avoid exposure to direct sunlight because the drug can cause photosensitivity.
- Advise the client to report possible side effects of the drug, such as rash, dizziness, or weakness.

EVALUATION
- Evaluate the effectiveness of the potassium-sparing diuretic such as triamterene. The presence of fluid retention (edema) is decreased or absent.
- Determine if urine output has increased and the serum potassium level is within normal range.

Diuretic: Potassium Sparing

Generic (Brand)	Route and Dosage	Preg Cat	Interaction	t1/2	PB	Onset	Peak	Duration
Single Agents								
Amiloride HCl (Midamor)	A: PO: 5 mg/d; may increase to 10–20 mg/d in 1–2 divided doses	B	*Increase* hyperkalemia with potassium supplements, ACE inhibitors, salt substitutes; *increase* effect of lithium, antihypertensives	6–9 h	23%	PO: 2 h	6–10 h	24 h
Spironolactone (Aldactone)	*Hypertension:* A: PO: 25–100 mg/d *Edema:* A: PO: 25–200 mg/d in divided doses C: PO: 3.3 mg/kg/d in divided doses	C	Similar to amiloride *Decrease* drug effect with aspirin	1.5–2 h	98%	PO: 24–48 h	48–72 h	48–72 h
Triamterene	See Prototype Drug Chart							

Combinations:						
Amiloride HCl and hydrochlorothiazide (Moduretic)	A: PO: 1–2 tab (amiloride 5 mg/hydrochlorothiazide 50 mg)	B	UK	UK	UK	UK
Spironolactone and hydrochlorothiazide (Aldactazide)	A: PO: 25/25 and 50/50 mg tab	B, C	UK	UK	UK	UK
Triamterene and hydrochlorothiazide (Dyazide, Maxzide)	A: PO: 1–2 cap b.i.d., p.c. (triamterene 50 mg/hydrochlorothiazide 25 mg)	B	UK	UK	UK	UK

KEY: For complete abbreviation key, see inside front cover.

Prototype: Antihypertensives: Beta Blockers

Metoprolol tartrate

Metoprolol tartrate
(Lopressor); ✤ Betaloc, Apo-Metoprolol
Adrenergic blocker, sympatholytic, beta$_2$ blocker
Pregnancy Category: C
Drug Forms:
Tab 50, 100 mg
Inj 1 mg/mL

Dosage

Hypertension:
A: PO: 50–100 mg/d in 1–2 divided doses; maint: 100–450 mg in divided doses; max: 450 mg/d in divided doses

Myocardial Infarction:
A: PO: 100 mg b.i.d.
IV: 5 mg q2min × 3 doses

Contraindications

Second- and third-degree heart block, cardiogenic shock, CHF, sinus bradycardia
Caution: Hepatic, renal, or thyroid dysfunction; asthma; peripheral vascular disease

Drug-Lab-Food Interactions

Increase bradycardia with digitalis; *increase* hypotensive effect with other antihypertensives, alcohol, anesthetics

Pharmacokinetics

Absorption: PO: 95%
Distribution: PB: 12%
Metabolism: t 1/2: 3–4 h
Excretion: In urine

Pharmacodynamics

PO: Onset: 15 min
　　Peak: 1.5 h
　　Duration: 10–19 h
IV: Onset: Immediate
　　Peak: 20 min
　　Duration: 5–10 h

Therapeutic Effects/Uses: To control hypertension.
Mode of Action: Promotion of blood pressure reduction via beta$_1$-blocking effect.

Side Effects

Fatigue, weakness, dizziness, nausea, vomiting, diarrhea, mental changes, nasal stuffiness

Adverse Reactions

Bradycardia, thrombocytopenia
Life-threatening: Complete heart block, bronchospasm, agranulocytosis

KEY: For complete abbreviation key, see inside front cover.

■ NURSING PROCESS: Antihypertensives: Beta Blockers

ASSESSMENT

- Obtain a medication history from the client. Report if a drug-drug interaction is probable.
- Obtain VS. Report abnormal blood pressure. Compare VS with baseline finding.
- Check laboratory values related to renal and liver function. An elevated BUN and serum creatinine may be caused by metoprolol or cardiac disorder. Elevated cardiac enzymes, such as AST and LHD, could result from use of metoprolol or from a cardiac disorder.

Antihypertensives: Beta Blockers

POTENTIAL NURSING DIAGNOSES
Decreased cardiac output
Noncompliance with drug regimen

PLANNING
- Client's blood pressure will be decreased and/or return to normal value.
- Client takes the medication as prescribed.

NURSING INTERVENTIONS
- Monitor VS, especially blood pressure and pulse.
- Monitor laboratory results, especially BUN, serum creatinine, AST, and LDH.

CLIENT TEACHING
General
- Instruct the client to comply with drug regimen: *abrupt discontinuation of the antihypertensive drug may cause rebound hypertension.*
- Suggest that the client avoid OTC drugs without first checking with the health care provider. Many OTC drugs carry warning against use in the presence of hypertension.
- Suggest that the client wear a Medic Alert bracelet or carry a card indicating the health problem and prescribed drugs.
- Instruct the client in a trauma situation to inform the physician of drugs taken daily, such as a beta blocker. Beta blockers block the compensatory effects of the body to the shock state. Glucagon may be needed to reverse the effects so that the client can be resuscitated.

Skill
- Instruct the client or family member how to take a radial pulse and blood pressure. Advise the client to report abnormal findings to the health care provider.

Diet
- Teach the client and family members nonpharmacologic methods to decrease blood pressure, such as a low-fat and low-salt diet, weight control, relaxation techniques, exercise, smoking cessation, and decreased alcohol ingestion (1–2 oz/d).
- Advise the client to report constipation. Foods high in fiber, a stool softener, and increased water intake (except in clients with CHF) are usually indicated.

Side Effects
- Advise the client that antihypertensives may cause dizziness due to orthostatic hypotension. Instruct the client to remain in a sitting position for several minutes before standing.
- Instruct the client to report dizziness, slow pulse rate, changes in blood pressure, heart palpitation, confusion, or GI upset to the health care provider.

EVALUATION
- Evaluate the effectiveness of the drug therapy, i.e., decreased blood pressure and the absence of side effects.
- Determine that the client is adhering to the drug regimen.

Antihypertensives: Beta Blockers and Central Alpha$_2$ Agonists

Generic (Brand)	Route and Dosage	Preg Cat	Interaction	t 1/2	PB	Onset	Peak	Duration
Beta-Adrenergic Blockers								
Acebutolol HCl (Sectral) Cardioselective beta$_1$	A: PO: 400–800 mg/d in 1 or 2 divided doses; max: 1,200 mg/d	B	*Increase* hypotensive effect with other antihypertensives and diuretics	3–13 h	26%	1 h	3–4 h	12–24 h
Atenolol (Tenormin) Cardioselective beta$_1$	A: PO: 25–100 mg/d	C	See acebutolol *Increase* absorption with anticholinergics; may *increase* lidocaine levels *Decrease* hypotensive effect with NSAIDs	6–7 h	6–16%	1 h	2–4 h	24 h
Betaxolol HCl (Kerlone) Cardioselective beta$_1$	A: PO: 10–20 mg /d Also for ophthalmic use: glaucoma	C	May *increase* hypotension with calcium channel blockers	14–22 h	UK	30 min	2 h	12 h
Bisoprolol fumarate (Zebeta) Beta$_1$ blocker	A: PO: Initially: 5 mg/d; maint: 2.5–20 mg/d	C	Similar to atenolol	9–12 h	<30%	UK	UK	UK
Carteolol HCl (Cartrol) Nonselective beta$_1$ and beta$_2$	A: PO: 2.5–5.0 mg/d	C	May *increase* hypoglycemia with insulin May *decrease* effect of theophylline; *decrease* blood pressure with aspirin and NSAIDs	4–6 h	23–30%	1 h	2–4 h	24–48 h

Metoprolol (Lopressor) Cardioselective beta$_1$	See Prototype Drug Chart					
Nadolol (Corgard) Nonselective beta$_1$ and beta$_2$	A: PO: 40–80 mg/d; max: 320 mg/d	C	Similar to acebutolol and atenolol	10–24 h	30%	1 h	2–4 h	18–24 h
Penbutolol SO$_4$ (Levatol)	A: PO: 10–20 mg /d; max: 80 mg/d	C	Similar to acebutolol Decrease hypoglycemic effect of glyburide	5 h	80–98%	1 h	2–3 h	20–24 h
Pindolol (Visken) Nonselective beta$_1$ and beta$_2$	A: PO: 5 mg b.i.d., t.i.d.; maint: 10–30 mg in divided doses; max: 60 mg/d in divided doses	B	Similar to acebutolol and atenolol	3–4 h	50%	3 h	1–2 h	24 h
Propranolol (Inderal) Nonselective beta$_1$ and beta$_2$	A: PO: Initially: 40 mg b.i.d. SR: 80 mg/d; maint: 120–240 mg/d in divided doses C: PO: Initially: 1 mg/kg/d in 2 divided doses; maint: 2 mg/kg/d	C	Similar to acebutolol and atenolol Increase effect with calcium channel blockers, phenothiazides Decrease absorption with antacid Lab: May increase AST, ALT, ALP, LDH, BUN	3–6 h	90%	0.5–1 h	1–1.5 h SR: 6 h	6–12 h
Timolol maleate (Blocadren) Nonselective beta$_1$ and beta$_2$	A: PO: Initially: 10 mg b.i.d.; maint: 20–40 mg/d in 2 divided doses; max: 60 mg/d Also for ophthalmic use: glaucoma	C	Similar to acebutolol	3–4 h	60%	1 h	2–4 h	12–24 h

continued

Antihypertensives: Beta Blockers and Central Alpha₂ Agonists—Continued

Generic (Brand)	Route and Dosage	Preg Cat	Interaction	t1/2	PB	Onset	Peak	Duration
Central Alpha₂ Agonists								
Clonidine HCl (Catapres)	A: PO: Initially: 0.1 mg b.i.d.; maint: 0.2–1.2 mg/d in divided doses max: 2.4 mg/d A: Transdermal patch: 100 µg (0.1 mg) b.i.d. or 200 µg (0.2 mg) q.d. or 300 µg (0.3 mg) q.d.	C	*Increase* hypotensive effect with diuretics, other anyihypertensives: *increase* CNS depression with alcohol, CNS depressants *Decrease* hypotensive effects with tricyclic antidepressants, MAOIs	6–20 h	20–40%	PO: 0.5–1 h Transdermal: 1–3 d	2–4 h 2–3 d	8 h 7 d
Guanabenz acetate (Wytensin)	A: PO: 4 mg b.i.d.; may increase to 4–8 mg/d q 1–2 wk; max: 32 mg b.i.d.	C	*Increase* CNS depression with alcohol, CNS depressants *Decrease* hypotensive effect with tricyclic antidepressants	4–14 h	90%	1 h	2–5 h	6–12 h
Guanfacine HCl (Tenex)	A: PO: 1 mg h.s.; may increase to 2–3 mg/d	B	Similar to guanabenz	>17 h	70%	1–2 h	2–6 h	24 h
Methyldopa (Aldomet)	A: PO: 250–500 mg b.i.d.; max: 3 g/d IV: 250 mg–1 g q6h C: PO: 10 mg/kg/d in 2–4 divided doses	C	May *increase* effect with tricyclic antidepressants, phenothiazides; *increase* hypotension with levodopa; *increase* risk of lithium toxicity *Decrease* effects of ephedrine	1.7 h	<15%	12–24 h	2–6 h	12–24 h

KEY: For complete abbreviation key, see inside front cover.

NOTES:

Prototype: Antihypertensives: Alpha-Adrenergic Blocker

Prazosin HCl

Prazosin HCl
 (Minipress)
Sympatholytic, selective alpha-adrenergic blocker
Pregnancy Category: C
Drug Forms:
Cap 1, 2.5 mg

Dosage

A: PO: 1 mg b.i.d./t.i.d.; maint: 3–15 mg/d; max: 20 mg/d in divided doses

Contraindications

Renal disease

Drug-Lab-Food Interactions

Increase hypotensive effect with other antihypertensives, nitrates, alcohol

Pharmacokinetics

Absorption: GI: 60% (5% to circulation)
Distribution: PB: 95%
Metabolism: t 1/2: 3 h
Excretion: 10% in urine; in bile and feces

Pharmacodynamics

IV: Onset: 0.5–2 h
 Peak: 2–4 h
 Duration: 10 h

Therapeutic Effects/Uses: To control hypertension, refractory CHF.

Mode of Action: Dilation of peripheral blood vessels via blocking the alpha-adrenergic receptors.

Side Effects

Dizziness, drowsiness, headache, nausea, vomiting, diarrhea, impotence, vertigo, urinary frequency, tinnitus, dry mouth, incontinence, abdominal discomfort

Adverse Reactions

Orthostatic hypotension, palpitations, tachycardia, pancreatitis

KEY: For complete abbreviation key, see inside front cover.

■ NURSING PROCESS: Antihypertensives: Adrenergic Blockers

ASSESSMENT

- Obtain a medication history from the client, including current drugs. Report if a drug-drug interaction is probable. Prazosin is highly protein-bound and can displace other highly protein-bound drugs.
- Obtain baseline VS and weight for future comparisons.
- Check urinary output. Report if it is decreased (<600 mL/d), because drug is contraindicated if renal disease is present.

Antihypertensives: Alpha-Adrenergic Blocker

POTENTIAL NURSING DIAGNOSES
High risk for activity intolerance
Knowledge deficit related to drug regimen
Altered sexuality patterns

PLANNING
- Client's blood pressure will decrease.
- Client will follow proper drug regimen.

NURSING INTERVENTIONS
- Monitor VS. The desired therapeutic effect of prazosin may not fully occur for 4 wk. A sudden marked decrease in blood pressure should be reported.
- Check daily for fluid retention in the extremities. Prazosin may cause sodium and water retention.

CLIENT TEACHING

General
- Instruct the client to comply with drug regimen. *Abrupt discontinuation of the antihypertensive drug may cause rebound hypertension.*
- Inform the client that orthostatic hypotension may occur. Explain that before arising, the client should dangle his or her feet.

Skill
- Instruct the client or family member how to take a blood pressure reading. A record for daily blood pressures should be kept.

Diet
- Encourage the client to decrease salt intake unless otherwise indicated by the health care provider.

Side Effects
- Caution the client that dizziness, lightheadedness, and drowsiness may occur, especially when the drug is first prescribed. If these symptoms occur, the health care provider should be notified.
- Inform the male client that impotence may occur if high doses of the drug are prescribed. This problem should be reported to the health care provider.
- Instruct the client to report if edema is present in the morning.
- Instruct the client not to take cold, cough, or allergy OTC medications without first contacting the health care provider.

EVALUATION
- Evaluate the effectiveness of the drug in controlling blood pressure and the absence of side effects.
- Evaluate the client's adherence to medication schedule.

Antihypertensives: Sympatholytics: Alpha-Adrenergic, Alpha-Beta, and Peripherally Acting Blockers; and Direct-Acting Vasodilators

Generic (Brand)	Route and Dosage	Preg Cat	Interaction	t1/2	PB	Onset	Peak	Duration
Selective Alpha-Adrenergic Blockers								
Doxazosin mesylate (Cardura)	A: PO: Initially: 1 mg/d; maint: 2–4 mg/d; max: 16 mg/d in divided doses	C	Similar to terazosin	22 h	98%	1.5–2 h	2–6 h	6–12 h
Prazosin HCl (Minipress)	See Prototype Drug Chart							
Terazosin HCl (Hytrin)	A: PO: Initially: 1 mg h.s.; maint: 1–5 mg/d; max: 20 mg/d	C	*Increase* hypotensive effect with diuretics, other antihypertensives, beta blockers, calcium channel blockers	9–12 h	95%	15 min	1–2 h	12–24 h
Alpha-Adrenergic Blockers								
Phenoxybenzamine HCl (Dibenzyline)	A: PO: Initially: 10 mg/d; maint: 20–40 mg/d C: PO: 0.2 mg/kg/d in 1–2 divided doses; may increase dose by 0.2 mg	C	Similar to phentolamine	24 h	UK	2 h	4–6 h	3–4 d
Phentolamine (Regitine)	A: IM/IV: 2.5–5 mg; repeat q5min until controlled; then q2–3h PRN C: IM/IV: 0.05–0.1 mg/kg; repeat if needed	C	*Increase* hypotensive effect with antihypertensives	20 min	UK	IM: 15–20 min IV: Immediate	IM: 20 min IV: 2 min	IM: 3–4 h IV: 15 min

Tolazoline HCl (Priscoline HCl)	NB: IV: Initially: 1–2 mg/kg; followed by 1–2 mg/kg/h for 24–48 h; expected effect within 30 min of initial dose A: IM/IV: 10–50 mg q.i.d.	C	*Increase* effect with alcohol, beta blockers, antihypertensives	3–10 h	UK	30 min	IM: 0.5–1 h	IM: 3–4 h

Peripherally Acting Sympatholytics

Guanadrel sulfate (Hylorel)	A: PO: Initially: 5 mg b.i.d.; maint: 20–75 mg/d in divided doses	B	Same as guanethidine	10–12 h	20%	1–2 h	4–6 h	6–12 h
Guanethidine monosulfate (Ismelin sulfate)	A: PO: Initially: 10 mg/d; maint: 25–50 mg/d; max: 300 mg/d C: PO: 0.2 mg/kg/d; max: 1–1.6 mg/kg/d	C	*Increase* hypotensive effect with diuretics, alcohol, antihypertensives, levodopa *Decrease* hypotensive effects with decongestants, tricyclic antidepressants, phenothiazides	5 d	UK	0.5–2 h	6–8 h	1–3 wk
Reserpine (Serpasil)	A: PO: Initially: 0.25–5.0 mg daily for 1–2 wk; maint: 0.1–0.25 mg/d	D	*Increase* hypotensive effect with diuretics, beta blockers antihypertensives; *increase* CNS depression with alcohol, narcotics, barbiturates; *increase* cardiac depression with antidysrhythmics	11–50 h	96%	Days to 2 wk	Initially: 2–4 h Later: 3–6 wk	1–6 wk

continued

Antihypertensives: Sympatholytics: Alpha-Adrenergic, Alpha-Beta, and Peripherally Acting Blockers; and Direct-Acting Vasodilators—*Continued*

Generic (Brand)	Route and Dosage	Preg Cat	Interaction	t1/2	PB	Onset	Peak	Duration
Direct-Acting Vasodilators								
Diazoxide (Hyperstat, Proglycem)	A & C: IV: 1–3 mg/kg in bolus (30 sec); repeat in 5–15 min as needed; max: 150 mg	C	*Increase* hypotensive hyperglycemia, hyperuricemia effect with thiazide diuretics	20–45 h	90%	1–2 min	5 min	3–12 h
Hydralazine HCl (Apresoline HCl)	A: PO: Initially: 10 mg q.i.d.; maint: 25–50 mg q.i.d. Severe hypertension: IM-IV: 10–40 mg; repeat as needed C: PO: 3–7.5 mg/kg/d in 4 divided doses	C	*Increase* hypotensive effects with diuretics, beta blockers, antihypertensives	2–8 h	87%	PO: 20–30 min IM: 10–30 min IV: 5–20 min	PO: 1–2 h IM: 1 h IV: 2–6 h	PO: 2–5 h IM: 2–6 h IV: 2–6 h

Drug	Dosage					
Minoxidil (Loniten, Rogaine, Minodyl)	A: PO: Initially: 5 mg/d; maint: 10–40 mg/d in single or divided doses; max: 100 mg/d C: PO: Initially: 0.2 mg/kg/d; max: 5 mg/d; maint: 0.25–1 mg/kg/d in divided doses; max: 50 mg/d *Topical for alopecia:* 2% sol b.i.d.	C	Similar to hydralazine *Lab:* May *increase* BUN, creatinine, ALP	3.5–4 h	0%	30 min	2–8 h	2–5 d
Sodium nitroprusside (Nipride, Nitropress)	A: IV: 1–3 µg/kg/min in D_5W; max: 10 µg/kg/min	C	None significant	2–7 d	UK	Immediate	2–5 min	10 min after infusion
Alpha- and Beta-Adrenergic Blocker								
Labetalol HCl (Trandate)	A: PO: Initially: 100 mg b.i.d.; maint: 200–800 mg/d in 2 divided doses A: IV: 2 mg/min in infusion; max: 300 mg as total dose	C	*Increase* hypotensive effect with diuretics, antihypertensives, nitrates, cimetidine, halothane; *increase* hypoglycemia with insulin, oral hypoglycemics *Decrease* effect with adrenergics, theophylline, lidocaine	4–8 h	50%	PO: 1–2 h IV: 2–5 min	PO: 2–4 h IV: 5–10 min	PO: 8–24 h IV: 2–4 h

KEY: For complete abbreviation key, see inside front cover.

Prototype: Antihypertensives: Angiotensin Antagonist

Captopril	Dosage
Captopril (Capoten); ✦ Apo-Captopril ACE inhibitor, angiotensin antagonist *Pregnancy Category:* C *Drug Forms:* Tab 12.5, 25, 50, 100 mg	A: PO: 12.5–25 mg b.i.d./t.i.d.; max: 450 mg/d; maint: 25–50 mg t.i.d.

Contraindications	Drug-Lab-Food Interactions
Heart block *Caution:* Leukemia, chronic obstructive pulmonary disease, renal or thyroid disease	*Increase* hypotensive effect with nitrates, diuretics, adrenergic blockers, vasodilators, other antihypertensives

Pharmacokinetics	Pharmacodynamics
Absorption: PO: 65% (food decreases absorption) *Distribution:* PB: UK *Metabolism:* t 1/2: 6–7 h *Excretion:* In urine	PO: Onset: 15 min Peak: 1 h Duration: 4–12 h

Therapeutic Uses/Effects: To reduce blood pressure; to control CHF.

Mode of Action: Suppression of the angiotensin-converting enzyme (ACE); inhibits angiotensin I conversion to angiotensin II.

Side Effects	Adverse Reactions
Dizziness, cough, nocturia, impotence, rash, polyuria, hyperkalemia, taste disturbance	Oliguria, urticaria, severe hypotension *Life-threatening:* Acute renal failure, bronchospasm, angioedema, agranulocytosis

KEY: For complete abbreviation key, see inside front cover.

■ NURSING PROCESS: Antihypertensives: Angiotensin Antagonist

ASSESSMENT

- Obtain a drug history from the client of current drugs that are being taken. Report if a drug-drug interaction is probable.
- Obtain baseline VS for future comparisons.
- Check the laboratory values for serum protein, albumin, BUN, and creatinine, and compare with future serum levels.

Antihypertensives: Angiotensin Antagonist

POTENTIAL NURSING DIAGNOSES
Knowledge deficit related to drug regimen
Anxiety related to hypertensive state

PLANNING
- Client's blood pressure will be within desired range
- Client is free of moderate to severe side effects

NURSING INTERVENTIONS
- Monitor laboratory tests related to renal function (BUN, creatinine, protein) and blood glucose levels. Caution: Watch for hypoglycemic reaction in a client with diabetes mellitus. Urine protein may be checked in the morning using a dipstick.
- Report to the health care provider occurrences of bruising, petechiae, and/or bleeding. These may indicate a severe adverse reaction to an angiotensin antagonist such as captopril.

CLIENT TEACHING
General
- Instruct the client not to abruptly discontinue use of captopril without notifying the health care provider. *Rebound hypertension could result.*
- Inform the client not to take OTC drugs (cold, allergy medications) without first contacting the health care provider.

Skill
- Teach the client how to take and record his or her blood pressure. Blood pressure chart should be established, and blood pressure changes should be reported.

Diet
- Instruct the client to take captopril 20 min–1 h before a meal. Food decreases 35% of captopril absorption.
- Inform the client that the taste of food may be diminished during the first month of drug therapy.

Side Effects
- Explain to the client that dizziness and/or lightheadedness may occur during the first week of captopril therapy. If dizziness persists, the health care provider should be notified.
- Instruct the client to report any occurrence of bleeding.

EVALUATION
- Evaluate the effectiveness of the drug therapy: in the absence of severe side effects and blood pressure return to desired range.

Antihypertensives: Angiotensin Antagonists and Calcium Blockers

Generic (Brand)	Route and Dosage	Preg Cat	Interaction	t1/2	PB	Onset	Peak	Duration
Angiotensin Antagonists (ACE Inhibitors)								
Benazepril HCl (Lotensin)	A: PO: Initially: 10 mg/d; maint: 20–40 mg/d in 2 divided doses	D	Similar to ramipril	10 h	97%	UK	1–2 h	20 h
Captopril (Capoten)	See Prototype Drug Chart							
Enalapril maleate (Vasotec)	A: PO: Initially: 5 mg/d; maint: 10–40 mg/d in 1–2 divided doses IV: 1.25 mg q6h infuse in 5 min	C	*Increase* hypotensive effects with diuretics, antihypertensives; may *increase* lithium levels; *increase* potassium levels with potassium-sparing diuretics, potassium supplements *Decrease* effect with antacids, NSAIDs, aspirin	1.5–2 h	50–60%	PO: 1 h IV: 15 min	PO: 4–8 h IV: 1–4 h	PO: 24 h IV: 6 h
Fosinopril (Monopril)	A: PO: 5–40 mg/d; max: 80 mg/d	C	Similar to enalapril	3–10 h	97%	1 h	2–6 h	24 h
Lisinopril (Prinivil, Zestril)	A: PO: Initially: 10 mg/d; maint: 20–40 mg/d; max: 80 mg/d	C	Similar to enalapril	12 h	0%	1 h	6–8 h	24 h

Quinapril HCl (Accupril)	A: PO: Initially: 10–20 mg; maint: 20–80 mg/d in 1–2 divided doses	D	Similar to enalapril	2 h	97%	1 h	2–4 h	24 h
Ramipril (Altrace)	A: PO: 2.5–5 mg/d; max: 20 mg/d	D	May *increase* effect with lithium; *increase* hypotension with diuretics; *increase* risk of hyperkalemia with potassium supplements, potassium-sparing diuretics	2–3 h	97%	2 h	6–8 h	24 h
Calcium Channel Blockers								
Diltiazem HCl (Cardizem, Cardizem CD or SR)	A: PO SR: Initially: 60–120 mg b.i.d.; max: 240–360 mg/d	C	May *increase* effects of theophylline, beta blockers, digoxin; *increase* effect with cimetidine	3.5–9 h	70–85%	PO SR: UK	PO SR: 6–11 h	PO SR: >12 h
Felodipine (Plendil)	A: PO: Initially: 5 mg; maint: 5–10 mg/d; max: 20 mg/d	C	*Increase* effect of beta blockers, digoxin; *increase* effect with histamine$_2$ blockers May *decrease* phenytoin, phenobarbital, carbamazepine *Lab:* May *increase* ALP, AST, ALT, CPK, LDH	10–16 h	99%	1–2 h	2–5 h	20–24 h

continued

Antihypertensives: Angiotensin Antagonists and Calcium Blockers —Continued

Generic (Brand)	Route and Dosage	Preg Cat	Interaction	t1/2	PB	Onset	Peak	Duration
Isradipine (DynaCirc)	*Hypertension:* A: PO: 1.25–10 mg b.i.d.; max: 20 mg/d	C	*Increase* effect of digoxin, cyclosporine	5–11 h	99%	1–2 h	2–3 h	12 h
Nifedipine (Procardia)	A: PO: 10–20 mg t.i.d. A: PO SR: 30–90 mg/d; max: 120 mg/d	C	*Increase* effect with cimetidine; *increase* effects of theophylline, beta blockers, antihypertensives	2–5 h	92–98%	PO: 20 min PO SR: UK	PO: 1–4 h PO SR: UK	PO: 6–8 h PO SR: 24 h
Verapamil (Calan SR, Isoptin SR)	A: PO SR: 120–240 mg/d in 2 divided doses; max: 480 mg/d	C	*Decrease* effect of lithium; other interactions similar to nifedipine	3–8 h	90%	PO SR: UK	PO SR: 4–8 h	PO SR: 24 h

KEY: For complete abbreviation key, see inside front cover.

NOTES:

Prototype: Anticoagulants

Warfarin sodium

Warfarin sodium
(Coumadin); ♦ Warfilone
Pregnancy Category: D
Drug Forms:
Tab 1, 2, 2.5, 5, 10 mg
Inj 50 mg/2 mL

Dosage

A: PO: LD: 10 mg/d for 2–3 d;
maint: 2–10 mg/d
Elderly: PO: 2.5 mg/d
IV: Dose is usually titrated according to PT or INR

Contraindications

Bleeding disorder, peptic ulcer, hepatic disease, blood dyscrasias, hemophilia, cerebral vascular accident (CVA), severe renal disease, eclampsia

Drug-Lab-Food Interactions

Increase effect with amiodarone, aspirin, NSAIDs, sulfonamides, thyroid drugs, allopurinol, histamine$_2$ blockers, oral hypoglycemics, metronidazole, miconazole, methyldopa, diuretics, oral antibiotics, vitamin E
Decrease effect with barbiturates, laxatives, phenytoin, estrogens, vitamins C and K, oral contraceptives, rifampin
Lab: May *increase* AST/ALT

Pharmacokinetics

Absorption: PO: Well absorbed
Distribution: PB: 99%
Metabolism: t 1/2: 0.5–3 d
Excretion: In urine and feces

Pharmacodynamics

PO: Onset: 12–24 h
Peak: 1–3 d
Duration: 2.5–5 d

Therapeutic Effects/Uses: To prevent blood clotting.

Mode of Action: Depression of hepatic synthesis of vitamin K–clotting factors (II, VII, IX, and X).

Side Effects

Anorexia, nausea, vomiting, diarrhea, abdominal cramps, rash, fever

Adverse Reactions

Bleeding, hematuria
Life-threatening: Hemorrhage, thrombocytopenia, agranulocytosis

KEY: For complete abbreviation key, see inside front cover.

Anticoagulants

■ NURSING PROCESS: Anticoagulants: Warfarin (Coumadin)

ASSESSMENT

- Obtain a history of abnormal clotting or health problems that affect clotting, such as severe alcoholism or severe liver or renal disease. Warfarin is contraindicated for clients with blood dyscrasias, peptic ulcer, cerebral vascular accident (CVA), hemophilia, or severe hypertension. Caution its use in a client with acute traumatic injury.
- Obtain a drug history of current drugs the client is taking. Report if a drug-drug interaction is probable. Warfarin is highly protein-bound and can displace other highly protein-bound drugs, or warfarin could be displaced, which may result in bleeding.
- Develop a flow chart that lists PT and warfarin dosages. A baseline PT should be taken before warfarin is administered.

POTENTIAL NURSING DIAGNOSES
High risk for injury (bleeding)
Knowledge deficit

PLANNING

- Client's PT will be 1.25 to 2.5 times the control level. For a client receiving heparin, the aPTT should be checked.
- Abnormal bleeding will be rapidly addressed while the client is taking an anticoagulant. The PT level will be closely monitored.

NURSING INTERVENTIONS

- Monitor VS. An increased pulse rate followed by a decreased systolic pressure can indicate a fluid volume deficit due to external or internal bleeding.
- Check PT for warfarin (Coumadin) and aPTT for heparin before administering the anticoagulant. The PT should be 1.25 to 2.5 times the control level. The platelet count should be monitored, because anticoagulants can decrease platelet count.
- Check for bleeding from the mouth, nose (epistaxis), urine (hematuria), and skin (petechiae, purpura).
- Check stools periodically for occult blood.
- Monitor elderly clients receiving warfarin closely for bleeding. Their skin is thin and capillary beds are fragile. PT should be frequently checked.
- Keep anticoagulant antagonists (protamine, vitamin K_1, or vitamin K_3) available when drug dose is increased or there are indications of frank bleeding. Fresh or frozen plasma may be needed for transfusion.

CLIENT TEACHING

General

- Instruct the client to inform the dentist when taking an anticoagulant. Contacting the health care provider may be necessary.
- Instruct the client to use a soft toothbrush to avoid causing the gums to bleed.
- Instruct the client to shave with an electric razor. Bleeding from shaving cuts may be difficult to control.
- Advise the client to have laboratory tests such as PT performed as ordered by the health care provider. Warfarin dose is regulated according to the PT.

Anticoagulants

• Instruct the client to carry or wear a medical identification card or jewelry (Medic Alert) listing the person's name, telephone number, and drug name.
• Encourage the client *not* to smoke. Smoking increases metabolism; thus, the warfarin dose may need to be increased. If the person insists on smoking, notify the health care provider.
• Instruct the client to check with the health care provider before taking OTC drugs. Aspirin should *not* be taken with warfarin because aspirin intensifies its action and bleeding is apt to occur. Suggest that the client use acetaminophen.
• Teach the client to control external hemorrhage (bleeding) from accidents or injuries by applying firm, direct pressure for at least 5–10 min with a clean, dry absorbent material.

Diet

• Advise the client to avoid alcohol, which could contribute to increased bleeding, and large amounts of green leafy vegetables, fish, liver, coffee, or tea (caffeine), which are rich in vitamin K.

Side Effects

• Advise the client to report bleeding, such as petechiae, ecchymosis, purpura, tarry stools, bleeding gums, or expectoration of blood.

EVALUATION

• Evaluate the effectiveness of drug therapy. Client's PT values are within the desired range, and client is free of significant side effects.

Anticoagulants, Antiplatelets, and Anticoagulant Antagonists

Generic (Brand)	Route and Dosage	Preg Cat	Interaction	t1/2	PB	Onset	Peak	Duration
Anticoagulants								
Dicumarol (Bishydroxycoumarin)	A: PO: LD: 200–300 mg/24 h; maint: 25–200 mg/d based on PT	D	*Increase* bleeding See warfarin	1–2 d	99%	Effect PT: 1–5 d	1–4 d	2–10 d
Enoxaparin sodium (Lovenox)	A: SC: 30 mg b.i.d.	B	*Increase* effect with other anticoagulants *Lab: Increase* AST, ALT	4.5 h	UK	UK	3 h	4–5 h
Heparin sodium (Lipo-Hepin)	A: SC: 5,000–7,500 units q6h or 8,000–10,000 units q8h A: IV: Bolus: 5,000 units Inf: 20,000–40,000 units over 24 h; dose varies according to APTT level C: IV: 50 units/kg bolus, 50–100 units/kg q4h or 20,000 units/m²/24 h	C	May *increase* bleeding with aspirin, NSAIDs *Decrease* effect with nitroglycerin, protamine *Lab: Increase* AST, ALT	1–1.5 h	95%	SC: 20–60 min IV: Rapid	SC: 5 min IV: 2 min	SC: 8–12 h IV: 2–6 h
Warfarin (Coumadin)	See Prototype Drug Chart							

continued

Anticoagulants, Antiplatelets, and Anticoagulant Antagonists—Continued

Generic (Brand)	Route and Dosage	Preg Cat	Interaction	t 1/2	PB	Onset	Peak	Duration
Dalteparin Na (Fragmin)	A: SC: 2500 IU/d for 5–10 d starting 1–2 h before surgery; repeat postop daily for 5–10 d	B	Similar to enoxaparin	UK	UK	1 h	4 h	UK
Antiplatelets								
Aspirin	A: PO: 325 mg/d or q.o.d.	D	*Increase* risk of bleeding with anticoagulant; *increase* risk of ulcer with glucocorticoids; *increase* risk of hypoglycemia with oral hypoglycemics *Lab: Decrease* potassium cholesterol, T_3, T_4	2–3 h	55%	15–30 min	1–2 h	4–6 h
Dipyridamole (Persantine)	A: PO: 50–100 mg t.i.d./q.i.d.	C	*Increase* effect with beta blockers, antidysrhythmics; *increase* antiplatelet effect with aspirin *Decrease* effect with phenytoin, rifampin	10–12 h	91–99%	0.5–1 h	1–2 h	6 h

Sulfinpyrazone (Anturane)	A: PO: 200–400 mg b.i.d.; max: 800 mg/d	C	*Increase* risk of hypoglycemia with oral hypoglycemics; *increase* PT with warfarin. *Decrease* effect with aspirin, theophyline	3 h	95–99%	<1 h	1–2 h	4–6 h
Anticoagulant Antagonists								
Protamine SO[4]	A: IV: Initially: 1 mg for 100 units heparin administered; 10–50 mg in 3–10 min slow push; max: 50 mg in any 10-min period	C	None significant	UK	UK	1–5 min	UK	2 h
Vitamin K$_1$, phytonadione (AquaMEPHYTON, Mephyton, Konakion)	A: PO/IM/IV: 2–10 mg q12–24 h as needed C: SC/IM: 5–10 mg	C	*Decrease* effects of warfarin, cholestyramine, colestipol	UK	UK	PO: 6–12 h SC/IM: 1–2 h IV: 15 min	SC/IM: 3–8 h Hemorrhage control	SC/IM 12–14 h
Vitamin K$_3$, menadiol sodium diphosphate	A: PO/SC/IM/IV: 5–10 mg/d C: PO: 50–100 µg/d	C: preterm, term, X	*Decrease* effects of warfarin; *decrease* absorption by mineral oil, sucralfate	UK	UK	SC/IM: 1–2	UK	8–24 h

KEY: For complete abbreviation key, see inside front cover.

Prototype: Thrombolytics

Streptokinase

Streptokinase
(Streptase, Kabikinase)
Thrombolytic enzyme
Pregnancy Category: C
Drug Forms:
Inj 250,000, 600,000, 750,000 IU

Dosage

Myocardial Infarction:
A: IV: 1,500,000 IU diluted in 45 mL; infuse over 60 min
Pulmonary Embolism (PE) and Deep Vein Thrombosis (DVT):
A: IV: LD: 250,000 IU
Inf: 100,000 IU/h for 24–72 h (24 h for PE; 72 h for DVT)

Contraindications

Recent CVA, cerebral neoplasm, active bleeding, severe hypertension, ulcerative colitis, anticoagulant therapy

Drug-Lab-Food Interactions

Increase risk of bleeding with heparin, oral anticoagulants, aspirin, antiplatelets, NSAIDs

Pharmacokinetics

Absorption: IV: Directly administered
Distribution: PB: UK
Metabolism: t 1/2: 20–80 min
Excretion: In urine and bile

Pharmacodynamics

IV: Onset: Immediate
Peak: Rapid
Duration: 4–12 h

Therapeutic Effects/Uses: To dissolve blood clots due to coronary artery thrombi, deep vein thrombosis, pulmonary embolism.

Mode of Action: Conversion of plasminogen to plasmin (fibrinolysis) for dissolving fibrin deposits.

Side Effects

Headache, nausea, flushing, rash, fever

Adverse Reactions

Bleeding, urticaria, unstable blood pressure
Life-threatening: Hemorrhage, bronchospasm, cardiac dysrhythmias, anaphylaxis

KEY: For complete abbreviation key, see inside front cover.

■ NURSING PROCESS: Thrombolytics: Streptokinase

ASSESSMENT

- Assess baseline VS and compare with future values.
- Check baseline PT value before administration of streptokinase.
- Obtain a medical and drug history. Contraindications for use of streptokinase include a recent CVA, active bleeding, severe hypertension, and anticoagulant therapy. It should be reported if the client is taking aspirin or NSAIDs. Thrombolytics are contraindicated for the client with a recent history of traumatic injury, especially head injury.

Thrombolytics

POTENTIAL NURSING DIAGNOSES
Decreased cardiac output
Anxiety related to severe health problem
Impaired tissue integrity

PLANNING
- The blood clot will be dissolved, and the client will be closely monitored for active bleeding.
- Client's VS will be monitored for stability during and after thrombolytic therapy.

NURSING INTERVENTIONS
- Monitor VS. Increased pulse rate followed by decreased blood pressure usually indicates blood loss and impending shock. Record VS and report changes.
- Observe for signs and symptoms of active bleeding from the mouth or rectum. Hemorrhage is a serious complication of thrombolytic treatment. Aminocaproic acid can be given as an intervention to stop the bleeding.
- Check for active bleeding for 24 h after thrombolytic therapy has been discontinued: q15min for the first hour, q30min until the eighth hour, and then hourly.
- Observe for signs of allergic reaction to streptokinase, such as itching, hives, flushing, fever, dyspnea, bronchospasm, hypotension, and/or cardiovascular collapse.
- Avoid administering aspirin or NSAIDs for pain or discomfort when the client is receiving a thrombolytic.
- Monitor the ECG for the presence of reperfusion dysrhythmias as the blood clot is dissolving; antidysrhythmic therapy may be indicated.

CLIENT TEACHING
General
- Explain the thrombolytic treatment to the client and family. Be supportive. If you cannot answer a question, refer the client or family to the health care provider.

Side Effects
- Instruct the client to report any side effects, such as lightheadedness, dizziness, palpitations, nausea, pruritus, or urticaria.

EVALUATION
- Determine the effectiveness of drug therapy. The client's clot has dissolved; VS are stable; there are no signs and symptoms of active bleeding; and the client is pain free.

Thrombolytics

Generic (Brand)	Route and Dosage	Preg Cat	Interaction	t1/2	PB	Onset	Peak	Duration
Thrombolytics								
Anistreplase (APSAC, Eminase)	A: IV: 30 U over 2–5 min	C	Similar to urokinase	1.5–2 h	UK	Immediate	45 min after injection	4–6 h
Streptokinase (Streptase, Kabikinase)	See Prototype Drug Chart							
Tissue-type plasminogen activator (t-PA, Alteplase)	*Acute Myocardial Infarction (AMI):* A: IV: Total: 100 mg over 1.5 h Bolus: 15 mg (over 2 min); then over 30 min: 0.75 mg/kg (not to exceed 50 mg) over 60 min: 0.5 mg/kg (not to exceed 35 mg) *Pulmonary embolism:* A: IV: 100 mg over 2 h	C	*Increase* risk of bleeding with aspirin, heparin, dipyridamole	30 min	UK	Rapid	10–45 min	UK

Urokinase (Abbokinase)	A: IV: LD: 4,400 IU/kg diluted over 10 min Inf: 4,400 IU/kg over 12–24 h *Occluded coronary artery:* Dose may be increased	B	*Increase* risk of bleeding with aspirin, NSAIDs, anticoagulants	10–20 min	UK	Rapid	3–4 h	4–12 h
Plasminogen Inactivator Aminocaproic acid (Amicar)	A: PO/IV: LD: 5 g first hour Inf: 1–1.25 g/h for 8 h; max: 30 g/d	C	*Increase* coagulation with estrogens, oral contraceptives; may *increase* serum potassium level	1–2 h	0%	0%	<2 h	UK

KEY: For complete abbreviation key, see inside front cover.

Prototype: Antilipemic

Lovastatin

Lovastatin
  (Mevacor)
Antilipemic, antihyperlipidemic
Pregnancy Category: X
Drug Forms:
Tab 20 mg

Dosage

A: PO: 20–80 mg/d in 1–2 divided doses with meals

Contraindications

Hepatic disease, pregnancy
Caution: Increase with alcohol consumption, seizure disorder, trauma

Drug-Lab-Food Interactions

Increase effect with other antilipemics; *increase* effect of Coumadin
Lab: May *increase* CPK, AST, ALT

Pharmacokinetics

Absorption: PO: 30%
Distribution: PB: 95%
Metabolism: t 1/2: 1–2 h
Excretion: 10% in urine, 80% in feces, bile

Pharmacodynamics

PO: Onset: 2–3 d
  Peak: UK
  Duration: UK

Therapeutic Effects/Uses: To control hypercholesterolemia; to decrease low-density lipoprotein (LDL); and to increase slightly high-density lipoprotein (HDL).

Mode of Action: Reduction of HMG-CoA reductase (enzyme), which inhibits cholesterol synthesis.

Side Effects

Nausea, diarrhea or constipation, abdominal pain or cramps, flatulence, dizziness, headache, blurred vision, rash, pruritus

Adverse Reactions

Hepatic dysfunction (elevated serum liver enzymes), myositis

KEY: For complete abbreviation key, see inside front cover.

Antilipemic

■ NURSING PROCESS: Antilipemics: Lovastatin (Mevacor) and Others

ASSESSMENT
- Assess VS and serum chemistry values (cholesterol, triglycerides, AST, ALT, CPK) for baseline values.
- Obtain a medical history. Lovastatin is contraindicated for clients with a liver disorder. Pregnancy category is X.

POTENTIAL NURSING DIAGNOSES
Impaired tissue integrity
Anxiety related to elevated cholesterol level

PLANNING
- Client's cholesterol level will be <200 mg/dL in 6–8 wk.
- Client will be taught to choose foods low in fat, cholesterol, and complex sugars.

NURSING INTERVENTIONS
- Monitor the client's blood lipid levels (cholesterol, triglycerides, low-density lipoprotein [LDL], and high-density lipoprotein [HDL] every 6–8 wk for the first 6 mo after lovastatin therapy and then every 3–6 mo. For lipid level profile, the client should fast for 12–14 h. Desired cholesterol value is <200 mg/dL; triglyceride value is <150 mg/dL (can vary); LDL is <130 mg/dL; and HDL is >60 mg/dL. Cholesterol levels of >240 mg/dL, LDL levels of >160 mg/dL, and HDL levels of >35 mg/dL can lead to severe cardiovascular or cerebral vascular accident.
- Monitor laboratory tests for liver function, such as ALT, ALP, and GGTP. Antilipemic drugs may cause liver disorder.
- Observe for signs and symptoms of GI upset. Taking the drug with sufficient water or with meals may alleviate some of the GI discomfort.

CLIENT TEACHING
General
- Advise the client that if there is a family history of hyperlipidemia, his or her children should have a baseline blood lipid level obtained and monitored. Instruct the client that children should decrease fatty foods in the diet.
- Emphasize the need to comply with the drug regimen to lower the blood lipids. Side effects should be reported to the health care provider.
- Inform the client that it may take several weeks before blood lipid levels decline. Explain that laboratory tests for blood lipids (cholesterol, triglycerides, LDL, and HDL) are usually ordered every 3–6 mo.
- Advise the client to have serum liver enzymes monitored as indicated by the health care provider. Lovastatin is contraindicated in acute hepatic disease and pregnancy.
- Instruct the client to have an annual eye examination and to report changes in visual acuity.

Clofibrate, Gemfibrozil, Probucol
- Advise the client taking clofibrate and probucol that decreased libido and impotence may occur and should be reported. Drug dosage can be changed or another antilipemic may be ordered.

Antilipemic

- Instruct diabetic or prediabetic clients to monitor blood glucose levels if they are taking gemfibrozil. Dietary changes or insulin adjustment may be necessary.
- Advise the client with cardiac dysrhythmias to tell the health care provider before starting probucol. Dysrhythmias should be monitored and reported.

Skill

Cholestyramine and Cholestipol

- Instruct the client to mix the powder well in water or juice.

Diet

- Explain to the client that GI discomfort is a common problem with most antilipemics. Suggest increasing fluid intake when taking the medication.
- Instruct the client to maintain a low-fat diet by eating foods that are low in animal fat, cholesterol, and complex sugars. Lovastatin and other antilipemics are not a substitute for a diet that is low in fat.

Nicotinic Acid

- Advise the client to take the drug with meals to decrease GI discomfort.

Side Effects

Cholestyramine, Cholestipol, and Nicotinic Acid (Niacin)

- Advise the client that constipation may occur with cholestyramine and cholestipol. Increasing fluid intake and food bulk should help in alleviating the problem.
- Explain to the client that flushing is common and should decrease with continued use of the drug. Usually, the drug is started at a low dose.

EVALUATION

- Evaluate the effectiveness of the antilipemic drug. The client's cholesterol level is within desired range.
- Determine that the client is on a low-fat, low-cholesterol diet.

Antilipemics

Generic (Brand)	Route and Dosage	Preg Cat	Interaction	t 1/2	PB	Onset	Peak	Duration
Cholestyramine resin (Questran)	A: PO: 4 g t.i.d. a.c. and hs; mix in 120–240 mL of fluid; max: 24 g/d	C	*Decrease* absorption of warfarin, digoxin, barbiturates, penicillins, tetracyclines, thyroid drugs, thiazides, iron, fat-soluble vitamins, folic acid *Lab: Increase* AST, ALT *Decrease* potassium and sodium levels	UK	UK	24–48 h	21 d	2–4 wk
Clofibrate (Atromid-S)	A: PO: 500 mg q.i.d.	C	*Increase* effects of insulin, oral hypoglycemics; *increase* risk of bleeding with warfarin; *increase* clofibrate effect with probenecid *Lab: Increase* AST, ALT, CPK	12–25 h	90–95%	UK	4–6 h	Weeks
Dextrothyroxine sodium (Choloxin)	A: PO: Initially: 1–2 mg/d; may increase monthly; maint: 4–8 mg/d; max: 8 mg/d C: PO: Initially: 0.05 mg/kg/d; max: 4 mg/d	C	May *alter* effects of oral anticoagulants	18 h	>90%	UK	UK	UK

continued

Antilipemics—Continued

Generic (Brand)	Route and Dosage	Preg Cat	Interaction	t 1/2	PB	Onset	Peak	Duration
Colestipol HCl (Colestid)	A: PO: 10–30 g/d in divided doses before meals	C	Same as cholestyramine	UK	UK	24–48 h	Within 1 mo	4 wk
Fenofibrate (Lipidil)	A: PO: 100 mg/d	UK	None known	UK	UK	UK	UK	UK
Fluvastatin (Lescol)	A: PO: Initially: 20 mg h.s.; maint: 20–40 mgs/d in 1 or 2 divided doses	B	*Decrease* effect with highly protein-bound drugs	UK	UK	UK	UK	UK
Gemfibrozil (Lopid)	A: PO: 600 mg b.i.d. before meals; max: 1,500 mg/d	B	*Increase* anticoagulant effect with warfarin *Lab:* May *increase* AST, ALT, ALP, LDH, bilirubin	1.5 h	90–95%	UK	1–2 h	UK
Lovastatin (Mevacor)	See Prototype Drug Chart							
Nicotinic acid (Niacin)	A: PO: Initially: 100 mg t.i.d.; maint: 1–3 g/d p.c. in 3 divided doses; max: 6 g/d	C	*Increase* hypotensive effect with antihypertensives	45 min	UK	Several days	0.5–1.2 h	UK
Pravastatin sodium (Pravachol)	A: PO: 10–40 mg/d	X	*Increase* effect of warfarin	1.5–2.5 h	55%	UK	1–1.5 h	UK

Probucol (Lorelco)	A: PO: 500 mg b.i.d. with meals	B	*Increase* risk of ventricular arrhythmia with tricyclic antidepressants, beta blockers, phenothiazines, digoxin, quinidine *Lab: Increase* AST, ALT, ALP, BUN, blood glucose	20 d	UK	UK	1–3 mo	6–8 mo
Simvastatin (Zocor)	A: PO: Initially: 5–10 mg/d in evening; maint: 20–40 mg/d in 1 or 2 divided doses; max 40 mg/d	X	May *increase* effect of digoxin; may *increase* bleeding with warfarin	UK	95%	Effect in 4 wk	1.3–2.4 h Max: 4 wk	UK

KEY: For complete abbreviation key, see inside front cover.

Prototype: Vasodilators

Isoxsuprine HCl

Isoxsuprine HCl
(Vasodilan, Voxsuprine)
Peripheral vasodilator,
beta-adrenergic agonist
Pregnancy Category: C
Drug Forms:
Tab 10, 20 mg

Dosage

A: PO: 10–20 mg t.i.d./q.i.d.

Contraindications

Arterial bleeding, severe hypotension, postpartum, tachycardia
Caution: Bleeding disorders, tachycardia

Drug-Lab-Food Interactions

Decrease blood pressure with antihypertensives

Pharmacokinetics

Absorption: PO: Readily absorbed
Distribution: BP: UK
Metabolism: t 1/2: 1.25–1.5 h
Excretion: In urine

Pharmacodynamics

PO: Onset: 0.5 h
    Peak: 1 h
    Duration: 3 h

Therapeutic Effects/Uses: To increase circulation due to peripheral vascular disease (Raynaud's disease, arteriosclerosis obliterans) are cerebrovascular insufficiency.
Mode of Action: Action is directly on vascular smooth muscle.

Side Effects

Nausea, vomiting, dizziness, syncope, weakness, tremors, rash, flushing, abdominal distention, chest pain

Adverse Reactions

Hypotension, tachycardia, palpitations

KEY: For complete abbreviation key, see inside front cover.

Vasodilators

■ NURSING PROCESS: Vasodilators: Isoxsuprine (Vasodilan)

ASSESSMENT
- Obtain baseline VS for future comparison.
- Assess for signs of inadequate blood flow to the extremities: pallor, coldness of extremity, and pain.

POTENTIAL NURSING DIAGNOSES
Impaired tissue integrity
Pain related to inadequate blood flow to extremity

PLANNING
- Client's blood flow to the extremities will improve, and the client's pain will be controlled.

NURSING INTERVENTIONS
- Monitor VS, especially blood pressure and heart rate. Tachycardia and orthostatic hypotension can be problematic with peripheral vasodilators.

CLIENT TEACHING
General
- Inform the client that a desired therapeutic response may take 1.5–3 mo.
- Advise the client not to smoke; smoking increases vasospasm.
- Instruct the client to use aspirin or aspirinlike compounds only with the health care provider approval. Salicylates help in preventing platelet aggregation.

Diet
- Advise the client with GI disturbances to take isoxsuprine with meals.
- Advise the client not to ingest alcohol with a vasodilator because it may cause a hypotensive reaction.

Side Effects
- Encourage the client to change position slowly but frequently to avoid orthostatic hypotension. Orthostatic hypotension is common when taking high doses of a vasodilator.
- Instruct the client to report side effects of isoxsuprine, such as flushing, headaches, and dizziness.

EVALUATION
- Evaluate the effectiveness of the isoxsuprine therapy; blood flow is increased in the extremities and pain has subsided.
- Client is experiencing no side effects from the prescribed drug.

Vasodilators (Peripheral)

Generic (Brand)	Route and Dosage	Preg Cat	Interaction	t1/2	PB	Action Onset	Action Peak	Action Duration
Alpha-Adrenergic Blocker								
Tolazoline HCl (Priscoline HCl)	A: SC/IM/IV: 10–50 mg q.i.d. NB: IV: Initially: 1–2 mg/kg, followed by 1–2 mg/kg/h for 24–48 h; initial dose effect: 30 min	C	May first *decrease* blood pressure, then *increase* with epinephrine, norepinephrine	Neonate: 3–10 h May be longer in adult	UK	30 min	1–2 h	3–4 h
Beta$_2$-Adrenergic Agonists								
Isoxsuprine HCl (Vasodilan)	See Prototype Drug Chart							
Nylidrin HCl (Arlidin)	A: PO: 3–12 mg t.i.d./q.i.d.	C	*Increase* hypotensive effect with antihypertensives, phenothiazines, other vasodilators	UK	UK	10 min	30 min	2h
Direct-Acting Peripheral Vasodilators								
Cyclandelate (Cyclospasmol)	A: PO: 20 mg q.i.d.; maint: 400–800 mg/d in 2–4 divided doses; dose may be reduced; max: 1,600 mg/d	C	May *increase* effects of alcohol, narcotics, tranquilizers (antipsychotics)	UK	UK	15 min	1–1.5 h	3–4 h

Ergoloid mesylates (Hydergine)	A: PO/SL: 1 mg t.i.d.; dose may increase to 4–12 mg/d	C	UK	3–12 h	UK	UK	1–3 h	UK
Nicotinyl alcohol (Ronigen)	A: PO: 150–300 mg b.i.d. (Canada only)	UK	UK	UK	UK	UK	UK	UK
Papaverine (Pavabid)	A: PO: 100–300 mg, 3–5 ×d SR: 150 mg q12h; max: 300 mg q12h IV: 30–120 mg q3h PRN	C	*Increase* hypotensive effect with antihypertensives, vasodilators, alcohol *Decrease* effect of levodopa	1.5 h	90%	15 min	1–2 h	3–6 h
Hemorrheologic Pentoxifylline (Trental)	A: PO: 400 mg t.i.d. with meals	C	*Increase* effect with cimetidine, other histamine$_2$ antagonists, warfarin Lab: *Decrease* calcium magnesium levels; *increase* theophylline levels	0.5–1 h	UK	UK	1–4 h	UK

KEY: For complete abbreviation key, see inside front cover.

GASTROINTESTINAL AGENTS

Antiemetics
Phenothiazines
Cannabinoids and Miscellaneous
Drugs for Motion Sickness

Emetics
Emetics and Adsorbent

Antidiarrheals
Opiates, Opiate-Related, and Adsorbents
Miscellaneous and Combinations

Laxatives
Osmotic and Contact
Bulk Forming, Emollients, and Evacuant

Antiulcers
Antacids
Anticholinergics
Histamine$_2$ Blockers
Pepsin Inhibitor, Gastric Acid Secretion Inhibitor, and Prostaglandin Analog

Prototype: Antiemetics: Phenothiazines

Perphenazine

Perphenazine
(Trilafon), ✤ Apo-Perphenazine
Phenothiazine antiemetic
Pregnancy Category: C
Drug Forms:
Tab 2, 4, 6, 8, 16 mg
Tab SR 8 mg
Sol 16 mg/5 mL
Inj 5 mg/mL

Dosage

A: PO: 8–16 mg/d in divided doses; max: 24 mg/d
IV: Max: 5 mg, diluted or slow IV drip
A&C >12 y: IM: 5–10 mg PRN; max: 15 mg ambulatory care; max: 30 mg acute care

Contraindications

Narrow-angle glaucoma, severe liver disease, intestinal obstruction, blood dyscrasias, bone marrow depression
Caution: Children <12 y, seizures, cardiovascular disease

Drug-Lab-Food Interactions

Increase effects of alcohol, sedative-hypnotics, beta-adrenergic blockers
Decrease levodopa, lithium, other phenothiazines
Toxicity with epinephrine
Lab: Increase liver and cardiac enzymes, cholesterol, blood sugar
Decrease hormones; false pregnancy test

Pharmacokinetics

Absorption: PO: Erratic absorption; liquid: absorption is increased
Distribution: PB: >90%
Metabolism: t 1/2: 8 h
Excretion: In urine and feces

Pharmacodynamics

PO: Onset: 2–6 h
    Peak: 2–4 h
    Duration: 6–12 h
IM: Onset: 10 min
    Peak: 1–2 h
    Duration: 6–12 h
IV: Onset: Rapid
    Peak: UK
    Duration: UK

Therapeutic Effects/Uses: To treat and prevent vomiting, especially from anticancer drug; to treat alcoholism.

Mode of Action: Effects of dopamine changed in CNS; inhibits medullary chemoreceptor trigger zone as antiemetic; anticholinergic blocking agent.

Side Effects

Anorexia, dry mouth and eyes, constipation, blurred vision, extrapyramidal symptoms, rash, photosensitivity, orthostatic hypotension, impotence, weight gain, amenorrhea, gynecomastia, transient leukopenia, pain at IM injection site

Adverse Reactions

Extrapyramidal syndrome (tardive dyskinesia, akathesia), tachycardia
Life-threatening: Agranulocytosis, respiratory depression, laryngospasm, allergic reactions, cardiac arrest

KEY: For complete abbreviation key, see inside front cover.

Antiemetics: Phenothiazines

■ NURSING PROCESS: Antiemetics: Phenothiazines

ASSESSMENT

- Obtain a history of the onset, frequency, and amount of vomiting and contents of the vomitus. If appropriate, elicit from the client possible causative factors such as food (seafood, mayonnaise).
- Obtain a history of present health problems. Clients with glaucoma should avoid many of the antiemetics.
- Assess VS for abnormalities and for future comparison.
- Assess urinalysis before and during therapy.

POTENTIAL NURSING DIAGNOSES

Altered nutrition: less than body requirements
High risk for fluid volume deficit related to vomiting

NURSING INTERVENTIONS

- Monitor VS. If vomiting is severe, dehydration may occur, and shocklike symptoms may be present.
- Monitor bowel sounds for hypoactivity or hyperactivity.
- Provide mouth care after vomiting. Encourage the client to maintain oral hygiene.

CLIENT TEACHING

General

- Instruct the client to store drug in tight, light-resistant container.
- Instruct the client to avoid OTC preparations.
- Instruct the client not to consume alcohol while taking antiemetics. Alcohol can intensify the sedative effect.
- Advise pregnant women to avoid antiemetics during the first trimester due to possible teratogenic effect on the fetus. Encourage them to seek medical advice about OTC or prescription antiemetics.

Side Effects

- Advise the client to report sore throat, fever, and mouth sores; notify health care provider and have blood drawn for a CBC.
- Instruct the client to avoid driving a motor vehicle or engage in dangerous activities because drowsiness is common with antiemetics. If drowsiness becomes a problem, a decrease in dosage may be indicated.
- Advise the client with a hepatic disorder to seek medical advice before taking phenothiazines. Instruct the client to report dizziness.
- Suggest to the client nonpharmacologic methods of alleviating nausea and vomiting such as flattened carbonated beverages, weak tea, crackers, and dry toast.

EVALUATION

- Evaluate the effectiveness of the nonpharmacologic methods or antiemetic by noting the absence of vomiting. Identify any side effects that may result from drug.

Antiemetics: Phenothiazines

Generic (Brand)	Route and Dosage	Preg Cat	Interaction	t½	PB	Onset	Peak	Duration
Chlorpromazine (Thorazine)	See Prototype Drug Chart for Antipsychotics							
Perphenazine (Trilafon)	See Prototype Drug Chart							
Prochlorperazine maleate (Compazine)	A: PO: IM: 5–10 mg, t.i.d./q.i.d., PRN SR: 10 mg q12h Rect: 5–25 mg PRN C: PO: Rect: 2.5 mg b.i.d./t.i.d.	C	*Increase* effect/toxicity with CNS depressants, anticonvulsants, epinephrine	23 h	≥90%	PO: 30–40 min SR: UK IM: 10–20 min Rect: 1h	UK	PO: 3–4 h SR: 12 h IM: 3–4 h Rect: 3–4 h
Thiethylperazine maleate (Torecan, Norzine)	A: PO/IM/PR: 10 mg q.d./t.i.d.	C	*Increase* anticholinergic effect with antidepressants *Decrease* absorption with antacids; *decrease* effects with barbiturates	UK	UK	PO: 30 min IM/PR: UK	UK UK	3–4 h UK
Triflupromazine (Vesprin)	A: PO: 20–30 mg/d A: IM: 5–15 mg q4–6h C: PO/IM: 0.2 mg/kg/d; max: 10 mg/d	C	Similar to chlorpromazine	UK	≥90%	20–40 min	UK	4 h

KEY: For complete abbreviation key, see inside front cover.

Antiemetics: Cannabinoids and Miscellaneous

Generic (Brand)	Route and Dosage	Preg Cat	Interaction	t 1/2	PB	Onset	Peak	Duration
Cannabinoids								
Dronabinol (Marinol) CSS II	*Chemotherapy-induced nausea:* A: PO: 5 mg/m² 1–3 h before chemotherapy; then q2–4h after; max: 15 mg/m²/dose	B	*Increase* drowsiness with alcohol, sedatives, CNS depressants	20–24 h	98%	UK	2h	6 h
Nabilone (Cesamet) CSS II	*Chemotherapy-induced nausea:* A: PO: 1–2 mg b.i.d. 1–3 h before chemotherapy, continue for 48 h after	B	*Increase* CNS depression with alcohol, other CNS depressants	2 h	UK	30–60 min	2h	8 h
Miscellaneous								
Benzoquinamide HCl (Emete-con)	A&C >12 y: IM: 50 mg q3–4h PRN IV: 25 mg or 0.2–0.4 mg/kg diluted in D_5W as one dose. Give remainder of doses as IM	C	*Increase* CNS depression with alcohol, sedative-hypnotics, antihistamines	30–45 min	60%	IM: 15 min IV: 15 min	30 min UK	3–4 h 3–4 h
Diphenidol HCl (Vontrol)	*Nausea, vomiting, vertigo:* A: PO:25–50 mg q4h C >6 y: PO: 0.9 mg/kg max: 5.5 mg/kg/d	C	None significant known	4 h	UK	30–45 min	1.5–3h	3–6 h
Droperidol (Inapsine)	A: IM/IV: 2.5–10 mg/0.5–1 h prior to surgery C 2–12 y: IM/IV: 0.88–0.165 mg/kg 0.5–1 h prior to surgery C <2 y: Not recommended	C	*Increase* effect/toxicity with CNS depressants, analgesics, epinephrine, atropine, lithium	2.5 h	UK	5–10 min	30 min	2–12 h

continued

Antiemetics: Cannabinoids and Miscellaneous—Continued

Generic (Brand)	Route and Dosage	Preg Cat	Interaction	t 1/2	PB	Onset	Peak	Duration
Granisetron (Kytril)	A: IV: 10 µg/kg 30 min before chemotherapy over 5 min	B	None significant	4–11 h	65%	1–3 h	UK	18–24 h
Hydroxyzine (Atarax, Vistaril)	See Antihistamines, p. 244							
Lorazepam (Ativan)	See Benzodiazepines, p. 75							
Metoclopramide monohydrochloride monohydrate (Reglan)	A: PO: 10 mg a.c. and h.s. IV: 2 mg/kg 30 min before chemotherapy; then repeat q2h for 2 doses; then q3h for 3 doses; infuse diluted solution over not less than 15 min	B	*Increase* effect with opiate analgesics	4–7 h	30%	PO: 30–60 min IV: 1–3 min	1–2 h 1–2 h	1–3 h 1–3 h
Ondansetron HCl (Zofran)	A: PO: 8 mg b.i.d. (1st dose 30 min before and 8 h after chemotherapy) IV: 0.15 mg/kg 30 min before chemotherapy; then 4 and 8 h after (total, 3 doses)	B	None significant	A: 4 h C: 2–3 h	70–75%	Rapid	15–30 min	4 h
Trimethobenzamide HCl (Tigan, Arrestin, Ticon)	A: PO: 250 mg t.i.d./q.i.d. IM/PR: 200 mg t.i.d./q.i.d. C >15 kg: PO/PR: 15–20 mg/kg/d divided in 3–4 doses or 100–200 mg t.i.d./q.i.d.	C	Similar to benzquinamide	UK	UK	PO: 10–40 min IM: 15–30 min PR: 10–40 min	UK UK UK	3–4 h 3–4 h 3–4 h

KEY: For complete abbreviation key, see inside front cover.

Antiemetics: Drugs for Motion Sickness

Generic (Brand)	Route and Dosage	Preg Cat	Interaction	t1/2	PB	Onset	Peak	Duration
Motion Sickness								
Buclizine HCl (Bucladin-S [Softab])	*Prophylaxis:* A: PO: 50 mg 0.5 h before travel; may repeat in 4–6 h	C	Increased toxicity with tricyclic antidepressants, MAOIs, CNS depressants	UK	UK	1 h	UK	4–6 h
Cyclizine HCl (Marezine)	A: PO: 50 mg 0.5 h before travel; may repeat in 4–6 h; max: 200 mg/d IM: 50 mg q4–6h PRN C 6–12 y: PO: 25 mg q.d./t.i.d. *Postoperative vomiting:* A: IM: 50 mg 0.5 h before surgery ends; may repeat q4–6h PRN	B	Increased toxicity with alcohol, CNS depressants	UK	UK	Rapid	UK	4–6 h
Dimenhydrinate (Calm-X, Dimetabs, Dramamine)	A: PO: 50–100 mg q4–6h; max: 400 mg/d; IM/IV: 50 mg PRN C 6–12 y: PO: 25–50 mg q6–8h; max: 150 mg/d C <6 y: Not recommended	B	Increased effects/toxicity with anticholinergics, tricyclic antidepressants, MAOIs, CNS depressants	UK	UK	PO: 15–30 min IV: Immediate IM: 20–30 min	1–2 h UK 1–2 h	3–6 h 3–6 h 3–6 h
Meclizine HCl (Antivert, Antrizine, Bonine)	A&C >12 y: PO: 25–50 mg 1 h before travel, after meal; may repeat q24h *Vertigo:* A: PO: 25–100 mg/d in divided doses	B	Increased toxicity with CNS depressants, anticholinergics, neuroleptics	6 h	UK	1–2 h	UK	8–24 h

KEY: *For complete abbreviation key, see inside front cover.*

Prototype: Emetics

Ipecac Syrup

Ipecac Syrup
Emetic
Pregnancy Category: C
Drug Forms:
Liq
Fluid/extract is 14 times more concentrated than syrup

Dosage

A: PO: 15–30 mL, followed by 200–300 mL tepid water
C: >1–12 y: PO: 15 mL, followed by 200–300 mL tepid water
C: <1 y: PO: 5–10 mL, followed by 100–200 mL tepid water
Repeat initial dose if > 1 yr if vomiting does not occur within 30 min

Contraindications

Hypersensitivity, depressed gag reflex, unconsciousness or semiconsciousness, poisoning with caustic or petroleum products, convulsions

Drug-Lab-Food Interactions

Decrease effect with activated charcoal, carbonated beverages, or milk

Pharmacokinetics

Absorption: Minimal
Distribution: PB: UK
Metabolism: t 1/2: UK
Excretion: GI

Pharmacodynamics

PO: Onset: 15–30 min
  Peak: UK
  Duration: 20–25 min

Therapeutic Effects/Uses: To induce vomiting after poisoning.

Mode of Action: Acts on chemoreceptor trigger zone (induces vomiting) and irritates gastric mucosa.

Side Effects

Diarrhea, sedation, lethargy, protracted vomiting

Adverse Reactions

Life-threatening: Cardiotoxicity if ipecac is not vomited (hypotension, tachycardia, chest pain)

KEY: For complete abbreviation key, see inside front cover.

■ NURSING PROCESS: Emetic: Ipecac Syrup

ASSESSMENT

- Determine the toxic substance ingested. Do *not* induce vomiting if caustics or petroleum products have been ingested.
- Determine the time elapsed since the ingestion; lavage may be indicated.
- Check the client's VS. Report abnormal findings.

Emetics

POTENTIAL NURSING DIAGNOSES
Potential risk for absorption of toxic substance
Potential risk for infection

PLANNING
- Toxic substance will be expelled before absorption. There will be no bodily harm due to the toxic substance.
- Client will be closely monitored for adverse effects of the toxic substance for 24–48 h depending on the substance.

NURSING INTERVENTIONS
- Call the poison control center to report the toxic ingestion and for instructions.
- Monitor VS. Report changes.
- Offer sufficient fluids with ipecac syrup; warm clear liquids are best: *no* milk or milk products. Have client in high Fowler's position. Fluids dilute the toxic substance and are vehicles for expelling the substance; avoid carbonated beverages as they cause abdominal distention. If emetic is unsuccessful, gastric lavage may be performed or activated charcoal given to adsorb the toxic substances.
- Do not offer ipecac syrup or fluids to a semiconscious or unconscious person because of the danger of aspiration. Gastric lavage is usually performed in such cases.
- Do not induce vomiting if the toxic substance is a caustic or a petroleum distillate.
- Prepare for forceful vomiting; have large basin ready, and move clothing to protected area.

CLIENT TEACHING
General
- Instruct the parent or other family member to have ipecac syrup on hand. Explain that ipecac syrup is an OTC drug.
- Explain to the parent that ipecac should be given with sufficient fluids. Advise that ipecac syrup is *not* given if the toxic substance is a caustic or petroleum product.
- Advise the client or parents to *never* remove toxic substances from original labeled containers. Instruct parents on the use of child safety caps for future prevention.
- Advise the parent to keep readily available the telephone numbers of the poison control center and all emergency services.

EVALUATION
- Evaluate the effectiveness of ipecac syrup for inducing vomiting.
- Continue monitoring VS.
- Continue monitoring for signs and symptoms related to effect of ingested substance.

Emetics and Adsorbent

Generic (Brand)	Route and Dosage	Preg Cat	Interaction	t 1/2	PB	Onset	Peak	Duration
Emetics								
Apomorphine CSS II	A: SC: 4–10 mg C: SC: 0.07–0.1 mg/kg; 100–200 mL of water or evaporated milk before injection; do not repeat	C	Do not use with iodines, iron preparations, tannins, oxidizing agents	UK	UK	A: 10–15 min C: 1–2 min	UK	Sedation: 2 h 2 h
Ipecac syrup (OTC preparation)	See Prototype Drug Chart							
Adsorbent								
Charcoal (Charcoaid, CharcoCaps)	*Charcoaid for poisonings:* 30 g/dose *CharcolCaps for flatulence:* 520 mg p.c.	C	Avoid sherbert, milk, ice cream *Decrease absorption of all PO meds*	NA	NA	UK	UK	UK

KEY: For complete abbreviation key, see inside front cover.

NOTES:

Prototype: Antidiarrheals

Diphenoxylate with atropine

Diphenoxylate with atropine (Lomotil)
Pregnancy Category: C
CSS V
Drug Forms:
Tab 2.5 mg (2.5 mg of diphenoxylate/0.025 mg atropine)

Dosage

A: PO: 2.5–5 mg b.i.d./q.i.d.
C: >2 y: PO: 0.3–0.4 mg/kg daily in 4 divided doses or 2 mg 3–5 × d; use liquid form only

Contraindications

Severe hepatic or renal disease, glaucoma, severe electrolyte imbalance, child <2 y

Drug-Lab-Food Interactions

Increase CNS depression with alcohol, antihistamines, narcotics, sedative-hypnotics; MAOIs may enhance hypertensive crisis

Lab: Increase serum liver enzymes, amylase

Pharmacokinetics

Absorption: PO: Well absorbed
Distribution: PB: UK
Metabolism: t 1/2: 2.5 h
Excretion: In feces and urine

Pharmacodynamics

PO: Onset: 45–60 min
  Peak: 2 h
  Duration: 3–4 h

Therapeutic Effects/Uses: To treat diarrhea by slowing intestinal motility.
Mode of Action: Inhibition of gastric motility.

Side Effects

Drowsiness, dizziness, constipation, dry mouth, weakness, flushing, rash, blurred vision, mydriasis, urine retention

Adverse Reactions

Angioneurotic edema
Life-threatening: Paralytic ileus, toxic megacolon, severe allergic reaction

KEY: For complete abbreviation key, see inside front cover.

■ NURSING PROCESS: Antidiarrheals

ASSESSMENT

- Obtain a history of any viral or bacterial infection, drugs taken, and foods ingested that could be contributing factors to diarrhea. Many of the antidiarrheals are contraindicated if the client has liver disease, narcotic dependence, ulcerative colitis, or glaucoma.
- Check VS to provide baseline for future comparison and to determine body fluid and electrolyte losses.
- Assess frequency and consistency of bowel movements.
- Assess bowel sounds. Hyperactive sounds can indicate increased intestinal motility.
- Report if the client has a narcotic drug history. If opiate or opiate-related antidiarrheals are given, drug misuse or abuse may occur.

Antidiarrheals

POTENTIAL NURSING DIAGNOSES
Diarrhea
Altered nutrition
Alteration in fluid volume

PLANNING
- Client's bowel movements will no longer be diarrhea.
- Client's body fluids will be restored.

NURSING INTERVENTIONS
- Monitor VS. Report tachycardia or a systolic blood pressure decrease of 10–15 mm Hg. Monitor respirations. Opiates and opiate-related drugs can cause CNS depression.
- Monitor the frequency of bowel movements and bowel sounds. Notify the health care provider if intestinal hypoactivity occurs when taking drug.
- Check for signs and symptoms of dehydration due to persistent diarrhea. Fluid replacement may be necessary. With prolonged diarrhea, check serum electrolytes.
- Administer antidiarrheals cautiously to clients with glaucoma, liver disorders, or ulcerative colitis or who are pregnant.
- Recognize that drug may need to be withheld if diarrhea continues for more than 48 h or acute abdominal pain develops.

CLIENT TEACHING

General
- Instruct the client not to take sedatives, tranquilizers, or other narcotics with drug. CNS depression may occur.
- Advise the client to avoid OTC preparations; they may contain alcohol.
- Instruct the client to take the drug only as prescribed. Drug may be habit forming; do not exceed recommended dose.
- Encourage the client to drink clear liquids. Advise the client not to ingest fried foods or milk products until after the diarrhea has stopped.
- Advise the client that constipation can result from the overuse of this drug.

EVALUATION
- Evaluate the effectiveness of the drug; diarrhea has stopped.
- Monitor long-term use of opiates and opiate-related drugs for possible abuse and physical dependence.
- Continue to monitor VS. Report abnormal changes.

Antidiarrheals: Opiates, Opiate Related, and Adsorbents

Generic (Brand)	Route and Dosage	Preg Cat	Interaction	t1/2	PB	Onset	Peak	Duration
Opiates								
Deodorized opium tincture CSS II	A: PO: 0.6 mL or 10 gtt q.i.d. mixed with water; max: 6 mL/d C: PO: 0.005–0.01 mL/kg/dose q3–4 h; max: 6 doses/d	B (D, at term in high doses or prolonged time)	*Increase* effects of CNS depressants, MAOIs, tricyclic antidepressants daily *Lab: Increase* ALT, AST daily	2–3 h	UK	UK	UK	4 h
Camphorated opium tincture (Paregoric) CSS III	Camphorated: 5–10 mL b.i.d./q.i.d. C: PO: 0.25–0.5 mL/kg daily—q.i.d.							
Opiate Related								
Diphenoxylate with atropine (Lomotil) CSS V	A: PO: 2.5–5 mg b.i.d.–q.i.d. C >2 y: 0.3–0.4 mg/kg daily in 4 divided doses or 2 mg 3–5 × d	C B	*Increase* effects with: MAOIs, alcohol, CNS depressants *Increase* effects with CNS depressants	2.5 h	UK	45–60 min	2 h	3–4 h

Drug	Dosage						
				7–12 h	98%	30–60 min	2 h	4–5 h
Loperamide HCl (Imodium)	A: PO: Initially: 4 mg; then 2 mg after each loose stool; max: 16 mg/d C 9–12 y: 2 mg t.i.d. 6–8 y: 2 mg b.i.d. 2–5 y: 1 mg t.i.d.							
Adsorbents								
Bismuth salts (Pepto-Bismol)	*Prevention of travelers' diarrhea:* A: PO: 2 tab q.i.d. a.c. and h.s. *Treatment:* A: PO: 2 tab or 30 mL q30–60 min PRN	UK	*Decrease* effects of tetracycline, aspirin	UK	UK	1 h	12 h	4 h
Kaolin-pectin (Kapectolin, Kaopectate)	A: 60–120 mL after each loose stool C 6–12 y: 30–60 mL after each loose stool	B	*Decrease* absorption of chloroquine, digitalis, tetracyclines, penicillamine	7–14 h	97%	30 min	UK	4 h

KEY: For complete abbreviation key, see inside front cover.

Antidiarrheals: Miscellaneous and Combinations

Generic (Brand)	Route and Dosage	Preg Cat	Interaction	t1/2	PB	Onset	Peak	Duration
Miscellaneous								
Colistin sulfate (Coly-Mycin S)	Infants & children: PO: 5–15 mg/kg/d in 3 divided doses q8h	C	*Increase* nephrotoxicity with vancomycin; amphotericin B; *increase* respiratory depression with aminoglycosides	3–5 h	UK	UK	1–2 h	8–12 h
Difenoxin and atropine (Motofen) CSS IV	A: PO: Initially: 2 mg; then 1 mg after each loose stool; max: 8 mg/d for 2 d C <2 y: Not recommended	C	*Increase* CNS depression with barbiturates, narcotics, CNS depressants, tranquilizers; avoid use with MAOIs	12–24 h	UK	45–60 min	2 h	3–4 h
Furazolidone (Furoxone)	A: PO: 100 mg q.i.d. C >1 mo: PO: 5–8 mg/kg/d in 4 divided doses; max: 400 mg/d	C	*Increase* toxicity of levodopa; *increase* effects with tricyclic antidepressants, MAOIs, narcotics, anorexiants Lab: False-positive for glucose with Clinitest	UK	UK	UK	UK	UK
Lactobacillus acidophilus and Lactobacillus bulgaricus (one or both) (Bacid [plus carboxymethylcellulose sodium], Lactinex, More-Dophilus)	A&C >3 y: PO: 2 cap 2–9×/d Granules: 1 pkg with cereal, food, water t.i.d/q.i.d. Powder: 1 tsp daily with fluid C <3 y: Not recommended	NR	None significant known	UK	UK	UK	UK	UK

Octreotide acetate (Sandostatin)	*Diarrhea related to carcinoid tumors:* A: SC: Initially: 0.05 mg/d in divided doses for 2 wk; then increase according to response; max: 0.75 mg/d	B	*Decrease* effects with cyclosporines	1.5 h	65%	UK	30 min	9–12 h
Combinations Diphenoxylate with atropine (Lomotil)	See Prototype Drug Chart							
*Kaolin, pectin, atropine SO$_4$, hyoscyamine SO$_4$, scopolamine hydrobromide (Donnagel)	A: PO: Initially: 30 mg; then 15–30 mg after each loose stool C: PO: 5–10 mg after each loose stool	C	Similar to diphenoxylate with atropine	UK	UK	UK	UK	UK
*Powdered opium, kaolin, pectin, hyoscyamine SO$_4$, atropine SO$_4$, scopolamine hydrobromide, alcohol (Donnagel-PG) CSS V	A: PO: 15 mg q3h	C	Similar to diphenoxylate with atropine	UK	UK	UK	UK	UK
Parapectolin CSS V	A&C >12 y: 15–30 mL after each loose stool; max: 120 mL/d C 6–12 y: 5–10 mL after each loose stool	C	*Increase* effect with depressants, MAOIs	UK	UK	UK	UK	UK

KEY: *For complete abbreviation key, see inside front cover.*
Not in common use due to atropine.

Prototype: Laxatives: Contact

Bisacodyl

Bisacodyl
  (Dulcolax), ✤ Apo-Bisacodyl
Contact laxative
Pregnancy Category: C
Drug Forms:
Enteric-coated tab 5 mg
Rectal supp 10 mg

Dosage

A: PO: 10–15 mg in A.M./P.M.; max: 30 mg
C: >3 y: PO: 5–10 mg; 0.3 mg/kg once daily
PO: Swallow whole; do not chew
A&C >6 y: Rectal supp: 5–10 mg
C <5 y & infants: 5 mg

Contraindications

Hypersensitivity, fecal impaction, intestinal/biliary obstruction, appendicitis, abdominal pain, nausea, vomiting, rectal fissures

Drug-Lab-Food Interactions

Decrease effect with antacids, histamine$_2$ blockers, milk

Pharmacokinetics

Absorption: Minimal absorption
Distribution: PB: UK
Metabolism: t 1/2: UK
Excretion: In bile and urine

Pharmacodynamics

PO: Onset: 10–15 min; act: 6–12 h
  Peak: UK
  Duration: UK
Rect: Onset: 15–25 min
  Peak: UK
  Duration: UK

Therapeutic Effects/Uses: Short-term treatment for constipation; bowel preparation for diagnostic tests.

Mode of Action: Increases peristalsis by direct effect on smooth muscle of intestine.

Side Effects

Anorexia, nausea, vomiting, cramps, diarrhea

Adverse Reactions

Dependence, hypokalemia
Life-threatening: Tetany

KEY: For complete abbreviation key, see inside front cover.

■ NURSING PROCESS: Laxatives: Contact

ASSESSMENT

- Obtain a history of constipation and possible causes such as insufficient water/fluid intake, diet deficient in bulk or fiber, or inactivity; a history of the frequency and consistency of stools; and the general health status.
- Obtain baseline VS for identification of abnormalities and for future comparisons.
- Assess renal function.
- Assess electrolyte balance of clients with frequent laxative use.

Laxatives: Contact

POTENTIAL NURSING DIAGNOSES
Constipation
Altered nutrition
High risk for fluid deficit
Knowledge deficit related to overuse of laxatives
Altered health maintenance

PLANNING
- Client will be free of constipation.
- Client will exercise, eat foods high in fiber, and have adequate fluid intake to avoid constipation.

NURSING INTERVENTIONS
- Monitor fluid intake and output. Note signs and symptoms of fluid and electrolyte imbalances that may result from watery stools. Habitual use of laxatives can cause fluid volume deficit and electrolyte losses.

CLIENT TEACHING

General
- Instruct the client to increase water intake, if not contraindicated, which will decrease hard, dry stools.
- Advise the client to avoid overuse of laxatives, which can lead to fluid and electrolyte imbalances and drug dependence. Suggest exercise to help increase peristalsis.
- Instruct the client not to chew the tablets; swallow them whole.
- Advise the client to store suppositories at <86°F.
- Advise the client to take the drug only with water to increase absorption.
- Instruct the client not to take drug within 1 h of any other drug.
- Remind the client that drug is not for long-term use; tone of bowel may be lost.
- Instruct the client to time administration of drug so as to not interfere with activities or sleep.

Diet
- Advise the client to increase foods rich in fiber such as bran, grains, and fruits.

Side Effects
- Instruct the client to discontinue use if rectal bleeding, nausea, vomiting, or cramping occurs.

EVALUATION
- Evaluate the effectiveness of nonpharmacologic methods for alleviating constipation.
- Evaluate the client's use of laxatives in managing constipation; constipation will be alleviated. Identify laxative abuse.

Laxatives: Osmotic and Contact

Generic (Brand)	Route and Dosage	Preg Cat	Interaction	t1/2	PB	Onset	Peak	Duration
Osmotics: Saline Glycerin	A: Supp: 3 g C <6 y: Supp: 1–1.5 g	C	None significant	30–45 min	UK	15–30 min	NA	NA
Lactulose (Cephulac, Cholac, Constilec, Enulose)	*Chronic Constipation:* A: PO: 30–60 mL/d PRN C: PO: 7.5 mL/d after breakfast	C	Do not give with other laxatives	UK	UK	24–48 h	UK	UK
Magnesium citrate (Citroma, Evac-Q-Mag)	A: PO: 120–240 mL C: PO: 4 mL/kg/dose or 1/2 adult dose	UK	*Increase* effects of neuromuscular blockers *Lab: Increase* magnesium level *Decrease* protein, calcium, potassium	UK	UK	0.5–3 h	UK	UK
Magnesium hydroxide (milk of magnesia)	A: PO: 20–60 mL/d C: PO: 0.5 mL/kg/dose	B	*Increase* effects of neuromuscular blockers *Decrease* absorption of digoxin, isoniazid, tetracyclines	UK	UK	4–8 h	UK	UK
Magnesium oxide (Maox, Mag-Ox)	A: PO: 2–4 g h.s. with 8 oz water Do not use in client with renal failure	B	*Decrease* effects of iron salts, digoxin, tetracyclines *Lab: Decrease* protein, calcium, potassium levels *Increase* magnesium level	UK	UK	4–8 h	UK	UK

Magnesium SO$_4$ (Epsom salts)	A: PO: 10–15 g in 8 oz water C: PO: 5–10 g in water	B	*Increase* CNS depression with barbiturates, anesthetics, CNS depressants	UK	UK	1–2 h	UK	UK
Sodium biphosphate (Fleet Phospho-Soda)	A: PO: 15–30 mL mixed in water	UK	None significant	UK	UK	PO: 0.5–3 h	UK	UK
Sodium phosphate with sodium biphosphate (Fleet enema)	*Enema:* A: 60–120 mL C: 30–60 mL	UK	None significant	UK	UK	Enema: 3–5 min	UK	UK
Contact							
Bisacodyl (Dulcolax)	See Prototype Drug Chart						
Cascara sagrada	A: PO: Tab: 325 mg/d Fluid extract: 1 mL/d Aromatic fluid extract: 5 mL/d	C	*Decrease* absorption of other oral medications	UK	UK	6–10 h	UK	UK
Castor oil (Emulsoil, Neoloid, Purge)	A: PO: 15–60 mL C 6–12 y: 5–15 mL	X	Similar to cascara sagrada	UK	UK	2–6 h	UK	UK
Phenolphthalein (Ex-Lax, Feen-A-Mint, Correctal)	A&C >12 y: 60–240 mg/d C 6–12 y: 30–60 mg	C	*Decrease* absorption of other oral medication	UK	UK	6–8 h	UK	2–3 d
Senna (Senokot)	A: PO: 1–4 tab or 1–4 tsp (granules) diluted in water	C	Similar to cascara sagrada	UK	UK	6–24 h	UK	UK

KEY: For complete abbreviation key, see inside front cover.

Prototype: Laxatives: Bulk Forming

Psyllium Hydrophilic Muciloid

Psyllium hydrophilic muciloid
 (Metamucil, Naturacil), ✤ Karasil
Bulk-forming laxative
Pregnancy Category: C
Drug Forms:
Chewable 1.7 g/piece
Powder 500, 600, 950 mg/g, 1 g/g

Dosage

A: PO: 1–2 tsp in 8 oz water/d
 followed by 8 oz water
C: >6 y: PO: 0.5–1 tsp in 4 oz water,
 followed by ≥4 oz water

Contraindications

Hypersensitivity, fecal impaction, intestinal obstruction, abdominal pain

Drug-Lab-Food Interactions

Decrease absorption of oral anticoagulants, aspirin, digoxin, nitrofurantoin

Pharmacokinetics

Absorption: Not absorbed
Distribution: PB: UK
Metabolism: t 1/2: UK
Excretion: In feces

Pharmacodynamics

PO: Onset: 10–24 h
 Peak: 1–3 d
 Duration: UK

Therapeutic Effects/Uses: To control chronic constipation.
Mode of Action: Bulk-forming laxative by drawing in water.

Side Effects

Anorexia, nausea, vomiting, cramps, diarrhea

Adverse Reactions

Esophageal and/or intestinal obstruction if not taken with adequate water
Life-threatening: Bronchospasm, anaphylaxis

KEY: For complete abbreviation key, see inside front cover.

■ NURSING PROCESS: Laxatives: Bulk Forming

ASSESSMENT

- Obtain a history of constipation and possible causes such as insufficient water/fluid intake, diet deficient in bulk or fiber, or inactivity; a history of the frequency and consistency of stools; and the general health status.
- Obtain baseline VS for identification of abnormalities and for future comparisons.
- Assess renal function, urine output, BUN, and serum creatinine.

Laxatives: Bulk Forming

POTENTIAL NURSING DIAGNOSES
Constipation
High risk for fluid deficit

PLANNING
- Client will be free of constipation.
- Client will exercise, eat foods high in fiber, and have adequate fluid intake to avoid constipation.

NURSING INTERVENTIONS
- Monitor fluid intake and output. Note signs and symptoms of fluid and electrolyte imbalances that may result from watery stools. Habitual use of laxatives can cause fluid volume deficit and electrolyte losses.
- Monitor bowel sounds.
- Identify the cause of constipation.
- Avoid inhalation of psyllium dust.

CLIENT TEACHING

General
- Instruct the client to mix drug with water immediately before use.
- Instruct the client to *not* swallow the drug in dry form.
- Advise the client to avoid overuse of laxatives, which can lead to fluid and electrolyte imbalances and drug dependence. Suggest exercise to help increase peristalsis.
- Advise the client to avoid inhaling psyllium dust; it may cause watery eyes, runny nose, and wheezing.

Diet
- Instruct the client to increase water intake, which will decrease hard, dry stools. Drink at least eight 8 oz glasses of fluids per day.
- Instruct the client to mix the drug in 8–10 oz of water, stir, and drink immediately. At least one glass of extra water should follow. Insufficient water can cause the drug to solidify and cause fecal impaction.
- Advise the client to increase foods rich in fiber such as bran, grains, and fruits.

Side Effects
- Instruct client to discontinue use if nausea, vomiting, cramping, or rectal bleeding occurs.

EVALUATION
- Evaluate the effectiveness of nonpharmacologic methods for alleviating constipation.
- Evaluate the client's use of laxatives in managing constipation. Identify laxative abuse.

Laxatives: Bulk Forming, Emollients, and Evacuants

Generic (Brand)	Route and Dosage	Preg Cat	Interaction	t1/2	PB	Action Onset	Action Peak	Action Duration
Bulk Forming								
Calcium polycarbophil (FiberCon, Fiberall, Mitrolan)	A: PO: 1 g, q.i.d. max: 6 g/d C 6–12 y: PO: 500 mg/d t.i.d.; max: 3 g C 2–5 y: PO: 500 mg/d b.i.d.; max: 1.5 g/d	C	*Decrease* absorption of tetracycline, digoxin, oral anticoagulants, potassium-sparing diuretics *Lab: Decrease* potassium	NA	NA	12–48 h	UK	UK
Methylcellulose (Cologel, Citrucel)	A: PO: 5–20 mL t.i.d. in 8–10 oz water C: 5–10 mL b.i.d. with 8 oz water	UK	*Decrease* absorption of salicylates, digitalis, antibiotics, oral anticoagulants	NA	NA	12–24 h	1–3 d	UK
Psyllium hydrophilic muciloid (Metamucil)	See Prototype Drug Chart							
Emollient: Stool Softeners								
Docusate calcium (Surfak)	A: PO: 240 mg/d C: PO: 60–120 mg/d	C	Similar to docusate sodium	NA	NA	12–72 h	UK	UK
Docusate potassium (Dialose)	A: PO: 100–300 mg/d	C	Similar to docusate sodium	NA	NA	12–72 h	UK	UK

Docusate sodium (Colace)	A: PO: 50–300 mg/d C >6 y: 40–120 mg/d	C	*Decrease* effect of aspirin, warfarin sodium *Increase* toxicity with mineral oil, phenolphthalein	NA	12–72 h	UK	UK
Docusate sodium with casanthranol (Peri-Colace)	A: PO: 1–2 cap/d C: PO: 1 cap/d	C	*Increase* absorption of mineral oil	NA	8–12 h	UK	UK
Emollient: Lubricant Mineral oil	A: PO: 15–45 mL/h.s. C 6–12 y: PO: 5–20 mL	UK	*Decrease* absorption of vitamins A, D, E, K	NA	6–8 h	UK	UK
Evacuant/Bowel Prep Polyethylene glycol–electrolyte solution (CoLyte, GoLYTELY)	Prep for GI exam requires 4 h; fasting for 3–4 h prior to dose A: PO: 240 mL q10–15 min for total of 4 L C: PO: 25–40 mL/kg/h for 4–10 h Administer via NGT to those unable or unwilling to drink solution (prepared with tap water and refrigerated)	C	Do not administer PO meds within 1 h of beginning drug	NA	30–60 min	UK	4 h

KEY: *For complete abbreviation key, see inside front cover.*

Prototype: Antiulcer: Antacids

Aluminum hydroxide	Dosage
Aluminum hydroxide (Amphojel, ALternaGEL, Alu-Tab) Antacid *Pregnancy Category:* C *Drug Forms:* Cap 475, 500 mg Tab 300, 500 mg Tab chewable 600 mg Liq 320 mg/5 mL, 600 mg/5 mL Susp (4%) 600 mg/5 mL	*Antacid:* A: PO: 600 mg 1 h p.c. and h.s.; chewed with water or milk Susp: 5–10 mL 1 h p.c. and h.s. *Hyperphosphatemia:* A: PO: 2 cap of 12.5 mL t.i.d./q.i.d. with meals

Contraindications	Drug-Lab-Food Interactions
Hypersensitivity to aluminum products, hypophosphatemia *Caution:* In elderly	*Decrease effects* with tetracycline, phenothiazine, isoniazid, phenytoin, digitalis, quinidine, amphetamines *Lab: Increase* urine pH

Pharmacokinetics	Pharmacodynamics
Absorption: PO: Small amount absorbed *Distribution:* PB: UK *Metabolism:* t 1/2: UK *Excretion:* In feces; small amount in urine	PO: Onset: 15–30 min Peak: 0.5 h Duration: 1–3 h

Therapeutic Effects/Uses: To treat hyperacidity, peptic ulcer, and reflux esophagitis; to reduce hyperphosphatemia.

Mode of Action: Neutralization of gastric acidity.

Side Effects	Adverse Reactions
Constipation	Hypophosphatemia, long term: GI obstruction

KEY: For complete abbreviation key, see inside front cover.

■ NURSING PROCESS: Antiulcer: Antacids

ASSESSMENT

- Assess the client's pain, including the type, duration, severity, and frequency.
- Assess the client's renal function.
- Assess for fluid and electrolyte imbalances, especially serum phosphate and calcium levels.
- Obtain drug history; report probable drug-drug interactions.

Antiulcer: Antacids

POTENTIAL NURSING DIAGNOSES
Pain
Knowledge deficit related to (mis)use of antacids

PLANNING
- Client will be free of abdominal pain after 1–2 wk of antiulcer drug management.

NURSING INTERVENTIONS
- Avoid administering antacids with other oral drugs, since antacids can delay their absorption. An antacid should definitely not be given with tetracycline, digoxin, or quinidine because it binds with and inactivates most of the drug. Antacids are given 1–2 h after other medications.
- Shake suspension well before administering: follow with water.
- Monitor urinary pH, calcium, and phosphate levels, and electrolytes.

CLIENT TEACHING
General
- Instruct the client to report pain, coughing, or vomiting of blood.
- Encourage client to drink 1 oz of water after antacid to ensure that the drug reaches the stomach.
- Advise the client to take the antacid 1–3 h after meals and at bedtime. Do not take antacids at mealtime; they slow gastric emptying time, causing increased GI activity and gastric secretions.
- Advise the client to notify the health care provider if constipation or diarrhea occurs; the antacid may have to be changed. Self-treatment should be avoided.
- Stress that antacids are not candy and that an unlimited amount is contraindicated.
- Advise the client to avoid taking acids with milk or foods high in vitamin D.
- Instruct the client to avoid taking antacids within 1–2 h of other oral medications since there may be interference with absorption.
- Advise the client to check antacid labels for sodium content if on a sodium-restricted diet.
- Alert the client to consult with the health care provider before taking self-prescribed antacids for longer than 2 wk.
- Instruct the client on the use of relaxation techniques.

Skill
- Instruct the client how to take antacids correctly. Chewable tablets should be thoroughly chewed and followed with water. With liquid antacid, 2–4 oz of water should follow the antacid.

Side Effects
- Advise the client to avoid foods and liquids that can cause gastric irritation, such as caffeine-containing beverages, alcohol, and spices.
- Advise that stools may become speckled or white.

EVALUATION
- Determine the effectiveness of the antiulcer treatment and the presence of side effects. The client should be free of pain, and healing should be progressing.

Antiulcer: Antacids

Generic (Brand)	Route and Dosage	Preg Cat	Interaction	t 1/2	PB	Onset	Peak	Duration
Aluminum carbonate (Basaljel)	A: PO: 10–30 mL or 2 tab/cap q2h Extra strength 5–15 mL	C	Similar to aluminum hydroxide	NA	NA	Slow	UK	Short
Aluminum hydroxide (Amphojel, ALternaGEL)	A: PO: 30 mL, 1–3 h p.c. and h.s. *Peptic ulcer disease:* A: PO: 15–45 mL 1–3 h p.c. and h.s. C: PO: 5–15 mL 1–3 h p.c. and h.s. *Prophylaxis GI bleeding:* A: PO: 30–60 mL qh C: PO: 5–15 mL q1–2h; maintain gastric pH >5	C	*Decrease* effects of digoxin, tetracyclines, isoniazid, corticosteroids, phenothiazine, histamine$_2$ antagonists	NA	NA	Slow	UK	Prolonged
Calcium carbonate (Tums, Dicarbosil)	A: PO: 2 tab or 10 mL q2h; max: 12 doses/d	C	*Decrease* absorption of tetracyclines *Lab:* Increase calcium level	UK	UK	UK	UK	UK
Dihydroxyaluminum sodium carbonate (Rolaids Antacid)	A: PO: Chew 1–2 tab PRN	C	*Decrease* absorption of quinolones, tetracyclines	UK	UK	Fast	UK	Moderate

Magaldrate (Riopan, Lowsium [plus simethicone])	A: PO: 5–15 mL PRN; max: 100 mL/d; or 1–2 tab PRN; max: 20 tab/d	C	*Decrease* absorption of phenothiazines, isoniazid, fluoroquinolones, tetracyclines	UK	UK	Immediate	UK	Prolonged
Magnesium hydroxide and aluminum hydroxide (Maalox)	A: PO: 2–4 tab PRN; max: 16 tab/d	UK	None significant known	UK	UK	Fast	UK	Short
Magnesium hydroxide, aluminum hydroxide, and calcium carbonate (Camalox)	A: PO: 10–20 mL PRN; max: 80 mL/d; or 2–4 tab PRN; max: 16 tab	UK	None significant known	UK	UK	Fast	UK	Prolonged
Magnesium hydroxide and aluminum hydroxide with simethicone (Aludrox, Mylanta, Mylanta III, Maalox Plus, Gelusil-I, Gelusil-II, Gelusil-M, Di-Gel)	A: PO: 10–20 mL PRN; max: 120 mL/d; or 2–4 tab PRN; max: 24 tab	UK	None significant known	UK	UK	UK	UK	UK
Magnesium trisilicate (Gaviscon)	A: PO: 1–2 tab PRN; max: 8 tab/d	UK	None significant known	UK	UK	Slow	UK	Prolonged
Sodium bicarbonate	A: PO: 0.5 tsp of powder in 8 oz water	C	*Increase* effects of amphetamines, quinidine, ephedrine *Decrease* effects of lithium, salicylates	UK	UK	Fast	UK	Short

KEY: For complete abbreviation key, see inside front cover.

Antiulcer: Anticholinergics

Generic (Brand)	Route and Dosage	Preg Cat	Interaction	t 1/2	PB	Onset	Peak	Duration
Belladonna tincture	A: PO: 0.3–1 mL t.i.d/q.i.d.	C	*Increase* cholinergic effects with MAOIs, antidepressants	18–36 h	UK	1–2 h	UK	4–6 h
Clidinium bromide and chlordiazepoxide HCl (Librax)	A: PO: 1–2 cap t.i.d/q.i.d. a.c., h.s.	C	Similar to belladonna	UK	UK	1 h	UK	3 h
Glycopyrrolate (Robinul)	A: PO: 1 mg b.i.d./t.i.d. IM/IV: 0.1–0.2 mg (100–200 µg) t.i.d/q.i.d.	B	Similar to belladonna	UK	UK	PO: 50 min IM: 20–45 min IV: 10–15 min	1 h 45 min 10–15 min	6 h 7 h 4 h
Propantheline bromine (Pro-Banthine)	A: PO: 15 mg t.i.d. a.c. and 30 mg h.s.	C	*Increase* cholinergic effects with antidepressants, atropine, antihistamines, phenothiazines	UK	UK	30–45 min	2–6 h	4–6 h
Tridihexethyl chloride (Pathilon)	A: PO: 25–50 mg t.i.d/q.i.d. a.c. and h.s.	C	Similar to belladonna	UK	UK	UK	UK	UK

KEY: *For complete abbreviation key, see inside front cover.*

NOTES:

Prototype: Antiulcer: Histamine$_2$ Blockers

Ranitidine

Ranitidine
 (Zantac)
Histamine$_2$ blocker
Pregnancy Category: B
Drug Forms:
Tab 150, 300 mg
Inj 25 mg/mL
OTC: 75 mg

Dosage

A: PO: 150 mg q12h or 300 mg h.s.;
 maint: 300 mg h.s.
IM: 50 mg q6–8 h
IV: 50 mg q6–8 h diluted 6.25
 mg/h over 24 h
C: PO: 2–4 mg/kg/d divided q12h
 IV: 1–2 mg/kg/d over 24 h
OTC: A: PO: 75 mg; max: 150 mg/d

Contraindications

Hypersensitivity, severe renal or liver disease
Caution: Pregnancy, lactation

Drug-Lab-Food Interactions

Decrease absorption with antacids; *decrease* absorption of ketoconazole; *toxicity* with metoprolol
Lab: Increase serum alkaline phosphatase

Pharmacokinetics

Absorption: PO: Well absorbed, 50%
Distribution: PB: 15%
Metabolism: t 1/2: 2–3 h
Excretion: In urine and feces

Pharmacodynamics

PO: Onset: 15 min
 Peak: 1–3 h
 Duration: 8–12 h
IM/IV: Onset: 10–15 min
 Peak: 15 min
 Duration: 8–12 h

Therapeutic Effects/Uses: To prevent and treat peptic ulcers, gastroesophageal reflux, and stress ulcers.

Mode of Action: Inhibition of gastric acid secretion by inhibiting histamine at histamine$_2$ receptors in parietal cells.

Side Effects

Headache, confusion, nausea, diarrhea or constipation, depression, rash, blurred vision, vertigo, malaise

Adverse Reactions

Life-threatening: Hepatotoxicity, cardiac dysrhythmias, blood dyscrasias

---

KEY: For complete abbreviation key, see inside front cover.

Antiulcer: Histamine$_2$ Blockers

■ NURSING PROCESS: Antiulcer: Histamine$_2$ Blockers

ASSESSMENT
- Assess the client's pain, including the type, duration, severity, frequency, and location.
- Assess GI complaints.
- Assess mental status.
- Assess fluid and electrolyte imbalances, including intake and output.
- Assess gastric pH (>5 is desired), BUN, and creatinine.
- Assess drug history; report probable drug-drug interactions.

POTENTIAL NURSING DIAGNOSES
Pain related to gastric dysfunction

PLANNING
- Client will no longer experience abdominal pain after 1–2 wk of drug therapy.

NURSING INTERVENTIONS
- Do not confuse drug with alprazolam (Xanax).
- Administer drug just before meals to decrease food-induced acid secretion.
- Be alert that reduced doses of drug are needed by the elderly, who have less gastric acid; need to prevent metabolic acidosis.
- Administer drug intravenously in 20–100 mL of IV solution.

CLIENT TEACHING
General
- Instruct the client to report pain, coughing, or vomiting of blood.
- Advise the client to avoid smoking because it can hamper the effectiveness of the drug.
- Remind the client that the drug must be taken exactly as prescribed to be effective.
- Instruct the client to separate ranitidine and antacid dosage by at least 1 h, if possible.
- Instruct the client not to drive a motor vehicle or engage in dangerous activities until stabilized on the drug.
- Tell the client that drug-induced impotence and gynecomastia are reversible.
- Instruct the client on the use of relaxation techniques to decrease anxiety.

Diet
- Advise the client to eat foods rich in vitamin B$_{12}$ to avoid deficiency as a result of drug therapy.
- Advise the client to avoid foods and liquids that can cause gastric irritation, such as caffeine-containing beverages, alcohol, and spices.

EVALUATION
- Determine the effectiveness of the drug therapy and the presence of any side effects or adverse reactions. The client should be free of pain, and healing should be progressing.

Antiulcer: Histamine₂ Blockers

Generic (Brand)	Route and Dosage	Preg Cat	Interaction	t1/2	PB	Onset	Peak	Duration
Cimetidine (Tagamet)	A: PO: 300 mg q.i.d. with meals and h.s. or 800 mg h.s.; maint: 300 mg h.s. IV: 37.5 mg/h (900 mg/d) over 24 h C: PO/IV: 10–40 mg/kg/d divided q6h	B	*Increase* effects of lidocaine, phenytoin, oral anticoagulants, theophylline *Decrease* effects of drug with smoking, antacids	1–2 h	20%	PO: 30 min IM/IV: 10–15 min	60–90 min 30 min	4–5 h 4–5 h
Famotidine (Pepcid)	A: PO: 20 mg q12h or 40 mg h.s.; maint: 20 mg h.s. IV: 20 mg q12h diluted C: PO: 1 mg/kg/d divided q8–12h C: IV: 0.6–0.8 mg/kg/d divided q8–12h Pepcid AC OTC	B	*Decrease* absorption with antacids; *decrease* effects of ketoconazole	2.5–4 h	15–20%	PO: 30–60 min IV: <1 h	1–4 h 1–3 h	6–12 h 8–15 h
Nizatidine (Axid)	A: PO: 150 mg q12h or 300 mg h.s.; maint: 150 mg h.s. Axid AR OTC 75 mg daily 30–60 min before eating; max: twice daily	B	*Increase* effects of salicylates *Decrease* effects with antacids	1.5 h	35%	UK	0.5–3 h	8–12 h
Ranitidine (Zantac)	See Prototype Drug Chart							

KEY: For complete abbreviation key, see inside front cover.

NOTES:

Prototype: Antiulcer: Pepsin Inhibitor

Sucralfate

Sucralfate
  (Carafate), ✢ Sulcrate
Antiulcer agent, pepsin inhibitor
Pregnancy Category: B
Drug Forms:
Tab 1 g

Dosage

Active Disease:
A: PO: 1 g q.i.d. 1 h a.c. and h.s.
Maintenance:
A: PO: 1 g b.i.d.

Contraindications

Hypersensitivity
Caution: Renal failure

Drug-Lab-Food Interactions

Decrease effects with tetracycline, phenytoin, fat-soluble vitamins, digoxin; *altered absorption* with ciprofloxacin, norfloxacin, antacids

Pharmacokinetics

Absorption: PO: Minimal absorption (<5%)
Distribution: PB: UK
Metabolism: t 1/2: 6–20 h
Excretion: In urine

Pharmacodynamics

PO: Onset: 30 min
  Peak: UK
  Duration: 5 h

Therapeutic Effects/Uses: To prevent gastric mucosal injury from drug-induced ulcers (aspirin, NSAIDs); to manage duodenal ulcers.

Mode of Action: In combination with gastric acid forms a protective covering on the ulcer surface.

Side Effects

Dizziness, nausea, constipation, dry mouth, rash, pruritus, back pain, sleepiness

Adverse Reactions

None significant

KEY: For complete abbreviation key, see inside front cover.

Antiulcer: Pepsin Inhibitor

■ NURSING PROCESS: Antiulcer: Pepsin Inhibitor

ASSESSMENT
- Assess the client's pain, including the type, duration, severity, and frequency. Ulcer pain usually occurs after meals and during the night.
- Assess the client's renal function. Report urine output of <600 mL/d or <25 mL/h.
- Assess for fluid and electrolyte imbalances.
- Assess gastric pH (>5 is desired).

POTENTIAL NURSING DIAGNOSES
Pain related to GI dysfunction

PLANNING
- Client will be free of abdominal pain after 1–2 wk of antiulcer drug management.

NURSING INTERVENTIONS
- Administer drug on empty stomach.
- Administer an antacid 30 min before or after sucralfate. Allow 1 to 2 h to elapse between sucralfate and other prescribed drugs; sucralfate binds with certain drugs such as tetracycline and phenytoin, thus reducing the effect of the other drugs.

CLIENT TEACHING

General
- Advise client to take drug exactly as ordered. Therapy usually requires 4–8 wk for optimal ulcer healing. Advise the client to continue to take drug even if feeling better.
- Increase fluids and dietary bulk, and exercise to relieve constipation.
- Instruct the client on the use of relaxation techniques.
- Monitor for severe, persistent constipation.
- Stress need for follow-up medical care.
- Emphasize cessation of smoking, as indicated.

Diet
- Advise the client to avoid foods and liquids that can cause gastric irritation, such as caffeine-containing beverages, alcohol, and spices.

Side Effects
- Instruct the client to report pain, coughing, or vomiting of blood.

EVALUATION
- Determine the effectiveness of the antiulcer treatment and the presence of any side effects. The client should be free of pain, and healing should be progressing.

Antiulcer: Pepsin Inhibitor, Gastric Acid Secretion Inhibitor, and Prostaglandin Analog

Generic (Brand)	Route and Dosage	Preg Cat	Interaction	t 1/2	PB	Onset	Peak	Duration
Pepsin Inhibitor Sucralfate (Carafate)	See Prototype Drug Chart							
Gastric Acid Secretion Inhibitor Lansoprazole (Prevacid)	*Duodenal ulcer:* A: PO: 15 mg/d for 4 wk a.c. *Erosive esophagitis:* A: PO: 30 mg/d for 8 wk a.c. *Zollinger-Ellison syndrome:* A: PO: Initially: 60 mg daily; increase as needed; daily doses > 120 mg in divided doses	B	*Decrease effects of digoxin, ketoconazole, theophylline Decrease effects with sucralfate*	30–90 min	95%	0.5–4 h	5 d	72–96 h
Omeprazole (Prilosec)	Gastroesophageal reflux disease (GERD) A: PO: 20 mg/d for 4–8 wk *Hypersecretory:* A: PO: Initially: 60 mg daily; may increase to 120 mg t.i.d. in divided doses up to 80 mg/d	C	*Increase levels of diazepam, warfarin, phenytoin*	1.5–3 h	97–99%	UK	0.5–3 h	UK
Prostaglandin Analog Misoprostol (Cytotec)	A: PO: 100–200 µg q.i.d. with food C <18 y: PO: Safety and efficacy not established	X	*Increase diarrhea with magnesium antacids*	1.5 h	85%	30 min	60–90 min	3–6 h

KEY: For complete abbreviation key, see inside front cover.

OPHTHALMIC AND OTIC AGENTS

Ophthalmic:
  Miotics: Cholinergics and
    Beta-Adrenergic Blockers
  Carbonic Anhydrase
    Inhibitors (CAIs)
  Osmotics
  Mydriatics and Cycloplegics
  Anti-Infectives
  Anti-Inflammatories

Otic:
  Anti-Infectives

Prototype: Miotics: Direct Acting

Pilocarpine

Pilocarpine
(Isopto Carpine, Pilopine HS, Ocusert Pilo-20 and -40)
Miotic
Pregnancy Category: C
Drug Forms:
Sol 0.25–10%
Ocusert Pilo-20 and -40 gel 4%

Dosage

A&C : sol: 1–2%, 1–2 gtt, t.i.d./q.i.d.
Gel: Apply 0.5-in ribbon in lower eyelid at bedtime
Ocusert: replaced q7 d

Contraindications

Retinal detachment, adhesions between iris and lens, acute ocular inflammation; must avoid systemic absorption of drug with coronary artery disease, obstruction of GI/GU tract, epilepsy, asthma

Drug-Lab-Food Interactions

Avoid use with carbachol and echothiophate
Decrease antiglaucoma effects with belladonna alkaloids; *decrease* dilation with phenylephrine

Pharmacokinetics

Absorption: Some systemic absorption
Distribution: PB: UK
Metabolism: t 1/2: UK; binds to ocular tissue
Excretion: UK

Pharmacodynamics

Miosis:
Ophthalmic: Onset: 10–30 min
Peak: 20 min
Duration: 4–8 h
Reduce IOP:
Ophthalmic: Onset: 45–60 min
Peak: 75 min
Duration: 4–14 h
Ocusert: Onset: 1 h
Peak: 1.5–2 h
Duration: 7 d
Gel: Onset: 1 h
Peak: 3–12 h
Duration: 18–24 h

Therapeutic Effects/Uses: To induce miosis; to decrease IOP in glaucoma.
Mode of Action: Stimulation of pupillary and ciliary sphincter muscles.

Side Effects

Blurred vision, eye pain, headache, eye irritation, brow ache, stinging and burning, nausea, vomiting, diarrhea, increased salivation and sweating, muscle tremors, contact allergy
Conjunctival irritation with Ocusert

Adverse Reactions

Dyspnea, hypertension, tachycardia, retinal detachment; long term: bronchospasm
Corneal abrasion and visual impairment potential with Ocusert

KEY: For complete abbreviation key, see inside front cover.

Miotics

■ NURSING PROCESS: Miotics

ASSESSMENT
- Obtain medical and drug history. Miotics are contraindicated in clients with narrow-angle glaucoma, acute inflammation of the eye, heart block, coronary heart disease, obstruction of the GI and/or GU tracts, and asthma. Report probable drug-drug interactions.
- Assess VS. Baseline VS can be compared with future findings.
- Assess the client's level of anxiety. The possibility of diminished vision or blindness increases anxiety.
- Assess the client's eye pigment. Heavily pigmented eyes may benefit from pilocarpine concentration of <4%.

POTENTIAL NURSING DIAGNOSES
Altered visual perception
High risk for injury

PLANNING
- Client will take miotics as prescribed.
- Client's intraocular pressure will decrease and be within the accepted range.

NURSING INTERVENTIONS
- Apply gentle pressure to the inner canthus when administering eye drops to prevent or minimize systemic absorption.
- Monitor VS. Heart rate and blood pressure may decrease with large doses of cholinergics.
- Monitor for side effects, such as headache, eye pain, and decreased vision.
- Monitor for postural hypotension. Instruct the client to arise slowly from a recumbent position.
- Check breath sounds for rales and rhonchi; cholinergics can cause bronchospasm and increase bronchial secretions.
- Maintain oral hygiene with excessive salivation.
- Have atropine available for antidote for pilocarpine.

CLIENT TEACHING

General
- Instruct the client not to use discolored solution.
- Instruct the client not to rinse the dropper; do not touch tip of dropper to any surface.
- Encourage the client not to close eyes tightly or blink frequently.
- Instruct the client on need for regular and ongoing medical supervision.
- Instruct the client to increase light for reading; dim light reduces acuity.
- Advise the client to avoid driving motor vehicles or engaging in dangerous activities while vision is impaired.
- Alert the client that long-term drug therapy is a possibility.
- Instruct the client on the use of relaxation techniques for decreasing anxiety, if indicated.
- Instruct the client with glaucoma to avoid atropinelike-drugs because they increase intraocular pressure. Clients should check drug label on OTC preparations.

Miotics

- Instruct the client not to suddenly stop medication without prior approval of health care provider.

Skill

- Instruct the client or family on correct administration of eye drops; include return demonstration.
  1. WASH HANDS.
  2. Instruct the client to lie or sit down and to look up toward the ceiling.
  3. Gently draw skin down below the affected eye to expose the conjunctival sac.
  4. Administer the prescribed number of drops into the center or outer aspect of the sac. Medication placed directly on the cornea can cause discomfort and/or damage. Do not touch eyelids or eyelashes with dropper.
  5. Gently press on lacrimal duct with sterile cotton ball or tissue for 1–2 min after instillation of drops to prevent systemic absorption through lacrimal canal.
  6. Client should keep eyes gently closed for 1–2 min after instillation to promote absorption.

Side Effects

- Advise the client that blurred vision after drug administration decreases with repeated use of drug.

OCULAR THERAPEUTIC SYSTEMS (OCUSERT)

- Instruct the client to follow directions related to insertion and removal.
- Wash hands with soap and water thoroughly before insertion.
- Store drug in refrigerator.
- Instruct the client to check for presence of disc in conjunctival sac at bedtime and when arising. Discard damaged or contaminated discs.
- Explain that myopia is minimized by bedtime insertion of drug in the upper conjunctival sac.
- Explain that temporary stinging is expected; notify health care provider if blurred vision or brow pain occurs.

EVALUATION

- Evaluate the effectiveness of drug.
- Intraocular pressure will be within the desired range.

Miotics: Cholinergics and Beta-Adrenergic Blockers

Generic (Brand)	Route and Dosage	Preg Cat	Interaction	t 1/2	PB	Onset	Peak	Duration
Direct-Acting Cholinergics								
Acetylcholine Cl (Miochol)	A: Intraocular: 5–20 mg of 1% sol injected in anterior chamber before or after suturing	C	*Decrease* effects with suprofen, flurbiprofen	NA	NA	Miosis: Prompt	UK	10 min
Carbachol Intraocular (Miostat)	A: Ophthalmic: 1–2 gtt 1–4 × d A: IO: 0.5 mL into anterior chamber before or after suturing	C	Similar to pilocarpine	NA	NA	Ophthalmic: 10–20 min IO: 2–5 min	UK	IOP: 4–8 h 24 h
Pilocarpine HCl (Isopto Carpine)	See Prototype Drug Chart							
Pilocarpine nitrate (Ocusert Pilo-20, Pilo-40)	See Prototype Drug Chart							
Echothiophate iodide (Phospholine Iodide)	A: 0.03–0.25% sol: 1 gtt q.d./b.i.d.	C	*Increase* toxicity with carbamate pesticides, succinylcholine	NA	NA	Miosis: 10–30 min IOP: 4–8 h	UK	1–4 wk
Indirect-Acting Cholinesterase Inhibitors: Short Acting								
Physostigmine salicylate (Isopto Eserine)	A&C: Oint 0.25%: 1/4 in up to 3 × d Sol 0.25–0.5%: 1–2 gtt q.d./q.i.d.	C	*Decrease* cholinergic effects with antidepressants, atropine, phenothiazines, antihistamines; atropine *decreases* optimal effects	NA	NA	Miosis: 20–30 min Decrease IOP: UK	UK 2–6 h	12–36 h 12–36 h

continued

Miotics: Cholinergics and Beta-Adrenergic Blockers — Continued

Generic (Brand)	Route and Dosage	Preg Cat	Interaction	t1/2	PB	Onset	Peak	Duration
Long-Acting								
Demecarium bromide (Humorsol)	A: Sol 0.125–0.25%: 1–2 gtt 2×wk or 1–2 gtt b.i.d.	X	Similar to physostigmine salicylate	NA	NA	Miosis: 15–60 min IOP: UK	2–4 h 24 h	3–10 d 7–28 d
Isoflurophate (Floropryl)	A&C: Oint 0.025%: 0.5 cm daily for 2 wk; then decrease to q2–7 d	X	Additive effects of anticholinesterase drugs	NA	NA	Miosis: 5–10 min Decrease IOP: UK	20–30 min 24 h	1–4 wk 1 wk
Beta-Adrenergic Blockers								
Betaxolol HCl (Betoptic)	0.25% susp or 0.5% sol: Usual dose: 1 gt b.i.d.	C	*Increase* effects with other ocular hypotensives *Lab:* Alters GTT	15–20 h	UK	30 min	2 h	12 h
Levobunolol HCl (Betagan Liquifilm)	0.25–0.5% sol: 1–2 gtt q.d./b.i.d.	C	Similar to betaxolol	60–90 min	UK	45–60 min	2–6 h	12–24 h
Timolol maleate (Timoptic)	A: Sol 0.25% or 0.5%: Initially: 1 gt b.i.d.; maint: 1 gt q.d. once response occurs with initial dosage	C	Additive effects with systemic beta blockers *Increase* effect of quinidine, verapamil *Decrease* effects of theophylline, isoproterenol *Lab: Increase* liver function tests, BUN, serum potassium *Decrease* hemoglobin, hematocrit	4 h	10%	30 min	1–2 h	12–24 h

KEY: For complete abbreviation key, see inside front cover.

Carbonic Anhydrase Inhibitors (CAIs)

Generic (Brand)	Route and Dosage	Preg Cat	Interaction	t 1/2	PB	Onset	Peak	Duration
Acetazolamide (Diamox)	A: PO: 250–1000 mg daily given in divided doses for amounts >250 mg; doses >1000 mg show no increased benefit	C	*Increase* toxicity of CAI with salicylates, cyclosporine *Decrease* effect with phenobarbital	2–6 h	UK	PO: SR 2 h IV: 2 min PO: 1–1.5 h	3–6 h 15 min 1–4 h	18–24 h 4–5 h 8–12 h
Dichlorphenamide (Daranide)	A: PO: Initially: 100–200 mg; then 100 mg q12h until desired results; maint: 25–50 mg q.d./t.i.d.; given with miotics	C	*Decrease* excretion of ephedrine, procainamide, tricyclic antidepressants *Increase* excretion of lithium, phenobarbital	UK	UK	1 h	2–4 h	6–12 h
Dorzolamide HCl (Trusopt)	A: 2% sol: 1 gt t.i.d.	UK	Avoid use of oral CAIs due to additive effect	UK	UK	UK	UK	UK
Methazolamide (Neptazane)	A: PO: 50–100 mg b.i.d./t.i.d.	C	May induce digitalis and salicylate toxicities due to hypokalemia	14 h	UK	2–4 h	6–8 h	10–18 h

KEY: For complete abbreviation key, see inside front cover.

Osmotics

Generic (Brand)	Route and Dosage	Preg Cat	Interaction	t 1/2	PB	Onset	Peak	Duration
Glycerin	A: PO: 1–1.5 g/kg 1–1.5 h before surgery	C	None significant reported	30–45 min	UK	Decrease IOP: 10–30 min Decrease ICP: 10–60 min	1–1.5 h	4–8 h
Isosorbide (Ismotic)	A: PO: 45% sol 1.5–3 g/kg b.i.d./q.i.d. IV: 15–25% sol 1.5–2 g/kg over 30–60 min	C	None significant reported	5–9.5 h	UK	10–30 min	1–1.5 h	2–3 h / 5–6 h
Mannitol (Osmitrol)	A: IV: 15–20% sol 1.5–2 g/kg over 30–60 min	C	*Decrease* effect with lithium	15–100 min	UK	30–60 min Decrease ICP: 15 min	1 h	6–8 h
Urea (Ureaphil)	A: IV: 30% sol 1–1.5 g/kg; over 1–3 h; max: 4 mL/min C >2 y: IV: 0.5-1.5 g/kg; max: 4 mL/min C <2 y: IV: 0.1 g/kg; max: 4 mL/min	C	*Decrease* effect with lithium	<60 min	UK	30–45 min	1–2 h	5–6 h

KEY: For complete abbreviation key, see inside front cover.

Mydriatics and Cycloplegics

Generic (Brand)	Route and Dosage	Preg Cat	Interaction*	t1/2	PB	Onset	Peak	Duration
Atropine sulfate (Isopto Atropine)	A: Sol 1%: 1–2 gtt up to q.i.d. C: Sol 0.5% 1–2 gtt up to t.i.d. 1% oint: Apply in lower eyelid sac up to t.i.d.	C	May *decrease* effects with miotics	NA	NA	M: 30–60 min C: 1–2 h	30–60 min 1–2 h	5–12 d 5–6 d
Cyclopentolate HCl (Cyclogyl)	A: Sol 0.5–2%: 1–2 gtt; then 1 gt in 5 min C: 1–2 gtt ×1; may repeat ×1 in 5–10 min with 0.5% or 1% sol	C	*Decrease* effect of cholinesterase inhibitors, carbachol	NA	NA	M&C: 10–15 min	25–60 min	6–24 h
Dipivefrin HCl (Propine)	A: Sol 0.1%; 1 gt q12h	B	*Increase* effects with other agents to decrease IOP	NA	NA	M: 30 min C: <30 min	1 h 1 h	6 h 12+ h
Epinephrine HCl (Epifrin, Glaucon)	A&C: Sol 0.1–2%: 1–2 gtt q.d./b.i.d.	C	Inactivates chymotrypsin, ophthalmic beta blockers Use with MAOIs may lead to hypertensive crises	NA	NA	<5 min	30 min	12 h
Epinephrine borate (Epinal, Eppy/N)	*Surgery:* A: 0.5–1% sol: Instill 1–2 gtt ≤3× *Open angle glaucoma:* A: 0.5% or 1.0% sol: Instill 1 gt in eye b.i.d.	C	*Increase* effect of lowering IOP with osmotics, carbonic anhydrase inhibitors	UK	UK	<1 h	4–8 h	24 h

continued

Mydriatics and Cycloplegics—Continued

Generic (Brand)	Route and Dosage	Preg Cat	Interaction*	t 1/2	PB	Onset	Peak	Duration
Homatropine hydrobromide (Isopto Homatropine)	A&C: Sol 2% and 5%: 1–2 gtt q3–4h *Cy: Use only 2%	C	None significant known	NA	NA	M: 10–15 min C: 30–60 min	40–60 min 30–60 min	1–3 d 1–3 d
Phenylephrine HCl (AK-Dilate, Ophthalmic)	*Mydriasis:* A&C: 2.5% or 10% sol: Instill 1 gt in eye before examination *Mydriasis with vasoconstriction:* A&C >12 y: Instill 1 gt in eye; repeat ×1 in 1h PRN C: 2.5% sol: Instill 1 gt in eye; repeat ×1 in 1h PRN	C	*Increase* effect with adrenergic and oxytocic drugs *Decrease* effect with alpha and beta blockers	UK	UK	Several minutes	10–90 min	3–7 h
Scopolamine hydrobromide (Isopto Hyoscine)	A: Sol: 0.25% 1–2 gtt 1 h before exam; 1–2 gtt for treatment up to q.i.d.	C	Similar to atropine sulfate	NA	NA	M&C: 15–30 min	30–60 min	3–7 d
Tropicamide (Mydriacyl Ophthalmic)	*Refraction:* 1%: 1–2 gtt; repeat in 5 min *Fundus exam:* 0.5%: 1–2 gtt 15–20 min before exam	C	None significant known	NA	NA	M&C: 10–15 min	20–40 min	6 h

KEY: *To minimize systemic absorption, apply gentle pressure to lacrimal duct. For complete abbreviation key, see inside front cover.
M: Mydriatic; Cy: Cycloplegic.

Ophthalmic: Anti-Infectives

Generic (Brand)	Route and Dosage	Preg Cat	Interaction*	t1/2	PB	Onset	Peak	Duration
Antibacterials								
Chloramphenicol (AK-Chlor, Chloromycetin Ophthalmic)	A&C: Ophthalmic: Instill 1–2 gtt or 1/2 in oint q3–4 h for 48 h; increase interval to b.i.d./t.i.d.	C	None significant reported	NA	NA	UK	UK	UK
Ciprofloxacin HCl (Cipro)	*Acute infections:* A&C: Instill 1–2 gtt q15–30 min; decrease frequency gradually as infection is controlled *Moderate infection:* A&C: Instill 1–2 gtt 4–6 ×d	C	None significant reported	NA	NA	UK	UK	UK
Erythromycin (Ilotycin)	Oint 0.5%: 0.5–1 cm q.d./q.i.d.	B	None significant reported	1.5 h	75–90%	UK	UK	UK
Gentamicin sulfate (Garamycin Ophthalmic)	A&C: Sol 0.3%: 1–2 gtt q4h; may increase to 2 gtt q1h Oint 0.3%: 1/2 in ribbon b.i.d./t.i.d.	C	None significant reported	NA	NA	UK	UK	UK
Norfloxacin (Chibroxin)	A&C >1 y: Sol 3%: Instill 1–2 gtt in affected eye(s) q.i.d. for ≤7 d	C	None significant reported	NA	NA	UK	UK	UK
Polymyxin B sulfate (Neomycin Sulfate, Bacitracin, Aerosporin)	A&C: Sol: 1–2 gtt b.i.d./q.i.d. for 7–10 d	B	None significant reported	4–6 h	UK	UK	UK	UK

continued

Ophthalmic: Anti-Infectives—Continued

Generic (Brand)	Route and Dosage	Preg Cat	Interaction*	t 1/2	PB	Onset	Peak	Duration
Antibacterials								
Silver nitrate 1% (Dey-Drop)	Neonate: Instill 2 gtt to each eye within 1 h of birth	C	None significant reported	NA	NA	UK	UK	UK
Tetracycline HCl (Achromycin Ophthalmic)	A: Instill 1–2 gtt b.i.d./q.i.d. A: Oint: 1/4–1/2 in q2–12h	D	None significant reported	NA	NA	UK	UK	UK
Antifungal								
Natamycin (Natacyn Ophthalmic)	A&C: Sol 5%: 1 gt q2h for 3–4 d; then 1 gt q3h for 14–21 d	C	Avoid ophthalmic glucocorticoids	NA	NA	2 d	2–4 wk	UK
Antiviral								
Idoxuridine (IDU, Herplex Liquifilm)	A&C: Sol 1%: Initially: 1 gt q1h during the day and q2h at night; after definite improvement, use 1 gt q2h during the day and q4h at night; continue 3–7 d after healing Oint 5%: q4h w.a.	C	Topical corticosteroids may be used concomitantly; avoid boric acid–containing products and systemic glucocorticoids	NA	NA	5–7 d	UK	
Trifluridine (Viroptic)	A: 1% sol: Instill 1 gt into infected eye q2h while awake; max: 9 gtt/d until corneal ulcer reepithelialized; then 1 gt q4h for 7 d; max: 21 d of treatment	C	Systemic absorption negligible	NA	NA	UK	UK	UK
Vidarabine (Vira-A Ophthalmic)	*Keratoconjunctivitis, herpes simplex keratitis:* A&C: Oint 3%: 1/2 in 5 ×d at 3-h intervals	C	Allopurinol increases neurologic side effects	UK	UK	UK	UK	UK

KEY: *To minimize systemic absorption, apply gentle pressure to lacrimal duct. For complete abbreviation key, see inside front cover.

Ophthalmic: Anti-Inflammatories

Generic (Brand)	Route and Dosage	Preg Cat	Interaction	t1/2	PB	Onset	Peak	Duration
Dexamethasone (AK-Dex Ophthalmic, Maridex Ophthalmic)	A&C: Oint: Apply into conjunctival sac t.i.d/q.i.d.; gradually decrease to discontinue Susp: Instill 2 gtt qh while awake and q2h during night; taper to q3–4h; then t.i.d./q.i.d.	C	None significant reported	NA	NA	UK	UK	UK
Diclofenac Na (Voltaren)	A: 1 gt to affected eye q.i.d. for 2 wk; start 24 h after cataract surgery	B	None significant reported	NA	NA	Rapid	UK	UK
Flurbiprofen Na (Ocufen)	A: Instill 1 gt q30 min 2 h before surgery; total dose is 4 gtt	C	None significant reported	NA	NA	UK	UK	UK
Ketorolac tromethamine (Acular)	A: 0.5% sol: Instill 1 gt q.i.d.	B	None significant reported	NA	NA	UK	UK	UK
Medrysone (HMS Liquifilm)	A&C: susp: Initially: Instill 1 gt in conjunctival sac q1–2h (1–2 d); then 1 gt b.i.d./q.i.d.	C	None significant reported	NA	NA	UK	UK	UK
Prednisolone acetate (Econopred, Predforte [Pred Forte])	A: Initially: Instill 1–2 gtt in conjunctival sac qh while awake, q2h during night until desired effect; maint: 1 gt q4h Susp: 0.125% and 1%	C	None significant reported	NA	NA	UK	UK	UK
Prednisolone Na phosphate (AK-Pred Inflamase)	Sol: 0.125% and 1%							
Suprofen (Profenal)	*Preoperative:* A: Instill 2 gtt in sac q4h w.a. on day before surgery and 3, 2, and 1 h before surgery	C	Decrease effects of ophthalmic acetylcholine or carbachol	NA	NA	UK	UK	UK

*KEY: *To minimize systemic absorption, apply gentle pressure to lacrimal duct. For complete abbreviation key, see inside front cover.*

Otic: Anti-Infectives

Generic (Brand)	Route and Dosage	Preg Cat	Interaction	t 1/2	PB	Onset	Peak	Duration
External								
Acetic acid and aluminum acetate (Otic Domeboro)	A&C: Sol 2%: Insert saturated wick, keep moist ×24h; instill 4–6 gtt q2–3h	UK	None significant reported	NA	NA	UK	UK	UK
Boric acid (Ear-Dry)	A&C >12 y: Instill 5–10 gtt b.i.d.; tilt head to unaffected side to keep gtt in ear or put cotton plug in outer ear	C	None significant reported	NA	NA	UK	UK	UK
Carbamide peroxide (Debrox)		C	None significant reported	NA	NA	UK	UK	UK
Chloramphenicol (Chloromycetin Otic)	A&C: Otic sol: Instill 2–3 gtt into ear t.i.d.	C	None significant reported	NA	NA	UK	UK	UK
Polymyxin B	A&C: 3–4 gtt t.i.d./q.i.d. for 7–10 d	B	None significant reported	NA	NA	UK	UK	UK
Tetracycline (Achromycin)	A&C: 1–2 gtt b.i.d./q.i.d.	D	None significant reported	NA	NA	UK	UK	UK
Trolamine polypeptide oleate-condensate (Cerumenex)	A&C: Fill ear canal and insert cotton plug for 15–30 min; flush ear with lukewarm water; repeat ×1 if needed	C	None significant reported	NA	NA	24 h	UK	UK

Internal

Amoxicillin (Amoxil, Augmentin)	A: PO: 250–500 mg q8h C: PO: 20–40 mg/kg/d in 3 divided doses	B	Similar to penicillin	1–1.5 h	20%	PO: 30 min	1–2 h	6–8 h
Ampicillin trihydrate (Polycillin)	A: PO: 250–500 mg q6h IM/IV: 2–8 g/d in divided doses C: PO: IM: IV: 50–200 mg/kg/d in divided doses	B	*Increase* risk for rash with allopurinol Similar to penicillin *Decrease* effect of oral contraceptives	1–2 h	15–25%	PO: Rapid IM: Rapid IV: Rapid	2 h 1 h 5 min	6–8 h 6–8 h 6–8 h
Cefaclor (Ceclor)	Usual dose: A: PO: 250–500 mg q8h; max: 4 g/d C: PO: 20–40 mg/kg/d in divided doses q8h; max: 1g/d	B	Similar to penicillin	30–60 min; *increase* to 2–3 h with renal dysfunction	25%	PO: Rapid	30–60 min	UK
Loracarbef (Lorabid)	A: PO: 200–400 mg q12h C: PO: 30 mg/kg/d in divided doses q12h; modify dose with renal dysfunction Take 1 h a.c. or 2 h p.c.	B	*Decrease* excretion of drug with probenecid; monitor for toxicity	45–60 min	25%	UK	30–60 min	UK

continued

Otic: Anti-Infectives—Continued

Generic (Brand)	Route and Dosage	Preg Cat	Interaction	t 1/2	PB	Onset	Peak	Duration
Erythromycin (E-Mycin)	A: PO: 250–500 mg q6h IV: 1–4 g/d in 4 divided doses C: PO: 30–50 mg/kg/d in 4 divided doses IV: 20–50 mg/kg/d in 4 divided doses	B	*Increase* effects of digitalis, theophylline; *increase* risk of toxicity with oral anticoagulants, carbamazepine	1–3 h; may *increase* to 5–6 h with renal dysfunction	70%	PO: 1 h IV: Rapid	1–4 h End of infusion	6 h UK
Penicillin (Pentids, Pen-V)	*Penicillin G:* A: PO: 200,000–500,000 U q6h IM: 500,000–5 million U/d in divided doses IV: 4–20 million U/in divided doses diluted in IV sol C: PO: 25,000–90,000 U/d in divided doses IV: 50,000–100,000 U/kg/d in divided doses	B	*Decrease* effects with erythromycin, tetracyclines; *decrease* effect of oral contraceptives	30–60 min	Pen V: 80% Pen G: 60%	PO: Rapid IM: Rapid IV: Rapid	1 h 15–30 min Rapid	6 h 6 h 6 h
Sulfonamides (Azulfidine [sulfasalazine], Gantrisin [sulfisoxazole], Bactrim [trimethoprim and sulfamethoxazole])	Dose and route vary See Antibacterials: Sulfonamides	Safety not established	*Increase* effect of anticoagulants, sulfonylureas; *increase* toxicity with methotrexate; may *increase* toxicity of cyclosporine *Decrease* effect of digoxin	6–10 h	68%	UK	UK	UK

KEY: For complete abbreviation key, see inside front cover.

ENDOCRINE AGENTS

Pituitary Hormones

Thyroid Hormone Replacements and Antithyroid Agents

Parathyroid Hormones: Replacements and Supplements

Adrenal Hormones: Glucocorticoids

Antidiabetics
Insulin
Sulfonylureas

Prototype: Pituitary: Adrenocorticotropic Hormone (ACTH)

Corticotropin

Corticotropin
(Acthar, Acthar gel, Cortrophin-Zinc)
Anterior pituitary hormone
Pregnancy Category: C
Drug Forms:
Inj 25, 40 U per vial

Dosage

Diagnostic testing:
A: SC/IM: 20 units q.i.d.
IV: 10–25 units in 500 mL D_5W q8h
C: SC/IM: 1.6 U/kg/d or
50 U/m^2/d in divided doses

Contraindications

Severe fungal infection, CHF, peptic ulcer
Caution: Hepatic disease, psychiatric disorder, myasthenia gravis

Drug-Lab-Food Interactions

Increase ulcer formation with aspirin; may *increase* effect of diuretics
Decrease effects of oral antidiabetics or insulin

Pharmacokinetics

Absorption: IM: Well absorbed
Distribution: PB: UK
Metabolism: t 1/2: 15–20 min
Excretion: In urine

Pharmacodynamics

IM: Onset <6 h
   Peak: 6–18 h
   Duration: 12–24 h
IV: Onset: UK
   Peak: 1 h
   Duration: UK

Therapeutic Effects/Uses: To diagnose adrenocortical disorders; acts as an anti-inflammatory agent; to treat acute multiple sclerosis (MS).

Mode of Action: Stimulation of the adrenal cortex to secrete cortisol.

Side Effects

Nausea, vomiting, increased appetite, mood swing (euphoria to depression), petechiae, water and sodium retention, hypokalemia, hypocalcemia

Adverse Reactions

Edema, ecchymosis, osteoporosis, muscle atrophy, growth retardation, decreased wound healing, cataracts, glaucoma, menstrual irregularities
Life-threatening: Ulcer perforation, pancreatitis

KEY: For complete abbreviation key, see inside front cover.

■ NURSING PROCESS: Pituitary Hormones

ASSESSMENT

- Obtain baseline VS for future comparison. Report abnormal results.
- Assess the client's urinary output and weight.
- Assess the client for an infectious process. Corticotropin can suppress signs and symptoms of infection.
- Assess the client's physical growth. Compare child's growth with reported standards. Report findings.

POTENTIAL NURSING DIAGNOSES

- Altered health maintenance
- Altered growth and development

Pituitary: Adrenocorticotropic Hormone (ACTH)

PLANNING
- Client will be free of pituitary disorder with appropriate drug regimen.

NURSING INTERVENTIONS

Antidiuretic Hormone (ADH)
- Monitor VS. Increased heart rate and decreased systolic pressure can indicate fluid volume loss due to decreased ADH production. With less ADH secretion, more water is excreted, decreasing vascular fluid (hypovolemia).
- Monitor urinary output. Increased output can indicate fluid loss due to a decrease in ADH.

Adrenocorticotropic Hormone (ACTH), Corticotropin
- Avoid administering corticotropin to clients with adrenocortical hyperfunction. Corticotropin stimulates the release of cortisol from the adrenal glands.
- Monitor the growth and development of a child receiving corticotropin.
- Monitor the client's weight. If a weight gain occurs, check for edema. A side effect of corticotropin (ACTH) is sodium and water retention.
- Monitor for adverse effects when corticotropin is discontinued. Dose should be tapered and not stopped abruptly because adrenal hypofunction may result.
- Check laboratory findings, especially electrolyte levels. Electrolyte replacement may be necessary.

Growth Hormone (GH)
- Monitor blood sugar and electrolyte levels in clients receiving GH. Hyperglycemia can occur with high doses.

Client Teaching
ACTH
- Advise the client to adhere to the drug regimen. Discontinuation of certain drugs, such as corticotropin, can cause hypofunction of the gland being stimulated.
- Advise the client to decrease salt intake to decrease or avoid edema. Potassium supplement may be needed.
- Instruct the client to report side effects, such as muscle weakness, edema, petechiae, ecchymosis, decrease in growth, decreased wound healing, and menstrual irregularities.

Growth Hormone
- Advise athletes not to take GH due to its side effects. GH can be effective for children whose height is markedly below the expected norm for their age. Because GH acts on the newly forming bone, it should be administered before the epiphyses are fused.
- Inform the diabetic client to closely monitor blood sugar levels. Insulin regulation may be necessary.
- Suggest that the client or family monitors the client's growth rate.

EVALUATION
- Evaluate the effectiveness of the drug therapy.

Anterior and Posterior Pituitary Hormones

Generic (Brand)	Route and Dosage	Preg Cat	Interaction	t1/2	PB	Onset	Peak	Duration
Anterior: Growth Hormone (GH)								
Sermorelin acetate (Geref)	*Diagnostic:* A&C: IV: 0.3–1 μg/kg	C	*Increase* effects with clonidine, levodopa	UK	UK	UK	UK	UK
Somatrem (Protropin)	*Growth hormone deficiency:* C: SC/IM: 100 μg/kg (0.1 mg/kg) 3×wk or 0.2 IU/kg 3×wk; 48-h interval is recommended between doses	C	*Increase* epiphyseal closure with androgens, estrogens, thyroid drugs *Decrease* somatrem effect with ACTH, glucocorticoids	20–30 min	UK	UK	UK	18–20 h
Somatropin (Humatrope)	C: SC/IM: 60 μg/kg (0.06 mg/kg) 3×wk or 0.16 IU/kg 3×wk; 48-h interval is recommended between doses	D	Same as somatrem	15–50 min	UK	UK	UK	18–20 h
Thyroid-Stimulating Hormone (TSH)								
Thyrotropin (Thytropar)	*Hypothyroidism and treatment of thyroid cancer:* A: SC/IM: 10 IU/d for 1–3 d; cancer treatment: 3–8 d	C	None significant reported	35 min with normal thyroid	UK	8 h	UK	24–28 h

Adrenocorticotropic Hormone (ACTH)						
Corticotropin (Acthar)	See Prototype Drug Chart		See Corticotropin, Prototype Drug Chart			
Corticotropin repository (Acthar gel)	A: SC/IM: 40–80 U/q24–48h					
Cosyntropin (Cortrosyn)	A: C >2 y: IM: 0.25–0.75 mg IV: 0.25 mg C <2 y: IM: 0.125 mg, IV: 0.125 mg (0.04 mg/h over 6 h)	C	May *increase* effect of spironolactone; may *increase* plasma cortisol level when taken with cortisone preparations	15 min (plasma)	UK	IM: 15–30 min IV: 5–15 min	1 h	2–4 h
Posterior: Antidiuretic Hormone (ADH)						
Desmopressin acetate (DDAVP)	A: Intranasal: 0.1–0.4 mL/d in divided doses C <12 y: Intranasal: 0.05–0.3 mL/d in divided doses	B	May *increase* ADH effect with carbamazepine, chlorpropamide May *decrease* ADH effect with other vasopressors, lithium	76 min	UK	0.5–1 h	1–5 h	5–20 h
Desmopressin (Stimate)	A: Inf: 0.3 µg/kg diluted in 50 mL of NSS admin over 20–30 min C <12 y: Inf: 0.3 µg/kg diluted in 10 mL of NSS over 15–30 min	B	Same as DDAVP	76 min	UK	0.5–1 h	1–5 h	5–20 h
Lypressin (Diapid)	*Diabetes insipidus*: A&C: Intranasal: 1–2 sprays per nostril q.i.d.	B	May *decrease* ADH effect with other vasopressors, lithium	15 min	UK	0.5–2 h	0.5–2 h	3–8 h

continued

Anterior and Posterior Pituitary Hormones—*Continued*

Generic (Brand)	Route and Dosage	Preg Cat	Interaction	t 1/2	PB	Onset	Peak	Duration
Vasopressin (aqueous) (Pitressin)	*Diabetes insipidus:* A: SC/IM: 5–10 units b.i.d./q.i.d. C: SC/IM: 2.5–10 units b.i.d./q.i.d.	X	May *increase* ADH effect with thiazides, carbamazepine, chlorpropamide May *decrease* ADH effect with alcohol, phenytoin, heparin, lithium	15 min	UK	UK	UK	2–8 h
Vasopressin tanate/oil (Pitressin Tannate)	A: IM: 1.5–5.0 units q2–3d C: IM: 1.25–2.5 units q2–3d	X	Same as aqueous vasopressin	10–20 min	UK	UK	UK	24–72 h

KEY: For complete abbreviation key, see inside front cover.

NOTES:

Prototype: Thyroid Hormone: Replacement

Levothyroxine Na

Levothyroxine sodium, T_4
(Synthroid, Levothroid), ✦ Eltroxin
Thyroid synthetic hormone
Pregnancy Category: A
Drug Forms:
Tab 25, 50, 75, 100, 125, 150, 200, 300 μg
Inj 200, 500 μg per vial

Dosage

A: PO: Initially: 50 μg/d (0.05 mg/d); maint: 50–200 μg/d (0.05–0.2 mg/d)
IV: 0.2–0.5 mg initial dose
C : >3 y: PO: 50–100 μg/d (0.05–0.1 mg/d)

Contraindications

Thyrotoxicosis, MI, severe renal disease
Caution: Cardiovascular disease, hypertension, angina pectoris

Drug-Lab-Food Interactions

Increase cardiac insufficiency with epinephrine; *increase* effects of anticoagulants, tricyclic antidepressants, vasopressors, decongestants
Decrease effects of antidiabetics (oral and insulin), digitalis products; *decrease* absorption with cholestyramine, colestipol

Pharmacokinetics

Absorption: PO: 50–75%
Distribution: PB: 99%
Metabolism: t 1/2: 6–7 d
Excretion: In bile and feces

Pharmacodynamics

PO: Onset: UK
  Peak: 24 h–1 wk
  Duration: 1–3 wk
IV: Onset: 6–8 h
  Peak: 24–48 h
  Duration: UK

Therapeutic Effects/Uses: To treat hypothyroidism, myxedema, and cretinism.
Mode of Action: Increase metabolic rate, oxygen consumption, and body growth.

Side Effects

Nausea, vomiting, diarrhea, cramps, tremors, nervousness, insomnia, headache, weight loss

Adverse Reactions

Tachycardia, hypertension, palpitations
Life-threatening: Thyroid crisis, angina pectoris, cardiac dysrhythmias, cardiovascular collapse

KEY: For complete abbreviation key, see inside front cover.

Thyroid Hormone: Replacement

■ NURSING PROCESS: Thyroid Hormone: Replacement and Antithyroids Drugs

ASSESSMENT
- Obtain baseline VS to compare with future data. Report abnormal results.
- Check serum T_3, T_4, and TSH levels. Report abnormal results.

THYROID REPLACEMENT
- Obtain a history of drugs the client is currently taking. Be aware that thyroid drugs enhance the action of oral anticoagulants, sympathomimetics, and antidepressants and decrease the action of insulin, oral hypoglycemics, and digitalis preparation. Phenytoin and aspirin can enhance the action of thyroid hormone.

ANTITHYROID DRUGS
- Assess for signs and symptoms of a thyroid crisis (thyroid storm), which includes tachycardia, dysrhythmias, fever, heart failure, flushed skin, apathy, confusion, behavioral changes, and later hypotension and vascular collapse. Thyroid crisis can result from a thyroidectomy (excess thyroid hormones released), abrupt withdrawal of antithyroid drug, excess ingestion of thyroid hormone, or failure to give antithyroid medication before thyroid surgery.

POTENTIAL NURSING DIAGNOSES
Altered health maintenance
Altered tissue perfusion

PLANNING
- Client's signs and symptoms of hypothyroidism will be alleviated within 2–4 wk with prescribed thyroid drug replacement, and the client will not experience side effects.
- Client's signs and symptoms of hyperthyroidism will be alleviated in 1–3 wk with the prescribed antithyroid drug.

NURSING INTERVENTIONS
- Monitor VS. With hypothyroidism, the temperature, heart rate, and blood pressure are usually decreased. With hyperthyroidism, tachycardia and palpitations usually occur.
- Monitor the client's weight. Weight gain commonly occurs in clients with hypothyroidism.

Client Teaching
Thyroid Drug Replacement for Hypothyroidism
- Instruct the client to take the drug at the same time each day, preferably before breakfast. Food will hamper absorption rate.
- Advise the client to check cautions on labels of OTC drugs. Avoid OTC drugs that caution against use by persons with heart or thyroid disease.
- Advise the client to report symptoms of hyperthyroidism (tachycardia, chest pain, palpitations, excess sweating) due to drug accumulation or overdosing.
- Suggest that the client carry a medical alert card, tag, or bracelet with health condition and thyroid drug listed.

Thyroid Hormone: Replacement and Antithyroid Drugs

Diet

- Instruct the client to avoid foods that can inhibit thyroid secretion, such as strawberries, peaches, pears, cabbage, turnips, spinach, kale, Brussels sprouts, cauliflower, radishes, and peas.

Antithyroid Drugs for Hyperthyroidism

- Instruct the client to take the drug with meals to decrease GI symptoms.
- Advise the client about the effects of iodine and its presence in iodized salt, shellfish, and OTC cough medicines.
- Emphasize the importance of drug compliance; abruptly stopping the antithyroid drug could bring on a thyroid crisis.
- Teach the client the signs and symptoms of hypothyroidism: lethargy, puffy eyelids and face, thick tongue, slow speech with hoarseness, lack of perspiration, and slow pulse. Hypothyroidism can result from treatment of hyperthyroidism.
- Advise the client to avoid antithyroid drugs if pregnant or breast feeding. Antithyroid drugs taken during pregnancy can cause hypothyroidism in the fetus or infant.

Skill

- Demonstrate to the client how to take a pulse rate. Instruct the client to monitor the pulse rate and report increases or marked decreases in pulse rate.

Side Effects

- Teach the client the side effects of antithyroid drugs, such as skin rash, hives, nausea, alopecia, loss of hair pigment, petechiae or ecchymoses, and weakness.
- Advise the client to contact the health care provider if a sore throat and fever occur while taking antithyroid drugs. А serious adverse reaction of antithyroid drugs is agranulocytosis (loss of WBCs). CBC should be monitored for leukopenia.

EVALUATION

Thyroid Replacement

- Evaluate the effectiveness of the thyroid drug and drug compliance.
- Continue monitoring for side effects from drug accumulation or overdosing.

Antithyroid Drugs

- Evaluate the effectiveness of the antithyroid drug in decreasing signs and symptoms of hyperthyroidism. If signs and symptoms persist after 2–3 wk of therapy, other methods for correcting hyperthyroidism may be necessary.

Thyroid Hormone: Replacement and Antithyroid Drugs

Generic (Brand)	Route and Dosage	Preg Cat	Interaction	t 1/2	PB	Onset	Peak	Duration
Thyroid Replacements: Hypothyroidism								
Levothyroxine Na (Synthroid)	See Prototype Drug Chart							
Liothyronine Na (Cytomel)	A: PO: Initially: 5–25 µg/d; maint: 25–100 µg/d C: PO: Initially: 5 µg/d > 3 y: 50–100 µg/d	A	Similar to thyroid	6–7 d	99%	UK	24–72 h	72 h
Liotrix (Euthroid, Thyrolar)	A: PO: Initially: 15–30 µg/d, *increase* q2–3wk; maint: 60–120 µg/d C: PO: Initially: same as adult C: 6–12 y: 75–150 µg/d	A	Similar to thyroid	6–7 d	99%	UK	24–48 h	72 h
Thyroglobulin (Proloid)	A: PO: Initially: 32 mg/d; maint: 32–200 mg/d Elderly: Initially: 16 mg/d	A	Similar to thyroid	6–7 d	99%	UK	12–24 h	UK
Thyroid (Armour Thyroid, Thyrar)	A: PO: Initially: 15–60 mg/d, *increase* monthly as needed; maint: 60–180 mg/d C: PO: 15 mg/d, *increase* q2wk as needed	A	May *increase* effects of anticoagulants, tricyclic antidepressants, adrenergics May *increase* dose requirement for insulin, oral hypoglycemics *Decrease* thyroid effect with cholestyramine, colestipol, phenytoin	6–7 d	99%	UK	1–3 wk	UK

continued

Thyroid Hormone: Replacement and Antithyroid Drugs—*Continued*

Generic (Brand)	Route and Dosage	Preg Cat	Interaction	t 1/2	PB	Action Onset	Action Peak	Action Duration
Antithyroid Drugs: Hyperthyroidism								
Methimazole (Tapazole)	A: PO: Initially: 15–60 mg/d in 3 divided doses; maint: 5–15 mg/d C: PO: Initially: 0.4 mg/kg/d in divided doses; maint: 0.2 mg/kg/d in divided doses	D	Similar to propylthiouracil	3–5 h	Not significant	0.5–1 h	1–2 h	2–4 h
Thioamide: Propylthiouracil (PTU)	A: PO: Initially: 300–400 mg/d in divided doses; maint: 100–300 mg/d C: 6–10 y: PO: 50–150 mg/d >10 y: PO: Same as adult or 150 mg/m^2/d	D	May *increase* effect of oral anticoagulants	1–2 h	80%	UK	1–1.5 h	UK
Iodine: strong iodine solution (Lugol solution, potassium iodide solution)	A&C: PO: 0.1–0.3 mL (3–5 gtt) t.i.d. *Thyroid crisis:* A & C: PO: 1 mL in water p.c. t.i.d.	D	*Increase* antithyroid effect with other antithyroid drugs *Lab:* May *increase* serum potassium level	UK	UK	24 h	10–15 d	UK

KEY: For complete abbreviation key, see inside front cover.

NOTES:

Prototype: Parathyroid Hormone

Calcitriol

Calcitriol
 (Rocaltrol)
Vitamin D analog
Pregnancy Category: C
Drug Forms:
Cap 0.25, 0.5 µg

Dosage

A: PO: 0.25 µg/d

Contraindications

Hypersensitivity, hypercalcemia, hyperphosphatemia, hypervitaminosis D, malabsorption syndrome
Caution: Cardiovascular disease, renal calculi

Drug-Lab-Food Interactions

Increase cardiac dysrhythmias with digoxin, verapamil
Decrease calcitriol absorption with cholestyramine
Lab: Increase serum calcium with thiazide diuretics, calcium supplements

Pharmacokinetics

Absorption: PO: Well absorbed
Distribution: PB: UK; crosses the placenta
Metabolism: t 1/2: 3–8 h
Excretion: Mostly in feces

Pharmacodynamics

PO: Onset: 2–6 h
  Peak: 10–12 h
  Duration: 3–5 d

Therapeutic Effects/Uses: To treat hypocalcemia in chronic renal failure.
Mode of Action: Enhancement of calcium deposits in bones.

Side Effects

Anorexia, nausea, vomiting, diarrhea, cramps, drowsiness, headache, dizziness, lethargy, photophobia

Adverse Reactions

Hypercalciuria, hyperphosphatemia, hematuria

KEY: For complete abbreviation key, see inside front cover.

Parathyroid Hormone

■ NURSING PROCESS: Parathyroid Hormone

ASSESSMENT
- Assess serum calcium level. Report abnormal results.
- Assess for symptoms of tetany in hypocalcemia: twitching of the mouth, tingling and numbness of the fingers, carpopedal spasm, spasmodic contractions, and laryngeal spasm.

POTENTIAL NURSING DIAGNOSES
High risk for impaired tissue integrity
Altered health maintenance

PLANNING
- The client's serum calcium level will be within the normal range.

NURSING INTERVENTIONS
- Monitor the serum calcium level. Normal reference value is 8.5–10.5 mg/dL, or 4.5–5.5 mEq/L. A serum calcium level <8.5 mg/dL, or <4.5 mEq/L, indicates hypocalcemia, and a serum calcium level >10.5 mg/dL, or >5.5 mEq/L, indicates hypercalcemia. Serum ionized calcium levels are usually used because much of the calcium is protein-bound and is nonionized and nonactive.

Client Teaching
Hypoparathyroidism
- Advise the client to report symptoms of tetany (see Assessment).

Hyperparathyroidism
- Advise the client to report signs and symptoms of hypercalcemia: bone pain, anorexia, nausea, vomiting, thirst, constipation, lethargy, bradycardia, and polyuria.
- Instruct women to inform their health care provider about pregnancy status before taking calcitonin preparation.
- Advise the client to check OTC drugs for possible calcium content, especially if the client has an elevated serum calcium level. Some vitamins and antacids contain calcium. Tell the client to contact the health care provider before taking drugs with calcium.

EVALUATION
- Monitor the effectiveness of drug therapy.
- Continue monitoring for signs and symptoms of hypocalcemia (tetany) when commercially prepared calcitonin has been given.

Parathyroid Hormones: Replacements and Supplements

Generic (Brand)	Route and Dosage	Preg Cat	Interaction	t 1/2	PB	Onset	Peak	Duration
Hypoparathyroidism and Hypocalcemia: Vitamin D Analogs								
Calcifediol (Calderol)	A: PO: Initially: 300–350 μg/wk PO: 50–100 μg/d or 100–200 μg q.o.d.	C	*Increase* cardiac dysrhythmias with digoxin; may *increase* hypercalcemia with thiazide diuretics *Decrease* absorption with cholestyramine, colestipol; *decrease* effect with glucocorticoids	12–22 d	Bound to specific alpha globulins for transport	UK	4 h	15–20 d
Calcitriol (Rocaltrol)	A: PO: 0.25 μg/d; may increase 0.25 μg q4wk; max: 1.0 μg/d IV: 0.5 μg 3×wk at end of dialysis C: PO: 0.014–0.041 μg/kd/d	C	Similar to calcifediol	3–6 h	Alpha globulins	2–6 h	7–12 h	1–5 d

Ergocalciferol (Drisdol Drops)	A&C: PO: 50,000–200,000 IU/d or 1.25–5.0 μg/d	C	Similar to calcifediol	12–24 h	Alpha globulins	12–24 h	4 wk	2–6 mo
Hyperparathyroidism and Hypercalcemia								
Calcitonin (human) (Cibacalcin)	A: SC: Initially: 0.5 mg/d; maint: 0.25 mg q.d.–0.5 mg b.i.d.	C	None significant reported	1 h	UK	15 min	4 h	8–24 h
Calcitonin (salmon) (Calcimar)	A: SC/IM: Initially: 4 IU/kg/d; maint: 4–8 IU/kg q12h	C	None significant reported	1–1.5 h	UK	15 min	4 h	8–24 h
Etidronate (Didronel)	A: PO: 5–10 mg/kg/d; max: 20 mg/kg/d	B	None significant reported	6 h	UK	UK	UK	UK

KEY: For complete abbreviation key, see inside front cover.

Prototype: Adrenal Hormone

Prednisone

Prednisone
(Deltasone, Meticorten, Orasone, Panasol-S), ♣ Apo-Prednisone, Winpred
Glucocorticoid
Pregnancy Category: C
Drug Forms:
Tab 2.5, 5, 10, 25, 50 mg
Liq 5 mg/5 mL
Syrup 5 mg/5 mL

Dosage

A: PO: 5–60 mg/d in divided doses
C : PO: 0.1–0.15 mg/kg/d in 2–4 divided doses or 4–5 mg/m^2/d in 2 doses

Contraindications

Hypersensitivity, psychosis, fungal infection
Caution: Diabetes mellitus

Drug-Lab-Food Interactions

Increase effect with barbiturates, phenytoin, rifampin, ephedrine, theophylline
Decrease effects of aspirin, anticonvulsants, isoniazid (INH), antidiabetics, vaccines

Pharmacokinetics

Absorption: PO: Well absorbed
Distribution: PB: UK; crosses the placenta
Metabolism: t 1/2: 3–4 h
Excretion: In urine

Pharmacodynamics

PO: Onset: UK
Peak: 1–2 h
Duration: 24–36 h

Therapeutic Effects/Uses: To decrease inflammatory occurrence; as an immunosuppressant; to treat dermatologic disorders.

Mode of Action: Suppression of inflammation and adrenal function.

Side Effects

Nausea, diarrhea, abdominal distention, increased appetite, sweating, headache, depression, flushing, mood changes

Adverse Reactions

Petechiae, ecchymosis, hypertension, tachycardia, osteoporosis, muscle wasting
Life-threatening: GI hemorrhage, pancreatitis, circulatory collapse, thrombophlebitis, embolism

KEY: For complete abbreviation key, see inside front cover.

Adrenal Hormone

■ NURSING PROCESS: Adrenal Hormone: Glucocorticoids

ASSESSMENT
- Obtain baseline VS for future comparison.
- Assess laboratory test results, especially serum electrolytes and blood sugar. Serum potassium level usually decreases and blood sugar level increases when a glucocorticoid such as prednisone is taken over an extensive period of time.
- Obtain the client's weight and urine output to use for future comparison.
- Assess the client's medical history. Report if the client has glaucoma, cataracts, peptic ulcer, psychiatric problems, or diabetes mellitus. Glucocorticoid can intensify these health problems.

POTENTIAL NURSING DIAGNOSES
Fluid volume excess
High risk for impaired tissue integrity

PLANNING
- The client's inflammatory process will abate. Side effects of glucocorticoid will be minimal.

NURSING INTERVENTIONS
- Monitor VS. Glucocorticoids such as prednisone can increase blood pressure and sodium and water retention.
- Administer glucocorticoids only as ordered. Routes of administration include PO, IM (not in the deltoid muscle), IV, aerosol, and topical. Topical glucocorticoid drugs should be applied in thin layers. Rashes, infection, and purpura should be noted and reported.
- Monitor weight. Report weight gain of 5 lb in several days; this would most likely be due to water retention.
- Monitor laboratory values, especially serum electrolytes and blood sugar. Serum potassium level would probably decrease to <3.5 mEq/L, and blood sugar level would probably increase.
- Observe for signs and symptoms of hypokalemia, such as nausea, vomiting, muscular weakness, abdominal distention, paralytic ileus, and irregular heart rate.
- Observe for side effects from glucocorticoid drugs when therapy has lasted >10 d and the drug is taken in high dosages. The cortisone preparation should not be abruptly stopped because adrenal crisis can result.
- Monitor older adults for signs and symptoms of increased osteoporosis. Glucocorticoids promote calcium loss from the bone.
- Report changes in muscle strength. High doses of glucocorticoids promote loss of muscle tone.

CLIENT TEACHING
General
- Advise the client to take the drug as prescribed. Instruct the client *NOT* to abruptly stop the drug. When the drug is discontinued, the dose is tapered over 1-2 wk.
- For short-term use of glucocorticoids such as prednisone or other cortisone preparations (<10 d), the drug dose still needs to be tapered. Prepare a

Adrenal Hormone

schedule for the client to decrease the dose over a period of 4–5 d. For example, take 1 tab q.i.d.; the next day take 1 tab t.i.d.; the next day, take 1 tab b.i.d.; and then take 1 tab q.d.

- Advise the client not to take cortisone preparations (PO or topical) during pregnancy unless necessary and prescribed by the health care provider. These drugs may be harmful to the fetus.
- Instruct the client to avoid persons with respiratory infections since these drugs suppress the immune system. This is especially important if the client is receiving a high dose of glucocorticoids.
- Advise the client receiving glucocorticoids to inform other health care providers of all drugs taken, especially before surgery.
- Advise the client to have a medical alert card, tag, or bracelet stating the glucocorticoid drug being taken.

Skill

- Teach the client how to use an aerosol nebulizer. Warn the client against overuse of the aerosol to avoid possible rebound effect.

Diet

- Instruct the client to take cortisone preparations at mealtime or with food. Glucocorticoid drugs can irritate the gastric mucosa and cause a peptic ulcer.
- Advise the client to eat foods rich in potassium, such as fresh and dried fruits, vegetables, meats, and nuts. Prednisone promotes potassium loss and, thus, hypokalemia.

Side Effects

- Teach the client to report signs and symptoms of drug overdose or Cushing's syndrome, including a moon face, puffy eyelids, edema in the feet, increased bruising, dizziness, bleeding, and menstrual irregularity.

EVALUATION

- Evaluate the effectiveness of glucocorticoid drug therapy. If the inflammation has improved, a change in drug therapy may be necessary.
- Continue monitoring for side effects, especially when the client is receiving high doses of glucocorticoids.

Adrenal Hormones: Glucocorticoids

Generic (Brand)	Route and Dosage	Preg Cat	Interaction	t 1/2	PB	Onset	Peak	Duration
Beclomethasone Dipropionate (Vanceril)	A: Inhal: 2 puffs b.i.d./q.i.d.	C	None significant reported	5–15 h	87%	UK	1–2 wk	UK
Betamethasone (Celestone, Celestone Phosphate)	A: PO: 0.6–7.2 mg/d in single or divided doses IM/IV: 1–9 mg/d; max: IM: 12 mg/d	C	*Increase* effect with aspirin, estrogens, oral contraceptives, erythromycin; *increase* risk of hypokalemia with diuretics, amphotercin B, ticarcillin; *increase* need of insulin, oral hypoglycemics *Decrease* effect with barbiturates, phenytoin, theophylline, rifampin, cholestyramine, ephedrine; *decrease* effects of anticoagulants, antidiabetics, aspirin	36–50 h (tissue)	80–90%	PO: 1 h IM/IV: Rapid	PO: 1–2 h IM/IV: 2–8 h	PO: 3 d IV: 1–3 d

continued

Adrenal Hormones: Glucocorticoids—Continued

Generic (Brand)	Route and Dosage	Preg Cat	Interaction	t1/2	PB	Onset	Peak	Duration
Cortisone acetate (Cortone Acetate, Cortistan)	A: PO/IM: 25–300 mg/d; decrease dose periodically	C	Same as betamethasone	0.5–12 h	UK	PO: UK IM: UK	PO: 2 h IM: 24–48 h	PO: 1.5 d IM: 1.5 d
Dexamethasone (Decadron)	*Inflammation:* A: PO: 0.25–4 mg b.i.d./q.i.d. IM: 4–16 mg q1–3wk C: PO: 0.2 mg/kg/d in divided doses *Shock:* A: IV: 1–6 mg/kg as a single dose	C	Same as betamethasone	3–4 h	80–90%	PO: UK IM: UK	PO: 1–2 h IM: 8 h	PO: 2–2.5 d IM: Days to 1–3 wk
Fludrocortisone acetate (Florinef Acetate)	A & C: PO: 0.1–0.2 mg/d	C	*Increase* potassium loss with thiazides, loop diuretics	≥3.5 h	92%	UK	1.5–2 h	1–2 d
Hydrocortisone (Cortef, Hydrocortone)	A: PO: 20–240 mg/d in 2–4 divided doses IV: 15–240 mg (phosphate) q12h Rectal supp: 10–25 mg	C	Similar to betamethasone	2–12 h	79%	PO: 1–2 h IV: Rapid	PO: 1 h IV: UK	PO: 1–1.5 d IV: 1–1.5 d
Methylprednisolone (Medrol, Solu-Medrol [sodium succinate], Depo-Medrol [acetate])	A: PO: 4–48 mg/d in one or more divided doses IM/IV: Succinate: 10–250 mg q6h IM: Acetate: 40–80 mg/wk	C	Similar to betamethasone	Tissue: 18–36 h	UK	PO: UK IM: Acetate: 6–48 h IV: Rapid	PO: 1–2 h IM: Acetate: 4–8 d IV: UK	PO: 1.5 d IM: Acetate: 1–5 wk IV: UK

Paramethasone acetate (Haldrone)	A: PO: 0.5–6 mg t.i.d./q.i.d. C: PO: 58–200 μg/kg/d in 3–4 divided doses	C	Similar to fludrocortisone May *change* PT with warfarin *Increase* risk of GI distress with NSAIDs, other steroids; *Decrease* effect with barbiturates, phenytoin, rifampin; *decrease* antibody response with toxoids, vaccines	3–4.5 h Tissue: 36–54 h	95%	UK	1–2 h	2 d
Prednisolone (Delta-Cortef, Hydeltrasol [phosphate])	A: PO: 2.5–15 mg b.i.d./q.i.d. IV: Phosphate: 2–30 mg q12h C: PO: 0.14–2 mg/kg/d in a single or divided doses	C	Similar to betamethasone	Tissue: 18–36 h	80–90%	PO: UK	PO: 1–2 h	PO: 1.5–2 d
Prednisone	See Prototype Drug Chart							
Triamcinolone (Aristocort, Kenacort, Kenalog)	A: PO: 4–48 mg/d in 2–4 divided doses Inhal: 2 puffs, t.i.d./q.i.d. Topical: cream, ointment	C	Similar to prednisone	2–5 h	65–90%	1 h	1–2 h	UK

KEY: For complete abbreviation key, see inside front cover.

Prototype: Antidiabetic: Insulins

Regular Insulin

Regular Insulin
  NPH Insulin
  Injectable insulins
Pregnancy Category: B
Drug Forms:
Inj 100 U/mL; 40 and 50 U/mL

Dosage

Varies according to client's blood sugar

Contraindications

Hypersensitivity to beef, zinc, protamine insulins

Drug-Lab-Food Interactions

Increase hypoglycemic effect with aspirin, oral anticoagulant, alcohol, oral hypoglycemics, beta blockers, tricyclic antidepressants, MAOIs, tetracycline

Decrease hypoglycemic effect with thiazides, glucocorticoids, oral contraceptives, thyroid drugs, smoking

Pharmacokinetics

Absorption: SC: Well absorbed
Distribution: PB: UK
Metabolism: t 1/2: Regular IV insulin: 5–9 min; varies with type of insulin
Excretion: Mostly in urine

Pharmacodynamics

Regular Insulin:
SC: Onset: 0.5–1 h
  Peak: 2–4 h
  Duration: 4–8 h
IV: Onset: 10–20 min
  Peak: 15–30 min
  Duration: 1–2 h
NPH Insulin:
SC: Onset: 1–2 h
  Peak: 6–12 h
  Duration: 18–24 h

Therapeutic Effects/Uses: To control diabetes mellitus; to lower blood sugar.
Mode of Action: Insulin promotes utilization of glucose by body cells.

Side Effects

Hunger, tremors, weakness, headache, lethargy, fatigue, redness, irritation or swelling at insulin injection site, flushing, confusion, agitation

Adverse Reactions

Urticaria, tachycardia, palpitations, hypoglycemic reaction, rebound hyperglycemia (Somogyi effect), lipodystrophy
Life-threatening: Shock; anaphylaxis

KEY: For complete abbreviation key, see inside front cover.

■ NURSING PROCESS: Antidiabetics: Insulin

ASSESSMENT

• Assess the drugs the client is currently taking. Certain drugs, such as alcohol, aspirin, oral anticoagulants, oral hypoglycemics, beta blockers, tricyclic antidepressants, MAOIs, and tetracycline, increase the hypoglycemic effect when taken with insulin. Note that thiazides, glucocorticoids, oral contraceptives, thyroid drugs, and smoking can increase blood sugar.

Antidiabetic: Insulins

- Assess the type of insulin and dosage. Note if it is given once or twice a day.
- Check VS and blood sugar levels. Report abnormal findings.
- Assess the client's knowledge of diabetes mellitus and the use of insulins.
- Assess for signs and symptoms of a hypoglycemic reaction (insulin shock) and hyperglycemia or ketoacidosis.

POTENTIAL NURSING DIAGNOSES
High risk for impaired tissue integrity
Altered nutrition: more or less than body requirements
High risk for injury

PLANNING
- Client's blood sugar will be within the normal values (70–110 mg/dL).

NURSING INTERVENTIONS
- Monitor VS. Tachycardia can occur during an insulin reaction.
- Monitor blood glucose levels and report changes. The reference value is 60–100 mg/dL for blood glucose and 70–110 mg/dL for serum glucose.
- Prepare a teaching plan based on the client's knowledge of the health problem, diet, and drug therapy.

CLIENT TEACHING
General
- Instruct the client to report immediately symptoms of a hypoglycemic (insulin) reaction, such as headache, nervousness, sweating, tremors, and rapid pulse, and symptoms of a hyperglycemic reaction (diabetic acidosis), such as thirst, increased urine output, and sweet fruity breath odor.
- Advise the client that hypoglycemic reactions are more likely to occur during the peak action time. Most diabetics know if they are having a hypoglycemic reaction; however, some have a higher tolerance to low blood sugar and can have a severe hypoglycemic reaction without realizing it.
- Explain that orange juice, sugar-containing drinks, and hard candy may be used when a hypoglycemic reaction begins.
- Instruct family members in administering glucagon by injection if the client has a hypoglycemic reaction and cannot drink sugar-containing fluid.
- Instruct the client about the necessity for compliance to prescribed insulin and diet.
- Advise the client to obtain a medical alert card, tag, and/or bracelet indicating the health problem and insulin dosage.

Skill
- Instruct the client how to check the blood sugar using Chemstrip bG test.
- Instruct the client in the care of the insulin bottle and syringes. Inform the client taking NPH or lente insulin with regular insulin that the regular insulin should be drawn up before the NPH or lente insulin.

Diet
- Advise the client taking insulin to eat the prescribed diet on schedule. The diet may be from the American Diabetic Association (ADA).

EVALUATION
- Evaluate the effectiveness of the insulin therapy by noting whether blood sugar level is within the accepted range.
- Evaluate the client's knowledge of the signs and symptoms of hypoglycemic or hyperglycemic reaction.

Antidiabetic: Insulins

Generic (Brand)	Route and Dosage	Preg Cat	Interaction	t 1/2	PB	Onset	Peak	Duration
Rapid-Acting								
Humulin R	Same as regular insulin							
Regular	A & C: SC/IV: 100 U/mL; dose is individualized according to blood sugar	B	May *increase* insulin effect with aspirin, beta blockers, tetracyclines, MAOIs, tricyclic antidepressants, oral anticoagulants. May *decrease* insulin effect with thiazides, glucocorticoids, thyroid drugs, oral contraceptives	10 min–1 h	UK	0.5–1 h	2–4 h	6–8 h
Semilente	A & C: SC: 100 U/mL; dose is individualized according to blood sugar	B	Same as all insulin	<13 h	UK	30–45 min	4–6 h	12–16 h

Intermediate Acting						
Humulin L Insulin	Same as lente	B	Similar to regular insulin	13 h	UK	1-2 h	8-12 h	18-28 h
Humulin N Insulin	Same as NPH insulin	B	Similar to regular insulin	13 h	UK	1-2 h	6-12 h	18-24 h
Lente Insulin	A & C: SC: 100 U/mL; dose is individualized according to blood sugar	B	Similar to regular insulin	13 h	UK	1-2 h	8-12 h	18-28 h
NPH Insulin	See Prototype Drug Chart	B	Similar to regular insulin	13 h	UK	1-2 h	6-12 h	18-24 h
Long Acting						
PZI Insulin	Same as lente	B	Similar to regular insulin	13 h	UK	4-8 h	14-20 h	24-36 h
Ultralente Insulin	Same as lente	B	Similar to regular insulin	13 h	UK	5-8 h	14-20 h	30-36 h

KEY: For complete abbreviation key, see inside front cover.

Prototype: Antidiabetics: Sulfonylurea

Acetohexamide

Acetohexamide
(Dymelor), ✽ Dimelor
Sulfonylurea, oral hypoglycemic drug
Pregnancy Category: C
Drug Forms:
Tab 250, 500 mg

Dosage

A: PO: 250–1,000 mg/d in 1 or 2 divided doses; max: 1.5 g/d

Contraindications

Diabetes mellitus (DM) type I; severe renal, hepatic, cardiac, or thyroid disease; unstable DM

Drug-Lab-Food Interactions

Increase hypoglycemic effect with aspirin, alcohol, anticoagulants, some NSAIDs, anticonvulsants, sulfonamides, oral contraceptives, MAOIs

Decrease hypoglycemic effect with glucocorticoids (cortisone), thiazide diuretics, estrogen, calcium channel blockers, phenytoin, thyroid drugs

Pharmacokinetics

Absorption: PO: Well absorbed
Distribution: PB: 90%
Metabolism: t 1/2: Drug: 1–1.5 h metabolite; 5–7 h
Excretion: Unchanged in urine

Pharmacodynamics

PO: Onset: 1 h
Peak: 2–6 h
Duration: 12–24 h

Therapeutic Effects/Uses: To control DM type II (maturity-onset diabetes); to lower blood sugar.

Mode of Action: Stimulation of beta cells to secrete insulin.

Side Effects

Nausea, vomiting, diarrhea, rash, pruritus, headache, photosensitivity

Adverse Reactions

Hypoglycemic reaction
Life-threatening: Aplastic anemia, leukopenia, thrombocytopenia

---

KEY: For complete abbreviation key, see inside front cover.

■ NURSING PROCESS: Antidiabetics: Sulfonylurea

ASSESSMENT

- Assess the drugs the client is currently taking. Aspirin, alcohol, sulfonamides, oral contraceptives, and MAOIs increase the hypoglycemic effect; decrease in oral hypoglycemic drug may be needed. Glucocorticoids (cortisone), thiazide diuretics, and estrogen increase blood sugar.
- Assess VS and blood sugar levels. Report abnormal findings.
- Assess the client's knowledge of diabetes mellitus and the use of oral antidiabetics (sulfonylurea).

Antidiabetics: Sulfonylurea

POTENTIAL NURSING DIAGNOSES
High risk for impaired tissue integrity
Altered nutrition: more or less than body requirements

PLANNING
- Client's blood sugar will be within normal serum levels (70–100 mg/dL).
- Client will adhere to prescribed diet, blood testing, and drug.

NURSING INTERVENTIONS
- Monitor VS. Sulfonylureas increase cardiac function and oxygen consumption, which can lead to cardiac dysrhythmias.
- Administer oral antidiabetics with food to minimize gastric upset.
- Monitor blood glucose levels and report changes. The reference value is 60–100 mg/dL for blood glucose and 70–110 mg/dL for serum glucose.
- Prepare a teaching plan based on the client's knowledge of health problems, diet, and drug therapy.

CLIENT TEACHING

General
- Advise the client that hypoglycemic (insulin) reaction can occur when taking an oral hypoglycemic drug. This drug stimulates the release of insulin from the beta cells of the pancreas. Oral antidiabetics are *not* insulin. Normally, clients with diabetes mellitus type I do not have functioning beta cells and should *not* take oral antidiabetics, only insulin. Sulfonylureas are prescribed for clients with diabetes mellitus type II.
- Instruct the client to recognize symptoms of hypoglycemic reaction (headache, nervousness, sweating, tremors, rapid pulse), and symptoms of hyperglycemic reaction (thirst, increased urine output, sweet fruity breath odor).
- Explain that insulin might be needed instead of an oral antidiabetic drug during stress, surgery, or serious infection. Blood sugar levels are usually elevated during stressful times.
- Instruct the client about the necessity for compliance to diet and drug.
- Advise the client to obtain a medical alert card, tag, and/or bracelet indicating the health problem and insulin dosage.

Skill
- Instruct the client how to check the blood sugar level using a Chemstrip bG test. Client should record and report abnormal results.

Diet
- To avoid a hypoglycemic reaction, instruct the client not to ingest alcohol with sulfonylurea drugs. Food taken with oral antidiabetics will decrease gastric irritation.
- Advise the client taking sulfonylurea to eat the prescribed diet on schedule. Delaying or missing a meal can cause hypoglycemia.
- Explain the use of orange juice, sugar-containing drinks, and hard candy when a hypoglycemic reaction begins.

Side Effects
- Instruct the client to report side effects, such as vomiting, diarrhea, rash.

EVALUATION
- Evaluate the effectiveness of drug therapy by noting whether blood sugar levels are within the accepted range.

Antidiabetic: Sulfonylurea

Generic (Brand)	Route and Dosage	Preg Cat	Interaction	t 1/2	PB	Onset	Peak	Duration
First Generation: Short Acting								
Tolbutamide (Orinase)	A: PO: 500–3,000 mg/d in 2–3 divided doses	C	*Increase* hypoglycemic effect with aspirin, NSAIDs, oral anticoagulants, insulin, cimetidine, sulfonamides, methyldopa *Decrease* effect with calcium channel blockers, glucocorticoids, estrogens, phenytoin, thyroid drugs, phenothiazines, thiazides	4–7 h	90–95%	1 h	3–5 h	6–12 h
First Generation: Intermediate Acting								
Acetohexamide (Dymelor)	See Prototype Drug Chart							
Tolazamide (Tolinase)	A: PO: 100–250 mg/d in 1–2 divided doses; max: 1 g/d	C	Similar to tolbutamide	7 h	90%	1–4 h	4–6 h	10–15 h

First Generation: Long Acting Chlorpropamide (Diabinese)	A: PO: Initially: 100–250 mg/d; maint: 100–500 mg/d in 1–2 divided doses; max: 750 mg/d	C	Similar to tolbutamide *Decrease* digoxin level with digoxin	36 h	95%	1 h	3–6 h	24 h
Second Generation: Glipizide (Glucotrol)	A: PO: Initially: 2.5–5.0 mg a.c. q.d./b.i.d.; maint: 10–15 mg/d (dose should be divided if >15 mg); max: 40 mg/d	C	Similar to tolbutamide	2.5–5 h	90–95%	0.5–1 h	1–2 h	10–24 h
Glyburide nonmicronized (DiaBeta, Micronase)	A: PO: Initially: 1.25–5 mg/d; maint: 1.25–20 mg q.d./b.i.d.; max: 20 mg/d	B	Same as tolbutamide *Decrease* digoxin level with digoxin; *decrease* effect with cimetidine	3–10 h	90–95%	0.5–1 h	1–2 h	10–24 h
Glyburide micronized (Glynase)	A: PO: 1.5–3 mg/d in AM; maint: 3–4.5 mg/d; max: 12 mg/d in 1–2 divided doses	B	Same as glyburide nonmicronized	3–10 h	90–95%	<1 h	1–2 h	10–24 h

KEY: For complete abbreviation key, see inside front cover.

REPRODUCTIVE AND GENDER-RELATED AGENTS

Beta-Adrenergic Agonists

Oxytocins

Estrogen Replacements

Oral Contraceptives

Androgens

Ovulation Stimulants

Prototype: Beta-Adrenergic Agonists: Ritodrine

Ritodrine HCl

Ritodrine HCl
 (Yutopar)
Adrenergic
Pregnancy Category: B
Drug Forms:
Tab 10 mg
Inj 10 mg/mL

Dosage

IV: Mix 150 mg in 500 mL D_5W and infuse at 10–20 mL/h; increase by 10 mL/h q15 min until contractions >15 min apart; max: 70 mL/h; decrease therapy as contractions taper off
Initiate PO therapy 10–20 mg 30 min before stopping IV drug; PO dose q1–6h until tocolysis not needed
Refer to specific protocol.

Contraindications

Before 20th week of gestation, condition in which maintenance of pregnancy is hazardous, e.g., antepartal hemorrhage and intrauterine fetal death; selected preexisting maternal conditions, e.g., uncontrolled hypertension or diabetes

Drug-Lab-Food Interactions

Increase effects of ritodrine with diazoxide, meperidine, potent general anesthetics, magnesium sulfate; *increase* effects of sympathomimetic amines
Decrease effects of ritodrine with beta blockers

Pharmacokinetics

Absorption: PO: 30%
Distribution: PB: 32%, crosses placenta; probably crosses blood–brain barrier
Metabolism: t 1/2: 15 h
Excretion: In urine

Pharmacodynamics

PO: Onset: 30 min
  Peak: 30–60 min
  Duration: 4–6 h
IV: Onset: Within 5 min
  Peak: 50–60 min
  Duration: 30 min

Therapeutic Effects/Uses: To inhibit uterine contractions.

Mode of Action: Stimulation of receptors in smooth muscles of uterus, thereby decreasing intensity and frequency of contractions.

Side Effects

Malaise, weakness, dyspnea, tachycardia (maternal and fetal), palpitations, increased systolic pressure, chest pain, nausea, vomiting, diarrhea, hyperglycemia, hypokalemia

Adverse Reactions

Ketoacidosis
Life-threatening: Long term: pulmonary edema, anaphylactic shock

KEY: For complete abbreviation key, see inside front cover.

Beta-Adrenergic Agonists: Ritodrine

■ NURSING PROCESS: Beta-Adrenergic Agonists: Ritodrine

ASSESSMENT
- Identify clients at risk for preterm labor early in pregnancy.
- Obtain a history, complete physical assessment, VS, fetal heart rate (FHR), and urine specimen for infection screening.

POTENTIAL NURSING DIAGNOSES
High risk for activity intolerance
Altered health maintenance

PLANNING
- Client's preterm contractions will be eliminated by resting in left side lying position, increasing fluid intake, and tocolytic therapy as needed.

NURSING INTERVENTIONS
- Monitor and assess uterine activity and FHR before, during, and for 1 h after discontinuing IV infusion.
- Maintain client in left lateral position as much as possible.
- Monitor maternal and fetal VS every 15 min when the client is receiving IV dose. Report if systolic blood pressure drops to <90 mm Hg or is >140 mm Hg, if diastolic blood pressure is <50 mm Hg, or if pulse increases to >120 beats per minute. If any of these occur, place client in Trendelenburg position and increase the infusion rate of primary IV (*not* of the piggyback IV containing the drug).
- Report auscultated cardiac dysrhythmias. An ECG may be ordered.
- Auscultate breath sounds every 4 h. Notify health care provider if respirations are >30/min or there is a change in quality (wheezes, rales, coughing).
- Monitor daily weight to assess fluid overload; monitor strict input and output every 8 h.
- Provide passive range of motion of legs every 1–2 h.
- Report fetal baseline heart rate >180 beats per min.
- Report persistence of frequent contractions despite tocolytic therapy.
- Report rupture of membranes, vaginal bleeding, or sudden complaints of rectal pressure, suggesting impending delivery.
- Be alert to presence of hypoglycemia and hypokalemia in the newborn delivered within 5 h of discontinued beta-sympathomimetic drugs.
- Administer only clear solutions of drugs if using IV form.
- Assist clients on home tocolytic therapy plan for assistance with self-care and family responsibilities.

CLIENT TEACHING

General
- Teach client the signs and symptoms of impending preterm labor (menstrual type cramps, sensation of pelvic pressure, low backache, and increased vaginal discharge).
- Instruct client that if she experiences preterm labor contractions at home, she should void, recline on her left side to increase uterine blood flow, drink extra fluids to decrease the release of antidiuretic hormone (ADH) and oxytocin from the posterior pituitary, rest for 30 min, and then attempt to resume her activities if asymptomatic. Stress that she should notify her health care provider if the contractions do not end or if they return.

Beta-Adrenergic Agonists: Ritodrine

- Tell client that she may return to her normal activities after 36–48 h without contractions; check with health care provider.
- Explain the effects of beta-sympathomimetic drugs; the contractions should be arrested. Report heart palpitations or dizziness.
- Instruct client to take the drug as directed.
- Advise the client to contact the health care provider before taking any other drugs while on tocolysis.
- Instruct the client that if she misses a dose and <1 h has elapsed, she should take the missed dose. However, if >1 h has elapsed, she should wait until the next regularly scheduled dose.

EVALUATION

- Evaluate the effectiveness of the tocolytic drug by noting the absence of six or more contractions in 1 h.
- Evaluate the client's understanding of nonpharmacologic measures for decreasing preterm contractions, such as increasing fluid intake and resting on the left side.
- Continue monitoring the client's and fetal VS. Report any change immediately.

Drugs Used to Decrease Uterine Motility

Generic (Brand)	Route and Dosage	Preg Cat	Interaction	t 1/2	PB	Onset	Peak	Duration
Beta-Adrenergic Agonists			Hypertensive crises with MAOIs *Decrease* effects of beta blockers	10–15 h	25%			
Ritodrine HCl (Yutopar)	See Prototype Drug Chart					PO: 30–45 min	1–2 h	4–8 h
Terbutaline SO$_4$ (Brethine)	SC: Initially: 0.25 mg (repeat as necessary); SC maint: 0.1 mg q4h followed with PO: 2.5–5 mg q4–6h starting with last SC dose; refer to protocol	B				SC: 5–15 min	0.5–1 h	1.5–4 h
Calcium Antagonist								
Magnesium sulfate	Follow protocol IV: Usual LD: 4–6 g in 50–100 mL over 20–30 min; maint: 40 g in 1 L IVF at 2–4 g/h; dose based on serum magnesium levels and deep tendon reflex assessment	A	Increased respiratory depression with neuromuscular blocking agents	UK	UK	Immediate	UK	30 min

KEY: For complete abbreviation key, see inside front cover.

Prototype: Oxytocins

Oxytocin

Oxytocin
  (Pitocin, Syntocinon)
Oxytocic
Pregnancy Category: X
Drug Forms:
Nasal sol 40 U/mL
Inj 10 U/mL

Dosage

A: IV: 10 U (1 amp) diluted in 1,000 mL lactated Ringer's to 10 mU/mL; connect to control IV line at the needle site of main IV line, as a secondary line; start at 0.5 mU/min (3 mL/h) and titrate at rate of 0.5–2.5 mU every 15–30 min until contractions are approximately 3 min apart and adequate
IV: 10 U added to 1 L electrolyte or dextrose solution; infuse at rate to control atony
(IM: 10 U after delivery of the placenta if no IV)
Nasal spray: 1 spray into 1 or both nostrils 2–3 min before nursing or pumping

Contraindications

Toxemia, cephalopelvic disproportionment, fetal distress, hypersensitivity, anticipated nonvaginal delivery, pregnancy (intranasal spray)

Drug-Lab-Food Interactions

Hypertension with vasopressors, cyclopropane anesthetics

Pharmacokinetics

Absorption: PO: Well absorbed
Distribution: PB: Low; widely distributed in extracellular fluid; minute amounts in fetal circulation
Metabolism: t 1/2: 1–9 min; rapidly metabolized by liver
Excretion: In urine

Pharmacodynamics

IM: Onset: 3–5 min
  Peak: UK
  Duration: 2–3 h
IV: Onset: Immediate
  Peak: UK
  Duration: 1 h
Intranasal: Onset: Few minutes
  Peak: UK
  Duration: 20 min

Therapeutic Effects/Uses: To induce/augment labor contractions; to treat uterine atony; milk letdown (intranasal spray).

Mode of Action: Action of myofibrils to stimulate letdown of milk and promote uterine contractions.

Side Effects

Maternal effects with IV use only: Hypotension, hypertension, nausea, vomiting, constipation, decreased uterine blood flow, rash, anorexia

Adverse Reactions

Seizures, water intoxication
Life-threatening: Intracranial hemorrhage, cardiac dysrhythmias, asphyxia; fetus: jaundice, hypoxia

KEY: For complete abbreviation key, see inside front cover.

Oxytocins

■ NURSING PROCESS: Oxytocins

ASSESSMENT
For induction or augmentation of labor:
- Collect accurate baseline data before beginning infusion, including maternal pulse and blood pressure, uterine activity, and fetal heart rate (FHR).
- Record assessment results on FHR monitor graph paper in addition to other agency records.

POTENTIAL NURSING DIAGNOSIS
Knowledge deficit

PLANNING
- Oxytocin will enhance uterine contractions without adverse effects.
- Client's VS will be within acceptable ranges during the therapy.

NURSING INTERVENTIONS
- Have magnesium sulfate and/or other tocolytic agents and oxygen readily available in case hypertonicity occurs.
- Monitor input and output every 2 h. Fluids should not exceed 1,000 mL/8 h.
- Monitor maternal pulse and blood pressure, uterine activity, and FHR before increasing oxytocin infusion.
- Maintain the client in the lateral recumbent position or sitting to promote placental infusion.
- Be alert for signs of uterine rupture (very infrequent), which include sudden increased pain, loss of contractions and decreased or absent FHR, hemorrhage, and rapidly developing hypovolemic shock.

CLIENT TEACHING
- Explain to the client that the drug is given intravenously to adjust dosage in response to contraction pattern.
- For milk letdown: Teach client timing and method of nasal administration.

EVALUATION
- Evaluate the effectiveness of the drug. Labor progresses.
- Continue monitoring VS. Report changes in VS or vaginal bleeding.

Oxytocic Drugs Used to Enhance Uterine Motility

Generic (Brand)	Route and Dosage	Preg Cat	Interaction	t 1/2	PB	Onset	Peak	Duration
Ergonovine maleate (Ergotrate)	PO: 0.2–0.4 mg q6–12 h over 48 h IM: 0.2 mg q2–4h; max: 5 doses IV: 0.2 mg (only for severe bleeding) over 1 min while blood pressure and contractions are monitored	X	*Increase* vasoconstriction with other vasopressors, smoking	UK	UK	PO: 5–15 min IM: 2–5 min IV: <5 min	60–90 min UK UK	3 h 3 h 45 min
Methylergonovine maleate (Methergine)	PO: 0.2–0.4 mg q6–12 h; max: 1 wk IM: 0.2 mg, after delivery of placenta, or postpartum; repeat q2–4h; oral doses may follow parenteral IV: Same as for IM; but slowly over 1 min with careful monitoring of blood pressure	C	Similar to ergonovine maleate	Initially: 1–5 min Terminal: 30–120 min	UK	PO: 5–15 min IM: 2–5 min IV: Immediate	0.5–3 h UK UK	3 h 3 h 0.5–3 h

Oxytocin (Pitocin, Syntocinon)	IV: 10 U diluted in 1,000 mL lactated Ringer's to 10 mU/mL; connect to control IV at needle site of main IV as a secondary line; start at 0.5 mU/min (3 mL/h) and titrate at rate of 0.5–2.5 mU q15–30 min until contractions are q2–3 min and adequate IV: 10 U added to 1 L electrolyte or dextrose solution (10 mU/mL); infuse at rate to control atony (IM: 10 U after delivery of placenta if no IV)	X	*Increase* vasoconstriction with other pressor drugs Hypotension with cyclopropane	1–5 min	30%	IV: 1 min IM: 3–5 min	UK	IV: <30 min IM: 30–60 min
Dinoprostone cervical gel (Prepidil gel) *(Oxytocic)*	Supplied in 3 g prefilled syringe applicators; 3 doses (1 dose q6h) 6 h after last dose IV oxytocin administration; max: 1.5 mg/24 h (7.5 mL or 3 syringes)	X	Avoid use of oxytocics, alcohol	UK	UK	10 min	UK	2–3 h
Carboprost tromethamine (Hemabate) *(Oxytocic)*	*Termination of pregnancy:* IM: 250 μg, then 250 μg at 1.5–4 h intervals based on uterine response; a 500 μg dose, if needed	X	None significant	UK	UK	15–60 min	UK	2–4 h

KEY: For complete abbreviation key, see inside front cover.

Prototype: Estrogen Replacements

Conjugated Estrogens

Conjugated estrogens
  (Premarin, PMB, Milprem-400), ✺
  C.E.S.
Hormone replacement therapy (HRT)
Pregnancy Category: X
Drug Forms:
Tab 0.3, 0.65, 0.9, 1.25, 2.5 mg
Cream 0.0623%
Inj 25 mg
Patch

Dosage

A: PO: 0.3–1.25 mg/d cyclically
  (with or without progestins); most
  often, 0.625 mg/d

Contraindications

Breast or reproductive cancer,
  undiagnosed genital bleeding,
  pregnancy, lactation,
  thromboembolitic disorders,
  smoking
Caution: Cardiovascular disease,
  severe renal or hepatic disease,
  smoking, diabetes mellitus

Drug-Lab-Food Interactions

Increase effects with corticosteroids
Decrease effects of anticoagulants,
  oral hypoglycemics; *decrease* effects
  with rifampin, anticonvulsants,
  barbiturates
Toxicity with tricyclic
  antidepressants

Pharmacokinetics

Absorption: PO: Well absorbed
Distribution: PB: Widely distributed;
  crosses placenta and enters breast
  milk
Metabolism: t 1/2: UK
Excretion: In urine and bile

Pharmacodynamics

PO/IV: Onset: Rapid
  Peak: UK
  Duration: UK
IM: Onset: Delayed
  Peak: UK
  Duration: UK

Therapeutic Effects/Uses: To relieve vasodilation, hot flashes, and vaginal dryness; to prevent cardiovascular disease and osteoporosis.

Mode of Action: Development and maintenance of female genital system, breasts, and secondary sex characteristics; increased synthesis of protein.

Side Effects

Nausea, vomiting, fluid retention,
  breast tenderness, leg cramps and
  breakthrough bleeding, chloasma

Adverse Reactions

Jaundice, thromboembolic disorders,
  depression, hypercalcemia, gall
  bladder disease
Life-threatening: Thromboembolism,
  cerebrovascular accident,
  pulmonary embolism, MI,
  endometrial cancer

KEY: For complete abbreviation key, see inside front cover.

■ NURSING PROCESS: Estrogen Replacements

ASSESSMENT

- Assess the client for baseline data, including height, weight, usual physical activity, diet, family history, and personal risk factors regarding osteoporosis,

Estrogen Replacements

family and personal risk of cardiovascular disease, and the nature of the family members' climacteric experience, the client's menstrual history, and current experience with the climacteric and the drugs the client is using.
- Assess the client's perception of menopause.
- Assess the client's attitude toward resumption of menstrual periods.

POTENTIAL NURSING DIAGNOSES
Sexual dysfunction
Body image disturbance
Health-seeking behaviors

PLANNING
- Client will know menopausal symptoms and the nonpharmacologic and pharmacologic measures that may aid in alleviating symptoms.

NURSING INTERVENTIONS
- Educate women about the nature of the climacteric, its potential effects, and nonpharmacologic as well as pharmacologic treatment. Place current educational materials in health and community sites.
- Indicate on the laboratory slip or specimen that the client is taking hormone replacement therapy (HRT).
- Administer IM route at bedtime to decrease adverse effects.
- Administer IV route slowly to avoid flushing reaction.

CLIENT TEACHING

General
- Review the risk-to-benefit ratio for deciding to use or not to use estrogen replacement therapy.
- Review the contraindications to this HRT.
- Advise the client to have a thorough breast examination, pelvic examination, Pap test, and endometrial biopsy before starting HRT.
- Tell the client that warm weather and stress exacerbate vasodilation/hot flashes.
- Advise the client to use a fan, drink cool liquids, wear layered cotton clothes, decrease intake of caffeine and spicy foods, and talk with her health care provider about the use of vitamin E to cope more comfortably with vasodilation. Individuals with diabetes, hypertension, or rheumatic heart disease should use vitamin E in low doses with the health care provider's approval.
- Encourage the client on HRT to have medical follow-up every 6–12 mo, including blood pressure check and breast and pelvic examinations.
- Suggest that the client carry sanitary pads or tampons for breakthrough bleeding or irregular periods.
- Stress the need to use nonhormonal birth control since irregular periods may create anxiety about pregnancy. Tell the client to plan to use birth control for 2 y. If she has progesterone-induced bleeding, the only way to determine whether she is truly menopausal is by hormone assay.
- Suggest to the client that she use a water-soluble vaginal lubricant to reduce painful intercourse (dyspareunia) and prevent trauma.
- Advise the client to decrease use of antihistamines and decongestants if she is experiencing vaginal dryness.
- Advise the client to wear cotton underwear and pantyhose with a cotton liner and to avoid douche and feminine hygiene products.

Estrogen Replacements

- Suggest that client take Premarin after meals together with progestin to avoid nausea and vomiting.
- Tell the client to report any heavy bleeding (flooding) and to have her hematocrit and hemoglobin evaluated for anemia.
- Tell the client to report bleeding that occurs between periods or return of bleeding after cessation of menstruation. A cancer work-up may be indicated.
- Advise the client starting on HRT that the withdrawal bleeding that occurs from days 25–30 is normal and not the same as the cyclic menstrual periods she had secondary to ovulation. Tell her that this bleeding will usually last only 2–3 d and that she will not experience the same degree of premenstrual symptoms she may have had with regular periods.
- Advise the client to report if bleeding occurs other than on days 25–30 once she has started on HRT.
- Tell her that the withdrawal bleeding does not signify that she can become pregnant (since she is not fertile).
- Advise the client that after HRT is discontinued, there may be a recurrence of menopausal signs and symptoms such as hot flashes.

Diet

- Discuss the use of yogurt containing *Acidophilus* or *Lactobacillus* as a way of maintaining normal bacterial flora in the vagina.
- Tell the client that she may experience an occasional hot flash on days 25–30 when she is going through withdrawal bleeding. Instruct the client to stop treatment and contact health care provider if she has headache, visual disturbances, signs of thrombophlebitis, heaviness in legs, chest pain, or breast lumps.
- Tell the client that if she wants to stop HRT, she should do so with guidance of her health care provider.
- Suggest that the client at risk for osteoporosis have consistent exercise such as walking or bicycling, eat a well-balanced diet (low in red meat and sugar) with 1,200 mg calcium/d if premenopausal or 1,200–1,500 mg/d if menopausal, and avoid smoking and alcohol.

Skill

- Teach the client to perform breast self-examination consistently.
- If the client is using vaginal cream, review the application procedure and suggest that she wear minipads.
- If the client is using the transdermal patch, tell her to open the package and apply it immediately, holding it in place for about 10 s; to check the edges to ensure adequate contact; to use the abdomen (except waistline) for the patch; to rotate the sites with at least 1 wk before reuse of a site; to not use the breast as a site; to not put the patch on an irritated or oily area; to reapply the patch if it loosens or put on a new one; and to follow the same cycle schedule.

EVALUATION

- Evaluate the effectiveness of the nonpharmacologic or pharmacologic measures for premenopausal symptoms.
- Determine whether side effects are occurring. Plan with the client alternative measures to control menopausal symptoms.

Estrogen Replacements

Estrogens and Progestins

Generic (Brand)	Route and Dosage	Preg Cat
Steroidal Estrogens		
Estradiol (Estrace, Estraderm)	*Menopausal/hypogonadism:* PO: 1–2 mg/d for 21 d; then, 7–10 d off cycle; may repeat cycle *Patch:* 10–20 cm^2 system 2×/wk, in above cycle *Breast cancer:* PO: 10 mg t.i.d. *Prostate cancer:* PO: 1–2 mg t.i.d. *Atrophic vaginitis:* Cream: 2–4 g/d for 1–2 wk; maint: 1 g 2×/wk	X
Estradiol cypionate (Depo-Estradiol Cypionate)	*Menopausal symptoms:* IM: 1–4 mg q3–4wk *Hypogonadism:* IM: 1.5–2 mg q mo	X
Esterified estrogens (Estratab, Menest)	*Menopausal symptoms:* PO: 0.3–1.25 mg/d for 3 wk; then 7–10 d off cycle *Breast cancer:* PO: 10 mg t.i.d. *Prostate cancer:* PO: 1.25–2.5 mg t.i.d.	X
Estrone (Theelin, Kestrone 5)	*Hypogonadism:* PO: 0.1–2 mg/wk *Prostate cancer:* PO: 2–4 mg 3×/wk	X
Estropipate SO$_4$ (Ogen, Ortho-Est)	*Hypogonadism:* PO: 1.25–7.5 mg/d for 3 wk; then 7–10 d off cycle	X
Nonsteroidal Estrogens		
Chlorotrianisene (Tace)	*Menopausal/hypogonadism:* PO: 12–25 mg/d for 21 d; then, 10 d off cycle; repeat cycle *Prostate cancer:* PO: 12–25 mg/d	X
Dienestrol (DV)	*Atrophic vaginitis:* Cream: Apply q.d./b.i.d. for 1–2 wk; maint: 1–3×/wk	X
Diethylstilbestrol	*Breast cancer:* PO: 15 mg/d *Prostate cancer:* PO: 1–3 mg t.i.d.	X
Quinestrol (Estrovis)	*Menopausal/hypogonadism:* PO: 100 μg daily for 7 d; then 7 d off cycle; maint: q wk	X
Progestins		
Progesterone	*DUB:* IM: 5–10 mg/d for 7 d *Amenorrhea:* IM: 5–10 mg/d for 6–8 d	X
Medroxyprogesterone acetate (Amen, Curretab, Provera, Cycrin, Depo-Provera)	*DUB/amenorrhea:* PO: 5–10 mg/d for 5–10 d *Endometriosis:* IM: 150 mg q3mon	X

continued

Estrogen Replacements

Estrogens and Progestins—*Continued*

Generic (Brand)	Route and Dosage	Preg Cat
Megestrol acetate (Megace)	*Breast cancer:* PO: 40 mg q.i.d. *Endometrial cancer:* PO: 40–320 mg/d in divided doses	X
Norethindrone (Norlutin)	*DUB/amenorrhea:* PO: 5–20 mg/d on days 5–25 of menstrual cycle	X

KEY: For complete abbreviation key, see inside front cover.

Oral Contraceptives

Product	Amount of Estrogen (μg)	Amount of Progestin (mg)
Combination Products: Listed by Decreasing Estrogen Content		
Monophasic Products		
Norinyl 1 + 50 (21 d)	50 mestranol	1 norethindrone
Genora 1/50	50 mestranol	1 norethindrone
Ovcon 50	50 ethinyl estradiol	1 norethindrone
Norlestrin 1/50	50 ethinyl estradiol	1 norethindrone acetate
Demulen 1/50	50 ethinyl estradiol	1 ethynodiol diacetate
Norlestrin 21 2.5/50	50 ethinyl estradiol	2.5 norethindrone acetate
Ovral	50 ethinyl estradiol	0.5 norgestrel
Genora 1/35	35 ethinyl estradiol	1 norethindrone
Norcept-E 1/35	35 ethinyl estradiol	1 norethindrone
Ortho-Novum 1/35	35 ethinyl estradiol	1 norethindrone
N.E.E. 1/35	35 ethinyl estradiol	1 norethindrone
Norethin 1/35 E	35 ethinyl estradiol	1 norethindrone
Norinyl 1 + 35	35 ethinyl estradiol	1 norethindrone
Modicon	35 ethinyl estradiol	0.5 norethindrone
Brevicon	35 ethinyl estradiol	0.5 norethindrone
Nelova	35 ethinyl estradiol	0.5 norethindrone
Ovcon 35	35 ethinyl estradiol	0.4 norethindrone
Demulen 1/35	35 ethinyl estradiol	1 ethynodiol diacetate
Desogen	30 ethinyl estradiol	0.15 desogestrel
Loestrin 21 1.5/30	30 ethinyl estradiol	1.5 norethindrone acetate
Lo/Ovral	30 ethinyl estradiol	0.3 norgestrel
Levlen	30 ethinyl estradiol	0.15 levonorgestrel
Nordette	30 ethinyl estradiol	0.15 levonorgestrel
Loestrin 21 1/20	20 ethinyl estradiol	1 norethindrone acetate
Biphasic Products		
Jenest-28	*Phase I:* 7 d 35 ethinyl estradiol *Phase II:* 14 d 35 ethinyl estradiol	0.5 norethindrone 1.0 norethindrone
N.E.E. 10/11	*Phase I:* 10 d 35 ethinyl estradiol *Phase II:* 11 d 35 ethinyl estradiol	0.5 norethindrone 1.0 norethindrone

Estrogen Replacements

Oral Contraceptives—*Continued*

Product	Amount of Estrogen (μg)	Amount of Progestin (mg)
Nelova 10/11	*Phase I:* 10 d; 35 ethinyl estradiol	0.5 norethindrone
	Phase II: 11 d; 35 ethinyl estradiol	1 norethindrone
Ortho-Novum 10/11	Same formulation as above but different colors for tablets	

Triphasic Products

Product	Amount of Estrogen (μg)	Amount of Progestin (mg)
Tri-Norinyl	*Phase I:* 7 d; 35 ethinyl estradiol	0.5 norethindrone
	Phase II: 9 d; 35 ethinyl estradiol	1 norethindrone
	Phase III: 5 d; 35 ethinyl estradiol	0.5 norethindrone
Ortho Tri-Cyclen	*Phase I:* 7 d; 35 ethinyl estradiol	0.18 norgestimate
	Phase II: 7 d; 35 ethinyl estradiol	0.215 norgestimate
	Phase III: 7 d; 35 ethinyl estradiol	0.25 norgestimate
Ortho-Novum 7/7/7	*Phase I:* 7 d; 35 ethinyl estradiol	0.5 norethindrone
	Phase II: 7 d; 35 ethinyl estradiol	0.75 norethindrone
	Phase III: 7 d; 35 ethinyl estradiol	1 norethindrone
Tri-Levlen	*Phase I:* 6 d; 30 ethinyl estradiol	0.05 levonorgestrel
	Phase II: 5 d; 40 ethinyl estradiol	0.075 levonorgestrel
	Phase III: 10 d; 30 ethinyl estradiol	0.125 levonorgestrel
Triphasil	Same as above	

Progestin-Only Products: Listed by Decreasing Progestin Content

Product	Amount of Progestin (mg)
Micronor	0.35 norethindrone
Nor-QD	0.35 norethindrone
Ovrette	0.075 norgestrel

Prototype: Androgens

Testosterone

Testosterone
(Andro-Cyp 100, depAndro 100, Depotest 100, Duratest 100, DEPO-Testosterone, Testred Cypionate 200, Virilon, depAndrogyn, Everone), 🍁 Malogen

Pregnancy Category: X
CSS III

Drug Forms:
Inj IM 25, 50, 100 mg/mL
Tab
Patch (transdermal system)

Dosage

Androgen Replacement:
PO: 10–40 mg daily
Buccal: 5–20 mg daily
SC: 150–450 mg q3–6mo
IM: 10–30 mg 2–3×/wk
Patch: Initially: Apply 2 Systems q.h.s. (5 mg/d)

Metastatic Carcinoma of the Breast:
PO: 200 mg daily
Buccal: 200 mg daily
IM: 100 mg 3×/wk

Contraindications

Pregnancy, nephrosis, hypercalcemia, pituitary insufficiency, hepatic dysfunction, benign prostatic hypertrophy, prostatic cancer, history of MI, prepubertal status, non–estrogen-dependent breast cancer

Caution: Hypertension, hypercholesteremia, coronary artery disease, gynecomastia, renal disease, seizure disorders, before puberty, older adults

Drug-Lab-Food Interactions

Increases effects of anticoagulants
Decreases effect with barbiturates, phenytoin, phenylbutazone
Antagonizes calcitonin, parathyroid
Corticosteroids exacerbate edema
Lab: Decreases blood glucose in diabetics; *increases* serum cholesterol, thyroid, liver function, hematocrit

Pharmacokinetics

Absorption: IM: Well absorbed
Distribution: PB: 98%
Metabolism: t 1/2: 10–100 min
Excretion: In urine and bile

Pharmacodynamics

IM: Onset: UK
Peak: UK
Duration: cypionate enanthate: 2–4 wk
base, propionate: 1–3 d

Therapeutic Effects/Uses: To achieve normal androgen levels; to slow progress of estrogen-dependent breast cancers.

Mode of Action: Development and maintenance of male sex organs and secondary sex characteristics.

Side Effects

Abdominal pain, nausea, diarrhea, constipation, hives, irritation at injection site, increased salivation, mouth soreness, increased or decreased libido, insomnia, aggressive behavior, weakness, dizziness, pruritus

Adverse Reactions

Acne, masculinization, irregular menses, urinary urgency, gynecomastia, priapism, red skin, jaundice, sodium and water retention, allergic reaction, depression

Life-threatening: Hepatic necrosis, hepatitis, hepatic tumors, respiratory distress

KEY: For complete abbreviation key, see inside front cover.

Androgens

■ NURSING PROCESS: Androgens: Testosterone

ASSESSMENT
- Assess the reason for androgen therapy and the client's perception of it. If delayed puberty is the indication, assess the client's and family's attitudes about the condition.
- Assess the client's weight, blood pressure, liver and thyroid function, hemoglobin, hematocrit, creatinine, clotting factors, glucose tolerance, serum lipids and electrolytes, and blood count before and throughout drug therapy.
- Assess the pregnancy status of fertile women. Concomitant anticoagulation therapy is recommended. When a prepubertal child is treated, assess x-rays before treatment and every 6 mo during and after treatment to monitor growth.
- Assess the client's affect during therapy, particularly aggressiveness in clients taking large doses. Self-concept is an important consideration with the client on androgen therapy, particularly in women and in children in whom puberty is delayed.

POTENTIAL NURSING DIAGNOSES
Sexual dysfunction
High risk for body image disturbance
High risk for situational low self-esteem

PLANNING
- Client adheres to prescribed drug regimen and monitoring.
- Medication is effective for intended purpose, and preventable side effects are avoided.
- Client maintains positive self-concept.

NURSING INTERVENTIONS
- Use lowest effective dose.
- Shake vial and warm to room temperature to dissolve crystals, as needed.
- Administer the IM form in a large muscle mass, such as the upper outer quadrant of the gluteus.
- Record body weight several times each week.
- Monitor muscle strength.
- Monitor bone maturation every 6 mo with x-rays of wrists and hands.

CLIENT TEACHING
General
- Instruct the client and family on the proper administration of the medication and potential undesired effects.
- Inform the client of effects that warrant prompt medical attention, such as urinary problems, priapism, and respiratory distress.
- Advise the client who is having an intermittent approach to treatment of the need for monitoring the endocrine status between courses of androgen therapy.
- Instruct the client to record body weight several times each week. Sodium may need to be restricted if edema develops.
- Advise the client with tissue wasting to reduce environmental stressors and promote rest and relaxation, since stress hormones are catabolic.

Androgens

- Instruct the client to take oral androgens with food to decrease gastric distress.
- Advise the family of normal development if the client is receiving treatment for delayed puberty.
- Instruct both prepubertal and adult female clients on good skin hygiene to control the severity of the acne.
- Instruct men to report priapism promptly; the drug dose needs to be reduced.

Diet

- Encourage adequate nutritional support with adequate intake of calories, proteins, vitamins, iron, and other minerals.

Side Effects

- Instruct the client with elevated serum calcium of the need for 3–4 L of fluid per day to prevent kidney stones. Individuals on bedrest need range-of-motion exercises, and ambulatory clients need to engage in active weight bearing. Hypercalcemia needs prompt medical attention because it can lead to cardiac arrest.

EVALUATION

- Evaluate the client's ability to adhere to treatment regimen.
- Identify therapeutic and side effects of drug.
- Determine the client's ability to cope with virilizing effects or acne and to maintain a positive self-concept.

Androgens

Generic (Brand)	Route and Dosage	Preg Cat	Interaction	t 1/2	PB	Onset	Peak	Duration
Natural Androgens Testosterone (Histerone, Tesamone, testosterone aqueous, testosterone powder) CSS III	*Replacement:* IM: 10–30 mg 2–3×wk PO: 10–40 mg daily Buccal: 5–20 mg daily SC: 150–450 mg q3–6 mo *Carcinoma of breast:* IM: 100 mg 3×wk PO: 200 mg daily Buccal: 100 mg daily See Prototype Drug Chart	X						
Testosterone cypionate (Andro-Cyp, depAndro, Depotest, DEPO-Testosterone, Duratest, Virilon, IM) CSS III	IM: 50–400 mg q2–6wk	X	*Increase* effects of oral hypoglycemics, insulin, glucocorticoids, anticoagulants *Lab:* May affect thyroid function tests	8 d	98%	UK	UK	2–4 wk
Testosterone enanthate (Andro L.A., Delatest Delatestryl, Everone) CSS III	IM: 50–400 mg q2–6wk	X	Similar to testosterone cypionate	UK	99%	UK	UK	2–4 wk
Testosterone propionate (Testex) CSS III	*Replacement:* IM: 10–25 mg 2–4×wk *Carcinoma of breast:* IM: 50 mg 3×wk	X	Similar to testosterone cypionate	UK	99%	UK	UK	1–4 d
Synthetic Androgens Danazol (Danocrine)	PO: 100–800 mg daily divided in 2 doses initially	X	May need increase in insulin dose *Lab:* Altered liver function tests	4.5 h	UK	3–4 wk	3–4 wk	2–6 mo

continued

Androgens—Continued

Generic (Brand)	Route and Dosage	Preg Cat	Interaction	t 1/2	PB	Onset	Peak	Duration
Fluoxymesterone (Halotestin) CSS III	*Replacement:* PO: 2–10 mg daily divided into 1–4 doses *Carcinoma of breast:* PO: 15–40 mg daily in divided doses	X	*Increase* effects of anticoagulants, oral antidiabetics *Lab:* Alters GTT, cholesterol, T_3, T_4, serum potassium, and calcium	20–100 min	98%	UK	UK	UK
Methyltestosterone (Android, Oreton-Methyl, Testred, Virilon) CSS III	PO: Initially: 10–50 mg daily in divided doses; maint: reduced Buccal: Initially: 5–25 mg daily in divided doses; maint: reduced *Carcinoma of breast:* PO: 50–200 mg daily Buccal: 25–100 mg daily	X	*Decrease* effect of insulin, oral anticoagulants	UK	UK	UK	PO: 2 h Buccal: 1 h	UK
Anabolic Steroids								
Nandrolone decanoate (Androlone-D, Deca-Durabolin, Hybolin Decanoate) CSS III	*Carcinoma of breast and osteoporosis:* A: IM: 50–200 mg q1–4wk C: IM: 25–50 mg q3–4wk	X	*Increase* effects of oral hypoglycemics, insulin, oral anticoagulants	UK	UK	UK	3–6 d	UK
Nandrolone phenpropionate (Durabolin) CSS III	*Carcinoma of breast and osteoporosis:* IM: 25–100 mg/wk C: IM: 12.5–25 mg q2–4wk	X	Similar to nandrolone decanoate	UK	UK	UK	1–3 d	UK

Oxandrolone (Oxandrin) CSS III	*Osteoporosis:* A: PO: 5–20 mg daily in divided doses C: PO: 0.1 mg/kg/d	X	Use with anticoagulants may *increase* PT *Decrease* need for insulin *Lab:* May alter urine, blood glucose	Phase I: 1 h Phase II: 9 h	UK	UK	UK	UK
Oxymetholone Anadrol-50 CSS III	A&C: PO: 1–5 mg/kg/d	X	Similar to oxandrolone	9 h	UK	UK	UK	UK
Stanozolol (Winstrol) CSS III	*Aplastic anemia:* A: PO: 2 mg t.i.d. C: 6–12 y: PO: 2 mg t.i.d. C <6 y: PO: 1 mg b.i.d.	X	Similar to oxandrolone	UK	UK	UK	UK	UK
Testolactone (Teslac)	*Carcinoma of breast:* PO: 250 mg q.i.d.	C	*Increase* effects of oral anticoagulants	UK	UK	UK	UK	UK

KEY: For complete abbreviation key, see inside front cover.

Prototype: Ovulation Stimulants

Clomiphene Citrate

Clomiphene Citrate
 (Clomid, Milophene, Serophene)
Ovulation stimulant
Pregnancy Category: X
Drug Forms:
Tab 50 mg

Dosage

A: PO: 50–250 mg/d for days 5–9 of cycle
If ovulation does not occur with 50 mg/d, increase next course to 100 mg/d.

Contraindications

Pregnancy, undiagnosed vaginal bleeding, depression, fibroids, hepatic dysfunction, thrombophlebitis, primary pituitary or ovarian failure

Drug-Lab-Food Interactions

None are significant; Danazol may inhibit response; *decrease* effects of ethinyl estradiol
Lab: Increase in serum thyroxine

Pharmacokinetics

Absorption: Readily absorbed from GI tract
Distribution: PB: UK
Metabolism: t 1/2: 5–8 d
Excretion: In feces

Pharmacodynamics

PO: Onset: 5–14 d
 Peak: UK
 Duration: UK

Therapeutic Effects/Uses: To stimulate ovarian follicle growth.

Mode of Action: Stimulates release of follicle-stimulating hormone (FSH) and luteinizing hormone (LH).

Side Effects

Breast discomfort, fatigue, dizziness, depression, anxiety, nausea, vomiting, constipation, increased appetite, headache, hot flashes, fluid retention, flatulence, multiple gestation

Adverse Reactions

Visual disturbances, abdominal pain, weight gain, hair loss, major congenital anomalies, ovarian hyperstimulation, anxiety, ovarian cysts

KEY: For complete abbreviation key, see inside front cover.

Ovulation Stimulants

■ NURSING PROCESS: Ovulation Stimulants: Clomiphene Citrate

ASSESSMENT
- Obtain general health history and physical examination of clients. Clients' reproductive and sexual histories are assessed, with attention to the timing and techniques of coitus.
- Perform pelvic exam for baseline data, including ovarian size.
- Assess liver function studies before start of drug therapy.
- Use an extensive series of diagnostic tests to assess the cause of infertility.
- Assess the couple's interpretation of their infertility and its impact on their relationship. Placing blame on each other or their families can be devastating.

POTENTIAL NURSING DIAGNOSES
Altered sexuality patterns
Body image disturbance
Situational low self-esteem

PLANNING
- Short term: Clients will adhere to drug therapy regimen with minimal adverse effects. Long term: Achievement of pregnancy or considerations of alternatives to pregnancy with the couple's self-esteem and relationship remaining intact.

NURSING INTERVENTIONS
- Interventions are aimed at helping clients to understand the interrelationships among and timing of menses, ovulation, and coitus as they relate to conception.

CLIENT TEACHING
General
- Advise the woman to take medication at the same time each day to maintain steady serum levels.
- Advise the woman to avoid driving motor vehicles and operating dangerous equipment until stabilized on medication.
- Notify health care provider immediately of suspected pregnancy.
- Alert clients that drug therapy increases the chance of multiple births.

Skill
- Instruct the clients how to evaluate and record basal body temperature and cervical mucus changes on a chart. The first day of menses is day 1 of the cycle. Ovulation is predicted by a 0.5°F drop in basal body temperature followed by a 1°F rise. In addition, OTC diagnostic kits for assessing ovulatory status can be used to time coitus. Coitus is recommended no more frequently than every other day from 4 d before to 3 d after ovulation to maximize the man's sperm count.

EVALUATION
- Client tolerates drug regimen.
- Client achieves pregnancy.

Ovulation Stimulants

Generic (Brand)	Route and Dosage	Preg Cat	Interaction	t 1/2	PB	Onset	Peak	Duration
Clomiphene citrate (Clomid)	See Prototype Drug Chart							
Bromocriptine mesylate (Parlodel) *Ovulation stimulant*	A: PO: up to 7.5 mg/d in divided doses	C	*Increase effects of antihypertensives; altered effects with oral contraceptives, phenothiazines, tricyclic antidepressants*	50 h	92%	1–2 h		4–8 h
Gonadorelin acetate (Lutrepulse) *Ovulation stimulant*	*Induction of ovulation in female with primary hypothalamic amenorrhea:* A: IV: 5 µg q 90 min for 21 d; increase dose as in protocol if no response from 3 treatment cycles (Lutrepulse pump is required)	B	None significant	10–40 min	UK	UK	UK	UK
Human chorionic gonadotropin (hCG) (A.P.L., Chorex, Glukor, Follutein, Gonic, Preznyl, Profasi HP)	IM: 5,000–10,000 U/d in presence of mature follicle (after last dose of menotropins)	C	None significant reported	23 h	UK	2 h	6 h	UK
Human menopausal gonadotropin (menotropins and FSH Pergonal)	IM: 1–2 ampules/d × 5–12 d until follicle maturation; next day, h.c. (5,000–10,000 IU IM) administered	X	None significant reported	UK	UK	UK	18 h	UK
Urofollitropin (Metrodin)		X	None significant reported	4–70 h	UK	UK	UK	UK

KEY: For complete abbreviation key, see inside front cover.

AGENTS FOR EMERGENCY TREATMENT

Cardiac States

Neurosurgical States

Poisoning

Shock

Hypertensive Crisis

Prototype: Emergency Treatment of Cardiac States: Antidysrhythmic

Lidocaine HCl

Lidocaine HCl
 (Xylocaine)
Antidysrhythmic, class IB
Pregnancy Category: C
Drug Forms:
IV: 20 mg/mL in 5-mL syringe
 (100 mg)

Dosage

A: IV: ETT*: 1–1.5 mg/kg; may repeat 0.5 mg/kg q5–10 min up to 3 mg/kg (max)
Drip: 1–4 mg/min
C : IV: ETT* or IO: Initially: 1 mg/kg; maint: 30–50 µg/kg/min is recommended after bolus
*Note: For *endotracheal* drug administration, dose should be 2 to 2.5 times IV dose in adults and up to 10 times the IV dose for pediatric arrest.
Therapeutic Range: 1.5–5 µg/mL

Contraindications

Hypersensitivity, advanced atrioventricular block
Caution: Liver disease, congestive heart failure, elderly

Drug-Lab-Food Interactions

Increase effects with phenytoin, quinidine, procainamide, propranolol; *increase* risk of toxicity with cimetidine, beta-adrenergic blockers

Pharmacokinetics

Absorption: IV
Distribution: PB: 60–80%; concentrates in adipose tissue
Metabolism: t 1/2: Initial: 7–30 min; terminal: 9–120 min
Excretion: Through the liver

Pharmacodynamics

PO: Onset: 45–60 s
 Peak: 45–60 s
 Duration: 10–20 min

Therapeutic Effects/Uses: Primary drug to treat ventricular dysrhythmias such as premature ventricular contractions (PVCs), ventricular tachycardia, and ventricular fibrillation.

Mode of Action: Decreases automaticity; increases electrical threshold of ventricle.

Side Effects

Drowsiness, confusion, dyspnea, lethargy, hypotension, nausea, vomiting

Adverse Reactions

Life-threatening: Seizures, cardiac arrest

KEY: For complete abbreviation key, see inside front cover.

Emergency Treatment of Cardiac States: Antidysrhythmic

■ NURSING PROCESS: Emergency Treatment of Cardiac States: Lidocaine

ASSESSMENT
- Assess health history. In clients with hepatic impairment, CHF, shock, or advanced age, client's lidocaine dose may need to be reduced by as much as 50%.
- Assess for chest pain.
- Assess mental status: baseline and ongoing.
- Assess ECG findings.
- Assess VS.

POTENTIAL NURSING DIAGNOSIS
Decreased cardiac output

PLANNING
- Client will be free of ventricular dysrhythmias.

NURSING INTERVENTIONS
- Continuous cardiac monitoring.
- Assess pulse for strength, rate, and rhythm.
- Assess for signs and symptoms of lidocaine toxicity (confusion, drowsiness, hearing impairment, muscle twitching, and seizures). If overdose occurs, stop infusion and monitor client closely; notify primary health care provider.
- Monitor serum lidocaine levels throughout therapy; desired range is 1.5–5 µg/mL.
- Monitor intake and output.
- Do not mix in same syringe with amphotericin B or cefazolin.
- Have dopamine readily available in the event of circulatory depression.

CLIENT TEACHING
General
- Advise the client and family of drug action.

Side Effects
- Instruct the client to be accompanied when ambulating due to drowsiness and dizziness.
- Instruct the client and family in use of automatic lidocaine injection device, if prescribed.

EVALUATION
- Determine the effectiveness of drug.
- Evaluate decrease in or absence of ventricular dysrhythmias.

Agents for Emergency Treatment of Cardiac States

Generic (Brand)	Route and Dosage	Preg Cat	Interaction	t1/2	PB	Onset	Peak	Duration
Adenosine (Adenocard)	A: IV: Initially: 6 mg; then 12 mg in 1–2 min if needed; may repeat 12 mg ×1	C	*Increase* effects with dipyridamole; may increase heart block with carbamazepine *Decrease* effects with theophylline, caffeine	<10 s	UK	3–5 s	UK	1–2 min
Atropine sulfate	IV: ETT: 0.5–1 mg: can repeat up to 0.03–0.04 mg/kg or 3 mg max	C	*Increase* cholinergic effects with tricyclic antidepressants, antihistamines	2–3 h	60–80%	Immediate	2–4 min	3–6 h
Bretylium tosylate (Bretylol)	IV: Initially: 5 mg/kg; then 10 mg/kg q10–30 min up to 30 mg/kg total (max) over 24 h	C	May *increase* hypotensive effects of beta blockers, other antihypertensives	4–18 h	1–6%	5 min	End of infusion	6–24 h
Epinephrine	IV: ETT: 0.5–1 mg; may be repeated q5min	C	Alkaline solutions inactivate catecholamines; do *not* push through an IV line containing sodium bicarbonate	UK	UK	Rapid	20 min	15–30 min
Lidocaine	See Prototype Drug Chart							
Morphine sulfate	IV: 1–3 mg q5–30 min	C	*Increase* CNS depression with alcohol, phenothiazines, antihistamines	2–2.5 h	35%	1–3 min	20 min	6–7 h

Nitroglycerin (Nitrostat, Tridil)	SL: 0.3–0.4 mg IV: Drip: 10–20 µg/min, increased 5–10 µg/min q5–10 min (titrated)	C	*Increase* effects with alcohol, beta blockers, calcium blockers, antihypertensives *Decrease* effects with heparin	1–4 min	60%	SL: 1–3 min IV: 1–3 min	4 min UK	20–30 min 0.5–2 h
Procainamide HCl (Pronestyl)	IV: 20–30 mg/min; max: 17 mg/kg *Recognize end points:* • Hypotension • QRS widens > 50% • Total dose of 17 mg/kg given Drip: 1–4 mg/min	C	*Increase* effects with histamine₂ blockers; *increase* hypotensive effects with antihypertensives, nitrates *Decrease* effects with barbiturates	3–4 h	20%	1–2 min	30–60 min	3–4 h
Sodium bicarbonate	IV: Initially: 1 mEq/kg; then 0.5 mEq/kg if needed	C	Alkaline solutions inactivate catecholamines; do *not* push through same line	UK	UK	15 min	UK	1–2 h
Verapamil HCl (Isoptin, Calan)	IV: Age- and weight-dependent dosages; should not exceed 5 mg; repeat doses may be needed	C	*Increase* effects with cimetidine; *increase* effects of theophylline, beta blockers, antihypertensives *Decrease* effects of lithium	3–8 h	90%	1–5 min	2–5 min	2 h

KEY: For complete abbreviation key, see inside front cover.

Prototype: Emergency Treatment of Neurosurgical States: Diuretic

Mannitol

Mannitol
  (Osmitrol)
Osmotic diuretic
Pregnancy Category: C
Drug Forms:
Inj IV 5%, 10%, 15%, 20%, 25%

Dosage

A: IV: Initially: 1.5–2.0 g/kg of D25% sol as a bolus
Highly individualized

Contraindications

Hypersensitivity, severe dehydration
Caution: Pregnancy, breast-feeding, current intracranial bleeding

Drug-Lab-Food Interactions

May *decrease* effectiveness with lithium

Pharmacokinetics

Absorption: IV
Distribution: PB: Confined to extracellular space
Metabolism: t 1/2: 100 min
Excretion: In urine

Pharmacodynamics

Decrease in Intracranial Pressure:
IV: Onset: 30–60 min
      Peak: 1 h
      Duration: 6–8 h

Diuresis: Onset: 1–3 h
          Peak: 1 h
          Duration: 6–8 h

Therapeutic Effects/Uses: To treat increased intracranial pressure, cerebral edema.

Mode of Action: Inhibition of reabsorption of electrolytes and water by affecting pressure of glomerular filtrate.

Side Effects

Temporary volume expansion, hypo/hypernatremia, hypo/hyperkalemia, dehydration, blurred vision, dry mouth

Adverse Reactions

Pulmonary congestion, fluid/electrolyte imbalances
Life-threatening: Convulsions

KEY: For complete abbreviation key, see inside front cover.

Emergency Treatment of Neurosurgical States: Diuretic

■ NURSING PROCESS: Emergency Treatment of Neurosurgical States: Mannitol

ASSESSMENT
- Assess VS, including intracranial pressure, level of consciousness, and neurologic function.
- Assess fluid and electrolyte balances.

POTENTIAL NURSING DIAGNOSES
Fluid volume excess
Fluid volume deficit

PLANNING
- Client's intracranial pressure will be reduced to the desired range.

NURSING INTERVENTIONS
- Monitor VS, output, and pulmonary artery (PA) pressures (if PA catheter is present) frequently during administration.
- Assess the client for signs and symptoms of dehydration or fluid overload.
- Maintain accurate intake and output records to assess fluid volume status because diuresis may be substantial.
- Monitor for signs and symptoms of electrolyte imbalance; notify health care provider of imbalances.
- Careful monitoring of IV line site; extravasation may cause tissue necrosis.
- Use a filter needle when administering drug as crystals may form in solution and be inadvertently injected. Do not administer solution if crystals remain undissolved after shaking bottle. Try warming bottle in warm water to dissolve crystals; cool to room temperature before administering drug.
- Monitor laboratory studies, especially serum osmolality. Administration of mannitol to clients with serum osmolality >310–320 mOsm/kg is contraindicated.
- Do not mix in solution or syringe with any other drug.
- Client should be reevaluated if urine is not >30–50 mL/h for 2–3 h after two doses.

CLIENT TEACHING
- Explain expected drug action to the client and family.

EVALUATION
- Evaluate the effectiveness of drug.
- Client will have reduction in intracranial pressure; level is within desired range.
- Client's urine output is >30–50 mL/h or established goal.
- Client's serum osmolality will be in the desired range (usually 290–310 mOsm/kg).

Agents for Emergency Treatment of Neurosurgical States

Generic (Brand)	Route and Dosage	Preg Cat	Interaction	t1/2	PB	Onset	Peak	Duration
Mannitol	See Prototype Drug Chart							
Methylprednisolone (Solu-Medrol)	*Acute spinal cord injury:* IV: Loading dose: 30 mg/kg in 100 mL NSS, then 5.4 mg/kg/h × 23h	C	*Decrease* effects of oral hypoglycemics, anticoagulants, phenobarbital, immunizations; *decrease* effects of drug with rifampin, barbiturates, ephedrine, theophylline	2–4 h	80–90%	IV: Rapid	UK	UK

KEY: For complete abbreviation key, see inside front cover.

NOTES:

Prototype: Emergency Treatment of Poisoning

Naloxone HCl

Naloxone HCl
  (Narcan)
Narcotic antagonist
Pregnancy Category: B
Drug Forms:
Inj 0.4, 1 mg/mL

Dosage

IV/IM/SC: 0.4–2 mg; repeat every 2–3 min, as indicated

Contraindications

Hypersensitivity, respiratory depression
Caution: Opiate-dependent clients, cardiac disease, breast-feeding, neonates

Drug-Lab-Food Interactions

Verapamil can precipitate withdrawal in a client dependent on narcotic analgesics
Lab: Urine VMA, 5-HIAA, urine glucose

Pharmacokinetics

Absorption: IM/SC: Well absorbed
Distribution: PB: UK
Metabolism: t 1/2: Adults: 1–4 h; neonates: 1–3 h
Excretion: In urine metabolites

Pharmacodynamics

SC/IM: Onset: 2–5 min
       Peak: UK
       Duration: 1–4 h
IV: Onset: 1–2 min
       Peak: UK
       Duration: 1–4 h

Therapeutic Effects/Uses: To treat respiratory depression caused by narcotics; to treat narcotic-induced depressant effects and narcotic overdose.
Mode of Action: Blocks effects of narcotics by competing for the receptor sites.

Side Effects

Negligible pharmacologic effect without narcotics in body

Adverse Reactions

Nausea, vomiting, tremulousness, sweating, tachycardia, elevated blood pressure
Life-threatening: Atrioventricular fibrillation, pulmonary edema (with overdose of morphine)

KEY: For complete abbreviation key, see inside front cover.

Emergency Treatment of Poisoning

■ NURSING PROCESS: Emergency Treatment of Poisoning: Naloxone

ASSESSMENT
- Assess VS and level of consciousness.
- Assess level of pain before administering drug to a client experiencing respiratory depression.
- Assess for signs and symptoms of withdrawal.
- Assess for improvement of symptoms; if improvement is not evident, symptoms are due to cause other than narcotic.

POTENTIAL NURSING DIAGNOSES
Ineffective breathing pattern
Altered comfort
Coping, ineffective individual

PLANNING
- Client will have respiratory depression reversed and have respiratory rate within the desired range.

NURSING INTERVENTIONS
- Have resuscitation equipment readily available to augment drug therapy if needed.
- Do *not* mix in the same syringe with heparin or benzquanamide.
- Monitor client closely for signs and symptoms of recurrent opiate effects, such as respiratory depression and hypotension. Effects of opiate may outlast effects of naloxone; a continuous naloxone infusion may be necessary.

CLIENT TEACHING
General
- Advise the client and family of drug action.

EVALUATION
- Determine the effectiveness of drug.
- Client's respiratory rate and VS (specifically, blood pressure) are within the desired range.

Agents for Emergency Treatment of Poisoning

Generic (Brand)	Route and Dosage	Preg Cat	Interaction	t1/2	PB	Onset	Peak	Duration
Activated charcoal	PO: 30 g (minimum dose)	C	*Decreases* absorption of laxatives, ipecac	NA	NA	<1 min	UK	4–12 h
Ipecac syrup	A&C >12 y: PO: 30 mL; can repeat in 20 min (see text for precautions) C >1 y: PO: 15 mL	C	*Decreased* effect with activated charcoal, carbonated beverages, or milk	UK	UK	15–30 min	UK	20–25 min
Magnesium citrate	PO: 5–10 oz	C	*Increased* effects of neuromuscular blockers Lab: increased Mg level; decreased protein, Ca, and K levels	UK	UK	0.5–3 h	UK	UK
Magnesium sulfate	PO: 5–15 g	C	*Increased* CNS depression with barbiturates, anesthetics, CNS depressants	UK	UK	1–2 h	UK	UK
Naloxone (Narcan)	See Prototype Drug Chart							

KEY: For complete abbreviation key, see inside front cover.

NOTES:

Prototype: Emergency Treatment of Shock

Dopamine HCl

Dopamine HCl
  (Intropin)
Adrenergic
Pregnancy Category: C
Drug Forms:
Inj 0.8, 1.6 mg/mL

Dosage

A: IV: Drip: 1–20 µg/kg/min (>10 µg/kg/min may be ordered if lower doses are ineffective)

Contraindications

Hypersensitivity, tachydysrhythmias, ventricular fibrillation, pheochromocytomas
Caution: Safety in children is not known

Drug-Lab-Food Interactions

Use within 2 wk of MAOIs may result in hypertensive crisis; concurrent IV administration of phenytoin may result in hypotension and bradycardia; sodium bicarbonate solutions inactivate dopamine—do *not* administer through the same IV line

Pharmacokinetics

Absorption: IV
Distribution: PB: UK
Metabolism: t 1/2: 2 min
Excretion: In urine

Pharmacodynamics

IV: Onset: 1–2 min
   Peak: <5 min
   Duration: <10 min

Therapeutic Effects/Uses: To treat hypotension in shock states not due to hypovolemia; to increase heart rate in atropine-refractory bradycardia. To increase urine output at a "renal dose" (<5 µg/kg/min).

Mode of Action: Stimulation of receptors to cause cardiac stimulation and renal vasodilation. Increase systemic vascular resistance at higher dose ranges.

Side Effects

Palpitations, tachycardia, hypertension, ectopic beats, angina, IV line site irritation, piloerection, nausea, vomiting

Adverse Reactions

Cardiac dysrhythmias, azotemia, tissue sloughing (from extravasation)
Life-threatening: MI, gangrene in extremities (from vasoconstriction)

KEY: For complete abbreviation key, see inside front cover.

Emergency Treatment of Shock

■ NURSING PROCESS: Emergency Treatment of Shock: Dopamine

ASSESSMENT
- Assess VS frequently.
- Assess ECG readings; monitor intake and output.

POTENTIAL NURSING DIAGNOSES
Shock
Altered tissue perfusion
Decreased cardiac output

PLANNING
- Client will have increase in blood pressure and/or hemodynamic parameters that are within the desired range.

NURSING INTERVENTIONS
- Monitor IV line site every 30–60 min for signs of infiltration. Extravasation can necessitate surgical debridement and skin grafting. If infiltration does occur, inject affected areas with phentolamine (Regitine) 5–10 mg SC diluted in 10–15 mL NSS to reduce or prevent tissue damage. Multiple injections may be necessary.
- Administer IV through a large vein; the central vein is preferable.
- Use an electronic infusion pump to ensure accurate IV rate.
- Monitor central venous pressure (CVP) or pulmonary artery catheter pressure readings to evaluate cardiovascular system response.
- Be alert that the solution appears slightly yellow. Any other color is indicative of decomposition; the solution should be discarded.
- Do not interrupt infusion; profound hypotension may result. Dopamine dose must be titrated downward slowly to avoid hypotensive response.

CLIENT TEACHING
General
- Advise the client and family of drug action.
- Alert the client to immediately report pain at the IV line site.

EVALUATION
- Determine the effectiveness of drug therapy and the presence of any side effects. The client should have blood pressure and/or other hemodynamic parameters (heart rate, cardiac output, urine output, systemic vascular resistance, and so on) within the desired range.

Agents for Emergency Treatment of Shock

Generic (Brand)	Route and Dosage	Preg Cat	Interaction	t½	PB	Onset	Peak	Duration
Dextrose 50%	A: IV: 50 mL C: IV: 0.5–1.0 g/kg of a D25% sol	C	Alters insulin and oral antidiabetic requirements of diabetics	UK	UK	Rapid	Rapid	Brief
Diphenhydramine (Benadryl)	IM/IV: 10–50 mg	C	*Increase* anticholinergic effects with tricyclic antidepressants, MAOIs, quinidine; *increase* CNS depression with sedative-hypnotics, alcohol, analgesics, antihistamines	3–8 h	98–99%	IV: Rapid IM: 20–30 min	UK 1–4 h	4–7 h 4–8 h
Dobutamine (Dobutrex)	IV: Drip: 2.5–10 μg/kg/min	C	*Increase* dysrhythmias with general anesthetics, MAOIs, tricyclic antidepressants; effects are antagonized by beta blockers	2 min	UK	IV: Within 2 min	10–20 min	Shortly after infusion terminated

Dopamine HCl (Intropin)	See Prototype Drug Chart					
Epinephrine	SC/IM: 0.1–0.5 mg (1:1,000 sol) IV: 0.1–0.25 mg (1:10,000 sol) Intratracheal: 0.1 mg/kg (q3–5 min)	C	*Increase* effects with other adrenergics; hypertensive crises with MAOIs; *increase* dysrhythmias with cardiac glycosides, general anesthetics	UK	UK	Intratracheal: <1 min SC: 3–5 min IV: Rapid	20 min 20 min	1–3 h 20–30 min
Glucagon	SC/IM/IV: 0.5–1 mg; may repeat ×1	B	Negates effects of insulin and oral antidiabetics; may *increase* effects of oral anticoagulants (large doses)	3–10 min	UK	Hyperglycemic: 5–20 min GI musculature: 1 min	30 min UK	1–2 h 9–25 min
Norepinephrine (Levophed)	IV: Drip: 2–12 μg/min	D	*Increase* effects with ergot alkaloids, tricyclic antidepressants, antihistamines, MAOIs, methyldopa	UK	UK	IV: Rapid	UK	1–2 min after infusion terminated

KEY: For complete abbreviation key, see inside front cover.

Prototype: Emergency Treatment of Hypertensive Crisis

Sodium Nitroprusside

Sodium Nitroprusside (Nipride)
Pregnancy Category: C
Drug Forms:
Inj IV 10 mg/mL in 5-mL vial

Dosage

A: IV: Drip: 0.5–10 μg/kg/min; begin at 0.1 μg/kg/min and titrate to desired effect up to 10 μg/kg/min

Contraindications

Hypersensitivity, hypertension (compensatory), decreased cerebral perfusion, coarctation of aorta
Caution: Increased intracranial pressure

Drug-Lab-Food Interactions

Antihypertensives, general anesthetics
Do not mix with any other drug in syringe or solution.
Lab: Decrease in carbonate, P_{CO_2}, pH

Pharmacokinetics

Absorption: IV only
Distribution: PB: UK
Metabolism: t 1/2: <10 min
Excretion: In urine

Pharmacodynamics

IV: Onset: 1–2 min
Peak: Rapid
Duration: 1–10 min

Therapeutic Effects/Uses: To treat hypertensive crisis; to produce controlled hypotension to reduce surgical bleeding; and to decrease systemic vascular resistance to improve cardiac performance.

Mode of Action: Stimulation of smooth muscle of veins and arteries; produces peripheral vasodilation.

Side Effects

Dizziness, headache, nausea, abdominal pain, sweating, palpitations, weakness, vomiting

Adverse Reactions

Tinnitus, dyspnea, blurred vision
Life-threatening: Severe hypotension, loss of consciousness, profound cardiovascular depression

KEY: For complete abbreviation key, see inside front cover.

Emergency Treatment of Hypertensive Crisis

■ NURSING PROCESS: Emergency Treatment of Hypertensive Crisis: Sodium Nitroprusside

ASSESSMENT
- Assess VS frequently.
- Assess serum thiocyanate and/or cyanide levels. Elevations are indicative of toxicity.

POTENTIAL NURSING DIAGNOSES
Altered tissue perfusion
Decreased cardiac output

PLANNING
- Client's hypertension and blood pressure will be controlled.

NURSING INTERVENTIONS
- Reconstitute drug using sterile water without preservative.
- Cover infusion bottle with aluminum foil immediately after reconstituting; do not cover IV tubing.
- Use drug within 24 h of preparation; new solution has slight brown color. Do not use solution if dark brown or blue.
- Administer via electronic infusion device to ensure accurate rate and dosage.
- Be attentive to avoiding extravasation (sloughing of tissue and severe pain).
- Do not interrupt infusion; alteration in blood pressure may result.
- If hypotension ensues, titrate drug downward; discontinuation of infusion may be necessary.

CLIENT TEACHING
General
- Alert the client to immediately report pain at the IV line site.

Side Effects
- Instruct client to immediately report dyspnea, dizziness, blurred vision, headache, or tinnitus.

EVALUATION
- Blood pressure is within desired range. Client is free of drug side effects.

BIBLIOGRAPHY

American Heart Association (1994). *Textbook of Advanced Cardiac Life Support*. Dallas, TX: American Heart Association.
American Society of Hospital Pharmacists (1996). *AHFS Drug Information*. Bethesda, MD: American Society of Hospital Pharmacists.
Bleck, T.P. (1990). Convulsive disorders: The use of anticonvulsant drugs. *Clinical Neuropharmacology*, 13 (3), 198–209.
Bobak, I.M. (1991). *Quick Reference for Maternity Nursing*. St. Louis: Mosby–Year Book, Inc.
Bortenschlager, L., and Zaloga, G.P. (1994). Vitamins. In B. Chernow (ed), *The Pharmacologic Approach to the Critically-Ill Patient* (3rd ed, pp. 3–17). Baltimore: Williams & Wilkins Co.
Chernecky, C. (1991). *Cancer Diagnostics and Chemotherapy*. Philadelphia: W.B. Saunders Co.
Chernow, B. (Ed.) (1994). *The Pharmacologic Approach to the Critically-Ill Patient* (3rd ed). Baltimore: Williams & Wilkins.
Clark, J., and Longo, D. (1986). Biological response modifiers. *Mediguide to Oncology*, 6 (2), 1–5, 9, 10.
Colfosceril (1995). *Drug Evaluation Monographs*, 1974–1995. Micromedex, Inc., 85, August 31, 1995.
Colucci, R.D., and Somberg, J.C. (1994). Treatment of cardiac arrhythmias. In B. Chernow (ed), *The Pharmacologic Approach to the Critically-Ill Patient* (3rd ed, pp. 445–463). Baltimore: Williams & Wilkins Co.
Davis, J.R., and Sherer, K. (1994). *Applied Nutrition and Diet Therapy for Nurses* (2nd ed.). Philadelphia: W.B. Saunders Co.
Drug Facts and Comparisons (1996, updated monthly). St. Louis: J.B. Lippincott Co.
Drug Information for Health Care Professionals, Vol 1 (14th ed). Taunton, MA.
Formulary and Drug Therapy Guide: 1995–1996. Medical Center of Delaware. Newark, DE: Lexi-Comp Inc. 1995–1996.
Gelone, S. (1995). *Therapy of Opportunistic Infections Associated with the Human Immunodeficiency Virus*. Philadelphia: Temple University Hospital.
Gilman, A.G., Goodman, L.S., and Gilman, A. (1991). *Goodman and Gilman's The Pharmacologic Basis of Therapeutics* (8th ed). New York: Pergamon Press Inc.
Green, M.R. (1991). *The Role of Colony-Stimulating Factors in Chemotherapy-Induced Neutropenia*. Seattle, WA: Immunex Corp.
Haeuber, D., and Dijulio, J.E. (1989). Hematopoietic colony-stimulating factors: An overview. *Oncology Nursing Forum*. 16 (2), 247–255.
Hodgson, B.B., Kizior, R.J., and Kingdon, R.T. (1996). *Nurse's Drug Handbook* (3rd ed). Philadelphia: W.B. Saunders Co.
Hoechst-Roussel Pharmaceuticals, Inc. (1991). *Myeloid Growth Factors*. Somerville, NJ: Hoechst-Roussel Pharmaceuticals, Inc.
Kee, J.L., and Paulanka, B.J. (1994). *Fluids and Electrolytes with Clinical Applications* (5th ed). New York: Delmar Publishers Inc.
Kee, J.L. (1995). *Laboratory and Diagnostic Tests With Nursing Implications* (4th ed). Norwalk, CT: Appleton and Lange.
Kuhn, M.M. (1991). *Pharmacotherapeutics* (2nd ed). Philadelphia: F.A. Davis Co.
Lehne, R. (1994). *Pharmacology for Nursing Care* (2nd ed). Philadelphia: W.B. Saunders Co.
McKenry, L.M., and Salerno, E. (1992). *Mosby's Pharmacology in Nursing* (18th ed). St. Louis: C.V. Mosby Co.
Nadler, J.L., and Rude, R.K. (1995). Disorders of magnesium metabolism. *Endocrinology and Metabolism Clinics of North America*, 24 (3), 623–637.
(1996). *Physicians' Desk Reference* (50th ed). Montvale, NJ: Medical Economics Co, Inc.
Rittenberg, C., Grallo, R., and Rehmeyer, T. (1995). Assessing and managing venous irritation associated with vinorelbine tartrate (Navelbine). *Oncology Nursing Forum*, 22 (4), 707–710.
Rogove, H.J., and Moore, K.A. (1993). *Critical Care Medicines: Handbook of Intravenous Pharmacotherapeutics*. Columbus, OH: Contemporary Critical Care Resources, Inc.
Schwertz, D.W. (1991). Basic principles of pharmacologic action. *Nursing Clinics of North America*, 26 (2), 245–262.
Seligman, M. (1994). Bronchodilators. In B. Chernow (ed), *The Pharmacologic Approach to the Critically-Ill Patient* (3rd ed, pp. 567–575). Baltimore: Williams & Wilkins Co.
Shannon, M.T., and Wilson, B.A. (1996). *Govoni and Hayes: Drugs and Nursing Implications* (9th ed). Norwalk, CT: Appleton and Lange.
Shaw, R.W. (1991). GrRH analogues in the treatment of endometriosis: Rationale and efficacy. In E. Thomas and J. Rock (eds), *Modern Approaches to Endometriosis* (pp. 257–274). Dordrecht, The Netherlands: Kluwer Academic Publishers.
Skidmore-Roth, L. (1996). *Mosby's 1996 Nursing Drug Reference*. St. Louis: Mosby–Year Book, Inc.
Spratto, G.R., and Woods, A.L. (1996). *Nurse's Drug Reference*. New York: Delmar Publishers, Inc.
Timmons, M.C. (1990). The use of estrogen replacement therapy. In R.C. Cefalo (ed), *Clinical Decisions in Obstetrics and Gynecology* (pp. 229–231). Rockville, MD: Aspen Publishers, Inc.
Trissel, L.A. (1994). *Handbook on Injectable Drugs*. Bethesda, MD: American Society of Hospital Pharmacists.
United States Pharmacopeia Drug Information (USP-DI) for the Health Care Professional (1995), Vol I, 15th ed. Rockville, MD: The US Pharmacopeial Convention, Inc.
Zaloga, G.P., and Chernow, B. (1994). Insulin and oral hypoglycemics. In B. Chernow (ed), *The Pharmacologic Approach to the Critically Ill Patient* (3rd ed, pp. 758–771). Baltimore: Williams & Wilkins Co.
Ziegler, M.G., and Ruiz-Ramon, P.F. (1994). Antihypertensive therapy. In B. Chernow (ed), *The Pharmacologic Approach to the Critically Ill Patient* (3rd ed, pp. 405–425). Baltimore: Williams & Wilkins Co.

APPENDIX A

Generic Drugs with Corresponding Canadian Trade Drug Names*

Generic Drug Names	Canadian Trade/Brand Names
Acebutolol	Monitan
Acetaminophen	Abenol, Atasol, Campain, Exdol, Robigesic, Rounox
Acetazolamide	Acetazolam, Apo-Acetazolamide
Acetohexamide	Dimelor
Acetylcysteine	Airbron
Albuterol	Novosalmol, Salbutamol
Allopurinol	Alloprin, Apo-Allopurinol, Novopurinol, Purinol
Aminophylline	Gorophyllin, Paladron
Aminosalicylate sodium	Parasal Sodium
Amitriptyline hydrochloride	Apo-Amitriptyline, Levate, Meravil, Novotriptyn, Rolavil
Amoxicillin	Apo-Amoxi, Amoxican
Amoxicillin clavulanate K	Clavulin
Ampicillin	Ampilean, Novo-Ampicillin, Penbritin
Ascorbic acid	Apo-C, Ce-Vi-Sol, Redoxon
Asparaginase	Kidrolase
Aspirin	Ancasal, Astrin, Entrophen, Novasen, Supasa, Triaphen-10
Atenolol	Apo-Atenolol
Atropine sulfate	Atropair
Bacampicillin hydrochloride	Penglobe
Benzalkonium chloride	Pharmatex
Benztropine mesylate	Apo-Benzotropine, Bensylate, PMS Benzotropine
Betamethasone	Beban, Betaderm, Betanelan, Betnesol, Betnovate, Celestoderm, Novobetamet
Bisacodyl	Apo-Bisacodyl, Bisco-Lax, Laxit
Bretylium tosylate	Bretylate
Carbamazepine	Apo-Carbamazepine, Mazepine, PMS Carbamazepine
Carbenicillin disodium	Pyopen
Cephalexin	Ceporex, Novolexin
Cephalothin sodium	Ceporacin
Chloral hydrate	Novochlorhydrate
Chloramphenicol	Novochorocap, Pentamycetin
Chlordiazepoxide hydrochloride	Medilium, Novopoxide, Solium
Chlorphenesin carbamate	Mycil
Chlorpheniramine maleate	Chlor-Tripolon, Novopheniram
Chlorpromazine hydrochloride	Chlorpromanyl, Largactil, Novochlorpromazine
Chlorpropamide	Apo-Chlorpropamide, Chloronase, Novopropamide
Chlorprothixene	Tarasan
Chlorthalidone	Novothalidone, Uridon
Cimetidine	Novocimetine, Peptol
Cisplatin	Abiplatin

continued

Appendix A

Generic Drugs with Corresponding Canadian Trade Drug Names*—Continued

Generic Drug Names	Canadian Trade/Brand Names
Clindamycin	Dalacin-C
Clofibrate	Claripen, Claripex, Novofibrate
Clonazepam	Rivotril
Clonidine hydrochloride	Dixarit
Clorazepate dipotassium	Novoclopate
Clotrimazole	Canesten
Cloxacillin sodium	Apo-Cloxi, Bactopen, Novocloxin, Orbenin
Codeine phosphate	Paveral
Colchicine	Novocolchine
Colestipol hydrochloride	Cholestabyl, Lestid
Co-trimoxazole	Apo-Sulfatrim
Cromolyn sodium	Fivent, Intal p, Rynacrom, Vistacrom
Cyanocobalamin	Anacobin, Bedoz, Cyanabin, Rubion
Cyclizine hydrochloride	Marzine
Cyclophosphamide	Procytox
Cyproheptadine hydrochloride	Vimicon
Danazol	Cyclomen
Dapsone	Avlosulfon
Dexamethasone	Deronil, Dexasone, Oradexon, Stress-Pam
Dextromethorphan	Balminil DM, Koffex, Ornex DM, Robidex, Sedatuss
Diazepam	Apo-Diazepam, Diazemuls, E-Pam, Meval, Novodipam, Vivol
Dicyclomine hydrochloride	Bentylol, Formulex, Lomine, Protylol, Viscerol
Diethylpropion hydrochloride	Nobesine
Diethylstilbestrol	Honval, Stilboestrol
Digitoxin	Digitaline, Purodigin
Dimenhydrinate	Apo-Dimenhydrinate, Gravol, Nauseatol, Novodimenate, Travamine
Dinoprostone	Prepidil Gel
Diphenhydramine hydrochloride	Allerdryl
Dipyridamole	Apo-Dipyridamole
Disopyramide	Rythmodan
Docusate sodium	Regulax
Dopamine hydrochloride	Revimine
Doxepin hydrochloride	Triadapin
Doxycycline hyclate	Doryx, Doxycin, Novodoxylin
Dyphylline	Protophylline
Econazole nitrate	Ecostatin
Epinephrine hydrochloride	SusPhrine, Eppy
Epinephrine racemic	Vaponefrin
Ergocalciferol	Ostoforte, Radiostol
Ergotamine tartrate	Gynergen
Erythromycin	Apo-Erythro Base, Erythromid, Novorythro, Ro-Mycin
Estradiol	Delestrogen
Estrogen, conjugated	C.E.S.
Estrogen, esterified	Climestrone, Neo-Estrone
Estrone	Femogen Forte
Ethambutol hydrochloride	Etibi
Ethopropazine hydrochloride	Parsitan
Fenfluramine hydrochloride	Ponderal
Ferrous fumarate	Neo-Fer-50, Novofumar, Palafer
Ferrous gluconate	Fertinic, Novoferrogluc
Ferrous sulfate	Novoferrosulfa
Flucytosine	Ancotil

Appendix A

Generic Drugs with Corresponding Canadian Trade Drug Names*—Continued

Generic Drug Names	Canadian Trade/Brand Names
Fluocinolone acetonide	Fluoderm
Fluocinonide	Lidemol, Lyderm, Topsyn
Fluoxymesterone	Ora T Estryl
Fluphenazine decanoate	Decanoate
Fluphenazine enanthate	Enanthate
Fluphenazine hydrochloride	Moditen HCl
Flurandrenolide	Drenison
Flurazepam	Apo-Flurazepam, Novoflupam, Somnol
Folic acid	Apo-Folic, Novofolacid
Furosemide	Fumide, Furomide, Luramide, Uritol
Gentamicin sulfate	Alcomicin, Cidomycin, Novosemide
Glyburide	DiaBeta, Euglucon
Griseofulvin, microsize	Grisovin-FP
Guaifenesin	Balminil, Resyl
Guanethidine sulfate	Apo-Guanethidine
Haloperidol	Haldol LA, Peridol
Heparin calcium	Calcilean, Calciparine
Heparin sodium	Hepalean
Hydrochlorothiazide	Apo-Hydro, Hydrozide, Neo-Codema, Urozide
Hydrocodone bitartrate	Hycodan, Robidone
Hydrocortisone	Cortamed, Cortiment, Rectocort
Hydroxocobalamin	Acti-B$_{12}$
Ibuprofen	Amersol
Imipramine hydrochloride	Impril, Novopramine
Indapamide	Lozide
Indomethacin	Indocid
Isoniazid (INH)	Isotamine
Isosorbide dinitrate	Coronex, Novosorbide
Iodoquinol	Diodoquin
Kaolin/pectin	Donnagel-MB, Kao-Con
Ketoprofen	Rhodis, Orudis E
Lactulose	Lactulax
Levothyroxine sodium (T$_4$)	Eltroxin
Lidocaine hydrochloride	Xylocard
Lithium carbonate	Carbolith, Duralith, Lithizine
Lorazepam	Apo-Lorazepam, Novolorazepam
Loxapine hydrochloride	Loxapac
Magaldrate	Antiflux
Meclizine hydrochloride	Bonamine
Mefenamic acid	Ponstan
Meperidine hydrochloride	Pethadol, Pethidine Hydrochloride
Meprobamate	Apo-Meprobamate, Novomepro
Mesalamine	Salofalk
Methohexital	Brietal
Methotrimeprazine	Nozinan
Methylclothiazide	Duretic
Methyldopa	Apo-Methyldopa, Dopamet, Novomedopa
Methyltestosterone	Metandren
Metoclopramide	Maxeran
Metoprolol	Apo-Metoprolol, Betaloc, Novometoprol
Metronidazole	Neo-Metric, Novonidazol, PMS Metronidazole
Miconazole	Monistat
Mineral oil	Kondremul, Lansoyl
Morphine sulfate	Epimorph, Statex
Naphazoline	Vasocon

continued

Appendix A

Generic Drugs with Corresponding Canadian Trade Drug Names*—Continued

Generic Drug Names	Canadian Trade/Brand Names
Naproxen	Apo-Naproxen, Naxen, Novonaprox
Niacin (vitamin B_3, nicotinic acid)	Novo-Niacin, Tri-B3
Nifedipine	Adalat P.A., Apo-Nifed, Novo-Nifedin
Nitrofurantoin	Apo-Nitrofurantoin, Nephronex, Novofuran
Norethindrone acetate	Aygestin, Norlutate
Nylidrin hydrochloride	Arlidin Forte, PMS Nylidrin
Nystatin	Nadostine, Nyaderm
Omeprazole	Losec
Oxazepam	Ox-Pam, Zapex, Apo-Oxazepam, Novoxapam
Oxtriphylline	Apo-Oxtriphylline, Novotriphyl
Oxycodone	Supeudol
Oxymetazoline hydrochloride	Nafrine
Oxymetholone	Anapolon
Penicillin G potassium	Megacillin, NovoPen-G, P-50, Crystapen
Penicillin G procaine	Ayercillin
Penicillin G sodium	Crystapen
Penicillin V	Apo-Pen-VK, Nadopen-V, Novopen-VK
Pentamidine isethionate	Pentacarinat
Pentobarbital	Novopentobarb
Perphenazine	Apo-Perphenazine, Phenazine
Phenazopyridine hydrochloride	Phenazo, Pyronium
Phentolamine mesylate	Rogitine
Phenazopyridine	Phenazo, Pyronium
Phenylephrine, ophthalmic	Minims Phenylephrine
Pilocarpine hydrochloride	Pilocarpine, Milocarpine
Piroxicam	Apo-Piroxicant
Potassium chloride	Apo-K, Kalium Durules, Klong, Novolente K, Roychlor 10% and 20%, Slo-Pot
Potassium gluconate	Potassium Rougier, Royonate
Potassium iodide	Thyro-Block
Pramoxine hydrochloride	Tronothane
Prednisone	Apo-Prednisone, Winpred
Primidone	Apo-Primidone, Sertan
Probenecid	Benuryl
Procarbazine hydrochloride	Natulan
Prochlorperazine maleate	Stemetil
Procyclidine hydrochloride	Procyclid
Progesterone	Progestilin
Promethazine hydrochloride	Histantil
Propantheline bromide	Propanthel
Propoxyphene hydrochloride	642, Novopropoxyn
Propranolol hydrochloride	Apo-Propranolol, Detensol, Novopranol
Propylthiouracil (PTU)	Propyl-Thyracil
Protriptyline hydrochloride	Triptil
Pseudoephedrine hydrochloride	Eltor, Eltor 120, Pseudofrin, Robidrine
Psyllium hydrophilic muciloid	Karasil
Pyrantel pamoate	Combantrin
Pyrazinamide	Tebrazid, PMS Pyrazinamide
Pyridostigmine	Mestinon Supraspan
Quinidine sulfate	APO-Quinidine, Novoquinidin
Quinine sulfate	Novoquinine
Reserpine	Novoreseroine, Reserfia
Rifampin	Rofact
Scopolamine	Transderm-V
Secobarbital	Novosecobarb
Silver sulfadiazine	Flamazine

Appendix A

Generic Drugs with Corresponding Canadian Trade Drug Names*—*Continued*

Generic Drug Names	Canadian Trade/Brand Names
Simethicone	Ovol
Sodium fluoride	Fluor-A-Day
Sotalol	Sotacor
Spironolactone	Novospiroton, Sincomen
Sucralfate	Sulcrate
Sulfasalazine	PMS Sulfasalazine, Salazopyrin, SAS-Enema, SAS Enteric-500, S.A.S.-500
Sulfinpyrazone	Antazone, Anturan, Apo-Sulfinpyrazone, Novopyrazone
Sulfisoxazole	Novosoxazole
Tamoxifen citrate	Nolvadex-D, Tamofen
Testosterone	Malogen
Testosterone enanthate	Malogex
Testosterone propionate	Malogen in oil
Tetracycline hydrochloride	Novotetra, Apo-Tetra, Tetralean
Theophylline	PMS Theophylline, Pulmopylline, Somophyllin-12
Thiamine HCl (vitamin B_1)	Bewon, Betaxin
Thioguanine (TG, 6-thioguanine)	Lanvis
Thioridazine hydrochloride	Novoridazine
Timolol maleate	Apo-Timol
Tolbutamide	Mobenol, Novobutamide
Tolnaftate	Pitrex
Trifluoperazine hydrochloride	Novoflurazine, Solazine, Terfluzine
Trihexyphenidyl hydrochloride	Aparkane, Apo-Trihex, Novohexidyl
Trimeprazine tartrate	Panectyl
Tripelennamine hydrochloride	Pyribenzamine
Valproic acid (divalproex sodium, sodium valproate)	Epival
Vinblastine sulfate	Velbe
Warfarin sodium	Warfilone

*Many of the trade or brand names are used in both the United States and Canada. This appendix lists selected trade or brand names that are specific to Canada.

APPENDIX B

Canadian Trade Drug Names with Corresponding Generic Drugs

Canadian Trade/Brand Names	Generic Drug Names
Abenol	Acetaminophen
Acetazolam	Acetazolamide
Acti-B$_{12}$	Hydroxocobalamin
Adalat P.A.	Nifedipine
Airbron	Acetylcysteine
Alcomicin	Gentamicin sulfate
Allerdryl	Diphenhydramine hydrochloride
Alloprin	Allopurinol
Amersol	Ibuprofen
Amoxican	Amoxicillin
Ampilean	Ampicillin
Anacobin	Cyanocobalamin
Anapolon	Oxymetholone
Ancasal	Aspirin
Ancotil	Flucytosine
Antazone	Sulfinpyrazone
Antiflux	Magaldrate
Anturan	Sulfinpyrazone
Aparkane	Trihexyphenidyl hydrochloride
Apo-Acetazolamide	Acetazolamide
Apo-Allopurinol	Allopurinol
Apo-Amitriptyline	Amitriptyline hydrochloride
Apo-Amoxi	Amoxicillin
Apo-Atenolol	Atenolol
Apo-Benzotropine	Benztropine mesylate
Apo-Bisacodyl	Bisacodyl
Apo-C	Ascorbic acid
Apo-Carbamazepine	Carbamazepine
Apo-Chlorpropamide	Chlorpropamide
Apo-Cloxi	Cloxacillin sodium
Apo-Diazepam	Diazepam
Apo-Dimenhydrinate	Dimenhydrinate
Apo-Dipyridamole	Dipyridamole
Apo-Erythro Base	Erythromycin
Apo-Flurazepam	Flurazepam
Apo-Folic	Folic acid
Apo-Guanethidine	Guanethidine sulfate
Apo-Hydro	Hydrochlorothiazide
Apo-Lorazepam	Lorazepam
Apo-Meprobamate	Meprobamate
Apo-Methyldopa	Methyldopa
Apo-Metoprolol	Metoprolol
Apo-Naproxen	Naproxen
Apo-Nifed	Nifedipine

continued

Appendix B

Canadian Trade Drug Names with Corresponding Generic Drugs—*Continued*

Canadian Trade/Brand Names	Generic Drug Names
Apo-Nitrofurantoin	Nitrofurantoin
Apo-Oxazepam	Oxazepam
Apo-Oxtriphylline	Oxtriphylline
Apo-PenVK	Penicillin V
Apo-Perphenazine	Perphenazine
Apo-Piroxicant	Piroxicam
Apo-Prednisone	Prednisone
Apo-Primidone	Primidone
Apo-Propranolol	Propranolol hydrochloride
Apo-Quinidine	Quinidine sulfate
Apo-Sulfatrim	Co-trimoxazole
Apo-Timol	Timolol maleate
Apo-Trihex	Trihexyphenidyl hydrochloride
Arlidin Forte	Nylidrin hydrochloride
Astrin	Aspirin
Atasol	Acetaminophen
Atropair	Atropine sulfate
Avlosulfon	Dapsone
Ayercillin	Penicillin G procaine
Aygestin	Norethindrone acetate
Bactopen	Cloxacillin sodium
Balminil	Guaifenesin
Beben	Betamethasone
Bedoz	Cyanocobalamin
Bensylate	Benztropine mesylate
Benuryl	Probenecid
Betaderm	Betamethasone
Betaloc	Metoprolol
Betanelan	Betamethasone
Betaxin	Thiamine hydrochloride
Betnesol	Betamethasone
Betnovate	Betamethasone
Bewon	Thiamine hydrochloride
Bisco-Lax	Bisacodyl
Bonamine	Meclizine hydrochloride
Bretylate	Bretylium tosylate
Brietal	Methohexital
Calcilean	Heparin calcium
Calciparine	Heparin calcium
Campain	Acetaminophen
Canesten	Clotrimazole
Carbolith	Lithium carbonate
Celestoderm	Betamethasone
Ceporacin	Cephalothin sodium
Ceporex	Cephalexin
C.E.S.	Estrogen, conjugated
Ce-Vi-Sol	Ascorbic acid
Chloronase	Chlorpropamide
Chlorpromanyl	Chlorpromazine hydrochloride
Chlor-Tripolon	Chlorpheniramine maleate
Cholestabyl	Colestipol hydrochloride
Cidomycin	Gentamicin sulfate
Claripen	Clofibrate
Claripex	Clofibrate
Clavulin	Amoxicillin clavulanate K
Climestrone	Estrogen, esterified

Appendix B

Canadian Trade Drug Names with Corresponding Generic Drugs—*Continued*

Canadian Trade/Brand Names	Generic Drug Names
Combantrin	Pyrantel pamoate
Coronex	Isosorbide dinitrate
Cortamed	Hydrocortisone
Cortiment	Hydrocortisone
Crystapen	Penicillin G sodium, penicillin G potassium
Cyanabin	Cyanocobalamin
Cyclomen	Danazol
Dalacin-C	Clindamycin
Decanoate	Fluphenazine decanoate
Delestrogen	Estradiol
Deronil	Dexamethasone
Detensol	Propranolol hydrochloride
Dexasone	Dexamethasone
DiaBeta	Glyburide
Diazemuls	Diazepam
Digitaline	Digitoxin
Dimelor	Acetohexamide
Diodoquin	Iodoquinol
Dixarit	Clonidine hydrochloride
Donnagel-MB	Kaolin/pectin
Doryx	Doxycycline hyclate
Doxycin	Doxycycline hyclate
Drenison	Flurandrenolide
Duralith	Lithium carbonate
Duretic	Methylclothiazide
Ecostatin	Econazole nitrate
Eltor, Eltor 120	Pseudoephedrine hydrochloride
Eltroxin	Levothyroxine sodium
Enanthate	Fluphenazine enanthate
E-Pam	Diazepam
Epimorph	Morphine sulfate
Epival	Valproic acid
Eppy	Epinephrine hydrochloride
Erythromid	Erythromycin
Etibi	Ethambutol hydrochloride
Euglucon	Glyburide
Exdol	Acetaminophen
Femogen Forte	Estrone
Fertinic	Ferrous gluconate
Flamazine	Silver sulfadiazine
Fluoderm	Fluocinolone acetonide
Fluor-A-Day	Sodium fluoride
Formulex	Dicyclomine hydrochloride
Fumide	Furosemide
Furomide	Furosemide
Gorophyllin	Aminophylline
Gravol	Dimenhydrinate
Grisovin-FP	Griseofulvin, microsize
Gynergen	Ergotamine tartrate
Haldol LA	Haloperidol
Hepalean	Heparin sodium
Histantil	Promethazine hydrochloride
Honval	Diethylstilbestrol
Hycodan	Hydrocodone bitartrate

continued

Appendix B

Canadian Trade Drug Names with Corresponding Generic Drugs—*Continued*

Canadian Trade/Brand Names	Generic Drug Names
Hydrozide	Hydrochlorothiazide
Impril	Imipramine hydrochloride
Indocid	Indomethacin
Isotamine	Isoniazid
Kalium Durules	Potassium chloride
Kao-Con	Kaolin/pectin
Karasil	Psyllium hydrophilic muciloid
Kidrolase	Asparaginase
Klong	Potassium chloride
Koffex	Dextromethorphan
Kondremul	Mineral oil
Lactulax	Lactulose
Lansoyl	Mineral oil
Lanvis	Thioguanine
Largactil	Chlorpromazine hydrochloride
Lestid	Colestipol hydrochloride
Lidemol	Fluocinonide
Lithizine	Lithium carbonate
Lomine	Dicyclomine hydrochloride
Losec	Omeprazole
Loxapac	Loxapine hydrochloride
Lozide	Indapamide
Lyderm	Fluocinonide
Malogen	Testosterone
Malogen in oil	Testosterone propionate
Malogex	Testosterone enanthate
Marzine	Cyclizine hydrochloride
Maxeran	Metoclopramide
Mazepine	Carbamazepine
Medilium	Chlordiazepoxide hydrochloride
Megacillin	Penicillin G potassium
Meravil	Amitriptyline hydrochloride
Mestinon Supraspan	Pyridostigmine
Metandren	Methyltestosterone
Meval	Diazepam
Milocarpine	Pilocarpine hydrochloride
Minims Phenylephrine	Phenylephrine, ophthalmic
Mobenol	Tolbutamide
Moditen HCl	Fluphenazine hydrochloride
Monistat	Miconazole
Monitan	Acebutolol
Mycil	Chlorphenesin carbamate
Nadopen V	Penicillin V
Nadostine	Nystatin
Nafrine	Oxymetazoline hydrochloride
Nauseatol	Dimenhydrinate
Naxen	Naproxen
Neo-Codema	Hydrochlorothiazide
Neo-Estrone	Estrogen, esterified
Neo-Fer-50	Ferrous fumarate
Neo-Metric	Metronidazole
Nephronex	Nitrofurantoin
Nobesine	Diethylproprion hydrochloride
Nolvadex-D	Tamoxifen citrate
Norlutate	Norethindrone acetate
Novasen	Aspirin

Appendix B

Canadian Trade Drug Names with Corresponding Generic Drugs—*Continued*

Canadian Trade/Brand Names	Generic Drug Names
Novo-Ampicillin	Ampicillin
Novobetamet	Bethamethasone
Novobutamide	Tolbutamide
Novochlorhydrate	Chloral hydrate
Novochlorpromazine	Chlorpromazine hydrochloride
Novochorocap	Chloramphenicol
Novocimetine	Cimetidine
Novoclopate	Clorazepate dipotassium
Novocloxin	Cloxacillin sodium
Novocolchine	Colchicine
Novodimenate	Dimenhydrinate
Novodipam	Diazepam
Novodoxylin	Doxycycline hyclate
Novoferrogluc	Ferrous gluconate
Novoferrosulfa	Ferrous sulfate
Novofibrate	Clofibrate
Novoflupam	Flurazepam
Novoflurazine	Trifluoperazine hydrochloride
Novofolacid	Folic acid
Novofumar	Ferrous fumarate
Novofuran	Nitrofurantoin
Novohexidyl	Trihexyphenidyl hydrochloride
Novolente K	Potassium chloride
Novolexin	Cephalexin
Novolorazepam	Lorazepam
Novomedopa	Methyldopa
Novomepro	Meprobamate
Novometoprol	Metoprolol
Novonaprox	Naproxen
Novo-Niacin	Niacin
Novonidazol	Metronidazole
Novo-Nifedin	Nifedipine
Novopentobarb	Pentobarbital
Novopen-VK	Penicillin V
Novopheniram	Chlorpheniramine maleate
Novopoxide	Chlordiazepoxide hydrochloride
Novopramine	Imipramine hydrochloride
Novopranol	Propranolol hydrochloride
Novopropoxyn	Propoxyphene hydrochloride
Novopurinol	Allopurinol
Novoquinidin	Quinidine sulfate
Novoquinine	Quinine sulfate
Novoreseroine	Reserpine
Novoridazine	Thioridazine hydrochloride
Novorythro	Erythromycin
Novosalmol	Albuterol
Novosecobarb	Secobarbital
Novosemide	Gentamicin sulfate
Novosorbide	Isosorbide dinitrate
Novosoxazole	Sulfisoxazole
Novospiroton	Spironolactone
Novotetra	Tetracycline hydrochloride
Novothalidone	Chlorthalidone
Novotriphyl	Oxtriphylline
Novotriptyn	Amitriptyline hydrochloride

continued

Appendix B

Canadian Trade Drug Names with Corresponding Generic Drugs—*Continued*

Canadian Trade/Brand Names	Generic Drug Names
Novoxapam	Oxazepam
Nyaderm	Nystatin
Ora T Estryl	Fluoxymesterone
Orbenin	Cloxacillin sodium
Ostoforte	Ergocalciferol
Ovol	Simethicone
Ox-Pam	Oxazepam
Paladron	Aminophylline
Palafer	Ferrous fumarate
Panectyl	Trimeprazine tartrate
Parasal Sodium	Aminosalicylate sodium
Parsitan	Ethopropazine hydrochloride
Paveral	Codeine phosphate
Penbritin	Ampicillin
Penglobe	Bacampicillin hydrochloride
Pentacarinat	Pentamidine isethionate
Pentamycetin	Chloramphenicol
Peptol	Cimetidine
Pethadol	Meperidine hydrochloride
Pethidine Hydrochloride	Meperidine hydrochloride
Pharmatex	Benzalkonium chloride
Phenazine	Perphenazine
Phenazo	Phenazopyridine hydrochloride
Pilocarpine	Pilocarpine hydrochloride
Pitrex	Tolnaftate
PMS Carbamazepine	Carbamazepine
PMS Metronidazole	Metronidazole
PMS Nylidrin	Nylidrin hydrochloride
PMS Pyrazinamide	Pyrazinamide
PMS Sulfasalazine	Sulfasalazine
PMS Theophylline	Theophylline
Ponderal	Fenfluramine hydrochloride
Ponstan	Mefenamic acid
Potassium Rougier	Potassium gluconate
Prepidil Gel	Dinoprostone
Procyclid	Procyclidine hydrochloride
Procytox	Cyclophosphamide
Progestilin	Progesterone
Propanthel	Propantheline bromide
Propyl-Thyracil	Propylthiouracil
Protophylline	Dyphylline
Protylol	Dicyclomine hydrochloride
Pseudofrin	Pseudoephedrine hydrochloride
Pulmophylline	Theophylline hydrochloride
Purinol	Allopurinol
Purodigin	Digitoxin
Pyopen	Carbenicillin disodium
Pyronium	Phenazopyridine
Radiostol	Ergocalciferol
Rectocort	Hydrocortisone
Redoxon	Ascorbic acid
Regulax	Docusate sodium
Resyl	Guaifenesin
Revimine	Dopamine hydrochloride
Rhodis	Ketoprofen
Robidex	Dextromethorphan

Appendix B

Canadian Trade Drug Names with Corresponding Generic Drugs—*Continued*

Canadian Trade/Brand Names	Generic Drug Names
Robigesic	Acetaminophen
Rofact	Rifampin
Rogitine	Phentolamine mesylate
Rolavil	Amitriptyline hydrochloride
Rounox	Acetaminophen
Royonate	Potassium gluconate
Rubion	Cyanocobalamin
Rythmodan	Disopyramide
Salbutamol	Albuterol
Salofalk	Mesalamine
SAS Enteric-500	Sulfasalazine
Sedatuss	Dextromethorphan
Sincomen	Spironolactone
Solazine	Trifluoperazine hydrochloride
Solium	Chlordiazepoxide hydrochloride
Somnol	Flurazepam
Somophyllin-12	Theophylline
Sotacor	Sotalol
Statex	Morphine sulfate
Stemetil	Prochlorperazine maleate
Stilboestrol	Diethylstilbestrol
Stress-Pam	Dexamethasone
Sulcrate	Sucralfate
Supasa	Aspirin
Supeudol	Oxycodone
SusPhrine	Epinephrine hydrochloride
Tamofen	Tamoxifen citrate
Tarasan	Chlorprothixene
Tebrazid	Pyrazinamide
Terfluzine	Trifluoperazine hydrochloride
Tetralean	Tetracycline hydrochloride
Thyro-Block	Potassium iodide
Travamine	Dimenhydrinate
Triadapin	Doxepin hydrochloride
Triaphen-10	Aspirin
Triptil	Protriptyline hydrochloride
Tronothane	Pramoxine hydrochloride
Uritol	Furosemide
Vaponefrin	Epinephrine racemic
Vasocon	Naphazoline
Velbe	Vinblastine sulfate
Vimicon	Cyproheptadine hydrochloride
Vistacrom	.Cromolyn sodium
Warfilone	Warfarin sodium
Xylocard	Lidocaine hydrochloride

APPENDIX C

Fat-Soluble and Water-Soluble Vitamins: RDA, Dosages for Vitamin Deficiencies, and Therapeutic Serum Ranges

Vitamin	RDA	Dosages for Vitamin Deficiencies	Therapeutic Serum Range
Fat-Soluble			
Vitamin A	Male: 1000 μg or 5000 IU Female: 800 μg or 4000 IU Preg: 1000 μg, 5000 IU Lact: 1200 μg, 6000 IU	10,000–20,000 IU or 3000–6000 μg/d	30–70 μg/dL *Deficit:* <20 μg/dL
Vitamin D	Male and female: 40–80 μg; 200–400 IU	*Mild:* 50–125 μg/dL *Moderate to severe:* 2.5–7.5 mg/d; 2500–7500 μg	Unknown
Vitamin E	Male: 10 mg/d; 15 IU Female: 8 mg/d; 12 IU Preg: 10–12 mg/d	*Malabsorption:* 30–100 mg/d *Severe deficit:* 1–2 mg/kg/d or 50–200 IU/kg/d	0.5–0.7 mg/dL *Deficit:* 0.5 mg/dL
Vitamin K	Male: 70–80 μg/d Female: 60–65 μg/d Taking broad-spectrum antibiotic: 140 μg/d Preg: 65 μg/d	5–15 mg/d	Based on PT results
Water-Soluble			
Vitamin C	Male and female: 60 mg/d Preg: 70 mg/dL Lact: 95 mg/dL	150–300 mg *Burns:* 500–2000 mg/d	Serum: >1.30 mg/dL WBC: >15 mg/dL *Deficit:* Serum: <0.2 mg/dL WBC: <7 mg/dL
Vitamin B₁ Thiamine	Male: 1.5 mg Female: 1.1 mg Preg: 1.5 mg Lact: 1.6 mg	30–60 mg/d	Urine: <50 μg/d
Vitamin B₂ Riboflavin	Male: 1.4–1.7 mg Female: 1.2–1.3 mg Preg: 1.6 mg Lact: 1.8 mg	5–25 mg/d *Prophylactic:* 3 mg/d	Urine: <50 μg/d

continued

Appendix C

Fat-Soluble and Water-Soluble Vitamins: RDA, Dosages for Vitamin Deficiencies, and Therapeutic Serum Ranges *Continued*

Vitamin	RDA	Dosages for Vitamin Deficiencies	Therapeutic Serum Range
Vitamin B_3 Nicotinic acid or niacin	Male: 15–19 mg/d Female: 13–15 mg/d Preg: 18 mg/d Lact: 20 mg/d	*Prevention:* 5–20 mg/d *Deficit:* 50–100 mg/d *Pellagra:* 300–500 mg in 3 divided doses *Hyperlipidemia:* 1–2 g/d in 3 divided doses	Unknown
Vitamin B_6 Pyridoxine	Male 2.0 mg/d Female: 1.6 mg/d Preg: 2.1 mg/d Lact: 2.2 mg/d	25–100 mg/d *Isoniazid therapy prophylaxis:* 25–50 mg/d *Peripheral Neuritis:* 50–200 mg/d	Serum: >50 ng/mL Urine: <1.0 mg/d
Folic acid Folate	Male and female: 400 μg/d Preg: 600–800 μg/d Lact: 600–800 μg/d	1–2 mg/d	Serum folate: 6–20 ng/mL RBC: 160–600 ng/mL *Deficit:* Serum: <3–4 ng/mL RBC: <140 ng/mL
Vitamin B_{12}	Male and female: 3 μg/d Preg: 4 μg/d	100 mg/d × 14 d *Pernicious anemia:* 50–100 μg/d or 1000 μg/wk × 3 wk	150–900 pg/mL *Deficit:* <100 pg/mL *Schilling test:* >30% normal

Key: Preg: pregnancy; Lact: lactation; d: day; wk: week; <: less than; >: greater than.

APPENDIX D

HINTS FOR MEDICATION USE IN THE COMMUNITY SETTING: Home, School, and Worksite

- Client's safety is of primary concern.
- Client's physical abilities require ongoing assessment. Capabilities may be temporarily impaired with the use of certain drugs (e.g., narcotics, selected eye medications, and psychotropics). Advise client not to operate hazardous machinery during such times and to use caution at all other times.
- Keep medications in original labeled containers with child-safe caps when needed.
- Provide client/family with written instructions (audio instructions if sight-impaired) about the drug regimen.
- Instruct client/family on all skills related to the medication regimen. Examples are: how to take pulse for clients taking digitalis preparations, correct use of inhalers, and techniques for successful administration of parenteral medications. Allow time for instruction and questions; include demonstration and return demonstration. Provide client/family with contact person and telephone number for questions and concerns.
- Advise client/family about the expected length of time to achieve therapeutic response from the medication. There is wide variation (e.g., narcotics within 30 minutes, many antibiotics within 24 hours, and some psychotropics within 6 weeks).
- Advise client/family about general side effects of the medication(s) and when to notify the health care provider.
- Advise client/family about possible drug–food and drug–laboratory test interactions. Detail which foods are to be avoided and which foods are encouraged for specific nutrient value. For example, tyramine-rich foods are contraindicated with monoamine oxidase inhibitors (MAOIs), and potassium-rich foods are recommended for clients taking potassium-wasting diuretics. Alcohol may be contraindicated with selected medications.
- Advise client/family to have adequate supply of necessary medications available at all times—at home, school, work, and while traveling. Order prescription refills in advance. Take extra medication with you when traveling. Drugs in original labeled containers are preferred for foreign travel.
- Caution against the use of over-the-counter (OTC) preparations without *first* contacting the health care provider.
- Reinforce the importance of follow-up appointments with health care provider(s). Encourage wellness check-ups, including preventive and restorative dental care. Complete laboratory studies in a timely manner.
- Encourage clients to wear Medic-alert ID band with medications and/or allergies indicated.
- Reinforce that community resources are available and need to be mobilized according to client's needs.

ADDITIONAL FDA APPROVED DRUGS

Acarbose
Acetophenazine maleate
Acetylcysteine
Aldesleukin
Amifostine
Amlodipine besylate
Anastrozole
Beclomethasone dipropionate
Bicalutamide
Capreomycin sulfate
Carvedilol
Ciprofloxacin
Cisapride
Clarithromycin
Clofazimine
Cycloserine
Dapiprazole HCl
Dexfenfluramine
Diethylcarbamazine citrate
Dihydrotachysterol
Diltiazem
Dirithromycin
Estramustine phosphate sodium
Ethionamide
Felbamate
Fluorometholone
Griseofulvin microsize
Ibutilide fumarate
Indinavir sulfate
Lamivudine
Leuprolide acetate
Losartan potassium
Magnesium citrate
Magnesium hydroxide
Magnesium oxide
Magnesium salicylate
Magnesium sulfate

Mebendazole
Mephentermine sulfate
Metformin HCl
Methysergide maleate
Metronidazole HCl
Miacalcin nasal spray
Midazolam HCl
Mivacurium Cl
Moexipril HCl
Moricizine HCl
Nabumetone
Nefazodone HCl
Niclosamide
Nisoldipine
Ofloxacin
Oxamniquine
Oxytocin nasal solution
Phenacemide
Primozide
Pipecuronium bromide
Piperazine citrate
Praziquantel
Pyrantel pamoate
Pyrazinamide
Rimexolone
Ritonavir
Saquinavir mesylate
Stavudine
Sulfacetamide sodium
Thiabendazole
Tobramycin ointment/solution
Tramadol HCl
Triamcinolone acetonide spray
Tubocurarine Cl
Valacyclovir HCl

Additional FDA Approved Drugs

Generic (Brand)	Route and Dosage	Preg Cat	Interaction	t 1/2	PB	Onset	Peak	Duration
Acarbose (Precose) *Oral antidiabetic/ nonsulfonylurea*	A: PO: 25 mg t.i.d.; max: 300 mg/d	C	Similar to metformin	2 h	UK	UK	1 h	UK
Acetophenazine maleate (Tindal) *Antipsychotic*	A: PO: 20 mg b.i.d./q.i.d.; max: 120 mg/d	C	*Increase* CNS depression with alcohol	10–20 h	>90%	UK	2–4 h	UK
Acetylcysteine (Mucomyst) *Mucolytic*	*Acetaminophen poisoning:* A&C: PO: 140 mg/kg; then 17 doses of 70 mg/kg q4h	B	*Admixture incompatibility:* Tetracycline, erythromycin; amphotericin B, ampicillin	2–5.5 h	50%	UK	5–10 min	UK
Aldesleukin (Interleukin-2, IL-2) *Biologic response modifier*	*Metastatic renal cell carcinoma:* A: IV: 600,000 IU/kg q8h × 5 d; repeat cycle after 9 d rest; may repeat course after 7 wk rest Refer to guidelines for discontinuation of this drug	C	*Increase* effects of antihypertensives; decrease effects with corticosteroids; use cautiously with psychotropic drugs	1.5 h	UK	UK	UK	Up to 12 mo
Amifostine (Ethyol) *Anticancer agent*	A: IV: 740–910 mg/m²/d in a 15 min IV infusion	C	*Increase* effects of antihypertensives	1–8 min	UK	5 min	15–20 min	UK
Amlodipine besylate (Lotrel) *Antihypertensive agent*	A: PO: 5 mg/d; max:10 mg/d	C	*Increase* effects with histamine₂ blockers	30–50 h	93%	UK	6–12 h	UK

Anastrozole (Arimidex) *Anticancer agent*	*Breast cancer:* A: PO: 1 mg/d	C	UK	50 h	40%	UK	UK	UK
Beclomethasone dipropionate (Beclovent, Vanceril) *Corticosteroid*	A&C >12 y: 1 spray q nostril b.i.d./q.i.d.; inhal: 2 t.i.d./q.i.d. max: 12 inhal/d C 6–12 y: Inhal: 1–2 t.i.d./q.i.d.; max: 10 inhal/d	NR	None significant reported	5–15 h	87%	UK	1–2 wk	UK
Bicalutamide (Casodex) *Anticancer agent, antiandrogen*	A: PO: 50 mg/d; may be taken with LHRH (luteinizing hormone-releasing hormone)	X	*Increase* effects of warfarin	5.8 d	UK	1–4 wk	UK	UK
Capreomycin sulfate (Capastat Sulfate) *Antitubercular agent*	A: IM: 1 g/d or 15 mg/kg/d for 24 mo; then 1 g, 2–3×wk; max: 20 mg/kg/d	C	May *increase* nephro-ototoxicity with aminoglycosides, antifungal drugs, vancomycin, cisplatin	4–6 h	UK	UK	31 h	UK
Carvedilol (Coreg) *Beta blocker, antihypertensive agent*	A: PO: 6.25 mg b.i.d.; may increase to 12.5 mg b.i.d.; max: 50 mg/d	C	*Increase* effect of antidiabetics, calcium blockers, digoxin, clonidine; *increase* effect with cimetidine, rifampin	7–10 h	98%	<1 h	1–2 h	UK
Ciprofloxacin (Cipro) *Urinary antiinfectives*	*Uncomplicated cystitis in females:* A: PO: 100 mg q12h for 3 d	C	*Increase* levels of drug with probenecid, theophylline; *decrease* absorption with antacids *Lab: increase* AST, ALT, BUN	4–6 h	20–40 %	UK	1–2 h	UK
						Rapid	1–2 h	6–8 h

continued

Additional FDA Approved Drugs—Continued

Generic (Brand)	Route and Dosage	Preg Cat	Interaction	t 1/2	PB	Onset	Peak	Duration
Cisapride (Propulsid) *GI stimulant*	*Heartburn and gastroesophageal reflux disease:* A: PO: 10 mg 15 min a.c. and h.s.	C	Alters effects of digoxin and drugs with narrow therapeutic range due to absorption rate; *decrease effects with anticholinergics* Lab: *Increase coagulation time with oral anticoagulants*	8–10 h	98%	30–60 min	1–1.5 h	Max effect: 8–12 wk
Clarithromycin (Biaxin) *Antiinfective, otic*	A: PO: 250–500 mg q12h for 10 d C: 7.5–15 mg/kg q12h for 10 d	C	*Increase effects of anticoagulants, carbamazepine, digoxin, terfenadine, theophylline; decrease effects of zidovudine*	3–5 h	65–75 %	<2 h	2–4 h	12 h
Clofazimine (Lamprene) *Antileprosy agent*	A: PO: 100 mg/d for 3 yr	C	May *decrease* effect with isoniazid Food: *increase absorption*	70 d	UK	UK	4–12 h	UK
Cycloserine (Seromycin) *Antitubercular agent*	*Antitubercular agent:* A: PO: 250 mg q12 h for 2 wk; then increase to 250 mg q8h for 2 wk; then increase to 250 mg q6h for 2 wk; max: 1 g/d *Urinary tract infection:* A: PO: 250 mg q12h for 2 wk	C	May increase risk of CNS toxicity (seizures) with alcohol or isoniazid	10 h	UK	UK	3–4 h	UK

Dapiprazole HCl (Rev-Eyes) *Mydriatic*	A: 2 gtt in sac, and 2 gtt in 5 min (conjunctival injection)	B	None significant reported	UK	UK	Rapid	UK	UK
Dexfenfluramine (Redux) *Anorexiant*	15 mg b.i.d. with meals; max: 30 mg/d Safety >1 y use not established	C	Avoid use with MAOIs or within 21 d of MAOI use	17–20 h	36%	UK	UK	UK
Diethylcarbamazine citrate (Hetrazan) *Anthelmintic drug*	A: PO: 2–3 mg/kg t.i.d.	C	None significant reported	UK	UK	UK	UK	UK
Dihydrotachysterol (DHT Intensol, Hytakerol) *Parathyroid hormone regulator*	A: PO: 0.75–2.5 mg/d × 3–4 d; maint: 0.2–1.5 mg/d *or* PO: 0.25 mg/d with calcium supplements C: PO: 1–5 mg/d × 4d; maint: 0.5–1.5 mg/d	A	None significant reported	1–2 d	UK	UK	1–2 wk	2–9 wk
Diltiazem *Emergency treatment of cardiac states*	IV: 0.25 mg/kg; repeat in 15 min at 0.5 mg/kg	C	*Increase* effects with beta blockers, cimetidine Lab: may *increase* serum digoxin level	2–5 h	80%	3 min	UK	Bolus: 0.5–3 h Inf: up to 10 h
Dirithromycin *Macrolide*	A&C>12y: PO: 500 mg/d × 10 d (take with food)	C	*Increase* effects with antacids, H₂ blockers	8–36 h	15–30 %	UK	4 h	UK
Estramustine phosphate sodium (Emcyt) *Anticancer/alkylating agent*	A: PO: 10–16 mg/kg/d in 3–4 divided doses; maint: 14 mg/kg/d	C	Food: dairy products *decrease* effects	20 h	UK	UK	2–3 h	UK
Ethionamide (Trecator-SC) *Antitubercular agent*	A: PO: 0.5–1 g/d in 2–3 divided doses C: PO: 12–15 mg/kg/d in 3–4 divided doses; max: 1 g/d	D	May *increase* CNS toxicity with isoniazid, cycloserine	3 h	UK	UK	1.8–3 h	9 h

continued

Additional FDA Approved Drugs—Continued

Generic (Brand)	Route and Dosage	Preg Cat	Interaction	t1/2	PB	Onset	Peak	Duration
						Action		
Felbamate (Felbatol) *Anticonvulsant, hydantoin*	*Partial seizures:* A: PO: Initially only: 1200 mg/d in 3–4 divided doses; increased by 600 mg q 2 wk if needed and tolerated; max: 3600 mg/d *Adjunctive therapy:* Initially: PO: 1200 mg/d in 3–4 divided doses as other drug reduced by 20%; increase felbamate 1200 mg/d in divided doses q wk until max of 3600 mg/d; reduce other drug concomitantly *Lennox-Gustaut syndrome:* C: PO: Initially: 15 mg/kg/d in 3–4 divided doses; may increase 15 mg/kg/d q wk; max: 45 mg/kg/d; reduce concomitant drug	C	*Increase* serum phenytoin and valproic acid level; *decreases* carbamazepine levels	20–24 h	25%	Therapeutic effect: 14 d	Serum: 1–6h	UK
Fluorometholone (FML Liquifilm Ophthalmic, Fluor-op) *Antiinflammatory*	A&C >2 y: Susp 0.1–0.25%, 1–2 gtt in sac b.i.d./t.i.d. (qh for 1st 48 h) Oint: 0.1%: 1.25 cm q4h; then daily/t.i.d. as condition improves	C	None significant reported	UK	UK	UK	UK	UK

Drug	Dose	Pregnancy Category	Interactions	t½	Protein Binding	Onset	Peak	Duration
Griseofulvin microsize (Grifulvin V, Grisactin, Fulvicin) *Antifungal agent*	A: PO: 500 mg/d in 1–2 divided doses (microsize); may increase to 1 g C: PO: 11 mg/kg/d (microsize)	C	May *increase* tachycardia with alcohol; may *decrease* effect of barbiturates, warfarin, oral contraceptives; may *increase* estrogen metabolism	9–24 h	UK	UK	4–8 h	UK
Ibutilide fumarate (Corvert) *Antidysrhythmic drug Class III*	A >60 kg: IV: 1–2 mg infusion over 10 min; repeat if necessary	C	None significant reported	6 h	40%	Immediate	5–10 min	UK
Indinavir sulfate *Antiviral agent (HIV)*	A: PO: 800 mg q8h	C	*Increase* effects of zidovudine (AZT), stavudine, oral contraceptives, isoniazid	1.8 h	60%	UK	1 h	UK
Lamivudine (Epivir) *Antiviral agent (HIV)*	A: PO: 4 mg/kg/d in 2 divided doses C: PO: 8 mg/kg/d in 2 divided doses	C	*Increase* effect of zidovudine (AZT); *increase* effect with trimethoprim-sulfamethoxazole	3.7 h	<36%	UK	UK	UK
Leuprolide acetate (Lupron) *Anticancer agent*	Advanced prostatic cancer: A: SC: 1 mg/d IM: 7.5 mg/mo	X	None significant reported	UK	UK	UK	1–2 mo	UK
Losartan potassium (Cozaar) *ACE inhibitor, antihypertensive agent*	A: PO: Initially 25–50 mg/d	C; D: last two trimesters	*Increase* effect with cimetidine; *decrease* effect with phenobarbital	2–9 h	95%	1 h	1–4 h	1 wk

continued

Additional FDA Approved Drugs—Continued

Generic (Brand)	Route and Dosage	Preg Cat	Interaction	t1/2	PB	Action Onset	Peak	Duration
Magnesium citrate (Citrate of magnesia) *Electrolyte*	*Laxative:* A: PO: 240 mL per dose C 6–12 y: PO: 50–100 mL per single dose	B	May *decrease* drug action of other drugs	UK	UK	2–6 h	UK	UK
Magnesium hydroxide (Milk of magnesia) *Electrolyte*	*Laxative:* A: PO: 30–60 mL/d in single or divided doses C 6–12 y: PO: 15–30 mL in single or divided doses	B	Same as magnesium citrate	UK	UK	3–6 h	UK	UK
Magnesium oxide (Mag-Ox 400, Maox) *Electrolyte*	*Antacid:* A: PO: cap: 420–560 mg/d in 3–4 divided doses; tab: 400–840 mg/d with water or milk in divided doses	B	Same as magnesium citrate	UK	UK	20 min	20–60 min	UK
Magnesium salicylate (Doan's Pills) *Electrolyte*	*Analgesic:* A: PO: 650 mg t.i.d/q.i.d	C	None significant reported	UK	UK	1.5–2 h	UK	UK
Magnesium sulfate (Epsom salts) *Electrolyte*	*Laxative:* A: PO: 10–30 g single dose *Preeclampsia, eclampsia:* A: IM/IV: 4 g (IV in D_5W 250 mL)	C	*Increase* respiratory depression with CNS depressants	UK	UK	PO: 1–2 h IM: 1 h IV: 1–2 min	UK	PO/IM: 3–4 h IV: 30 min

Mebendazole (Vermox) *Anthelmintic drug*	A: PO: 100 mg b.i.d. ×3d, repeat in 2–3 wk if necessary C >2 y: PO: same as adult	C	*Increase* effect with cimetidine	UK	UK	UK	2–5 h	UK
Mephentermine sulfate (Wyamine) *Adrenergic agent*	A: IM/IV: 30–45 mg 10–20 min prior to anesthesia C: IM/IV: 0.4 mg/kg *Spinal anesthesia hypotension:* A: IV: 15 mg; may be repeated	D	None significant reported	UK	UK	IM: 5–15 min IV: immediate	UK	IM: 1–4 h IV: 15–30 min
Metformin HCl (Glucophage) *Oral antidiabetic/ nonsulfonylurea*	A: PO: Initially: 500 mg daily b.i.d.; increase dose gradually; max: 2500 mg/d	B	May *increase* hyperglycemia with calcium channel blockers, estrogens, corticosteroids, oral contraceptives, phenothiazides	6.2 h	0%	UK	1 h	UK
Methysergide maleate (Sansert) *Adrenergic blocker, antimigraine agent*	A: PO: 4–8 mg/d in divided doses with food	C	None significant reported	10 h	UK	1 d	UK	1–2 d
Metronidazole HCl (Flagyl, Protostat, MetroGel) *Antifungal agent*	*Trichomoniasis:* A: PO: Initially: 2 g in 1–2 divided doses; then 250 mg q8h ×7d *Bacterial infections:* A: PO: 500 mg q6–8h; max: 4 g/d	B	May *increase* effect of warfarin, lithium *Lab:* may *increase* AST, ALT, LDH	6–8 h	UK	UK	1–3 h	UK
Miacalcin nasal spray (calcitonin) *Parathyroid stimulant*	200 IU intranasally daily, alternating nostrils	C	UK	45 min	UK	UK	30–40 min	UK

Additional FDA Approved Drugs—Continued

Generic (Brand)	Route and Dosage	Preg Cat	Interaction	t 1/2	PB	Action Onset	Action Peak	Action Duration
Midazolam HCl (Versed) CSS IV *Anxiolytic*	*IV induction general anesthesia:* A: IV: 0.15–0.25 mg/kg over 30 sec; effects in 2 min *Conscious sedation:* A: IM: 0.07–0.08 mg/kg 0.5–1 h before event IV: 1–1.5 mg; repeat in 2 min PRN	D	*Increase* effects with other opiates or CNS depressants; *increase* risk of apnea with CNS depressants, alcohol	1–4 h	97%	IM: <15 min IV: 2–5 min	15–60 min rapidly	2–6 h
Mivacurium Cl (Mivacron) *Skeletal muscle relaxant*	A: IV: Initially: 0.15 mg/kg infuse over 5–15 sec; maint: 0.1 mg/kg Continuous infusion: Initially: 9–10 μg/kg/min then reduce to 4 μg/kg/min C 2–12 y: IV: Initially: 0.2 mg/kg	C	Similar to atracurium besylate	2 min	UK	Immediate	2–6 min	30 min
Moexipril HCl (Univasc) *ACE inhibitor, antihypertensive agent*	A: PO: Initially: 10 mg/d; maint: 20–40 mg/d	C; D: last 2 trimesters	Similar to enalapril	2–9 h	50%	1 h	2–6 h	UK
Moricizine HCl (Ethmozine) *Antidysrhythmia drug*	A: PO: 200–300 mg q8h; dose decreased with renal and hepatic dysfunction	B	May *increase* effect of warfarin, cimetidine; may *decrease* theophylline concentration	10 h	92–95%	2 h	10 h	10–24 h

Drug	Dose	Preg. Cat.	Interactions	Half-life	PB	Onset	Peak	Duration
Nabumetone (Relafen) *Antiinflammatory agent*	A: PO: 1000 mg (1 g) in 1–2 divided doses; max: 2 g/d	C	*Increase* effect with warfarin *Food: Increase* effect	24 h	99%	UK	2–6 h	UK
Nefazodone HCl (Serzone) *Antidepressant*	A: PO: Initially: 200 mg/d in 2 divided doses; maint: 300–600 mg/d in divided doses	C	*Increase* effects of alprazolam, triazolam, digoxin; avoid MAOIs	11–24 h	>97%	1 wk	3–5 wk	UK
Niclosamide (Niclocide) *Anthelmintic drug*	A: PO: 2 g single dose, then may give 2 g/d × 1 wk C >34 kg: PO: 1.5 g single dose, then 1 g/d × 6 d C <34 kg: PO: 1 g single dose	B	None significant reported	UK	UK	UK	UK	UK
Nisoldipine (Sular) *Calcium blocker, antihypertensive agent*	A: PO: 20 mg/d; may increase 10 mg per wk; maint: 20–40 mg/d	C	Similar to amlodipine besylate	7–12 h	99%	UK	6–12 h	UK
Ofloxacin (Floxin) *Urinary antiinfective*	A: PO/IV: 200 mg q12h × 10 d	C	*Increase* effect of warfarin; *increase* effect with cimetidine, probenecid; *decrease* effect with antacids, sucralfate nitrofurantoin	5–7.5 h	20–32 %	1 h	1–2 h	UK
Oxamniquine (Vansil) *Anthelmintic drug*	A: PO: 15 mg/kg single dose, then 15 mg/kg b.i.d. for 1–2 d C <30 kg: PO: 10 mg/kg; may repeat 2–8 h later	C	None significant reported	1–2.5 h	UK	<1 h	1–2 h	UK
Oxytocin synthetic nasal solution *Oxytocic*	*Milk let-down:* 1 spray into 1 or both nostrils 2–3 min before nursing or pumping breasts	X	Avoid use with sympathomimetic pressors to prevent severe hypertension	15 min	UK	Several min	UK	20 min

continued

Additional FDA Approved Drugs—Continued

Generic (Brand)	Route and Dosage	Preg Cat	Interaction	t 1/2	PB	Onset	Peak	Duration
Phenacemide (Phenurone) *Anticonvulsant, hydantoin*	*Severe epilepsy refractory to other drugs:* A: PO: Initially: 500 mg t.i.d.; increased q wk by 500 mg/d; max: 5 g/d C 5–10 y: PO: Initially: 250 mg t.i.d.; increase q wk by 250 mg/d; max: 2.5 g/d	D	*Increase risk of toxicity with other anticonvulsants; contraindicated for those achieving seizure control with other drugs*	UK	UK	UK	Serum 1–2 h	5 h
Pimozide *Antipsychotic*	*Treatment of severe tics of Tourette's disorder refractory to standard treatment:* A: PO: Initially: 1–2 mg/d in divided doses; increase q.o.d.; maint: max: 0.2 mg/kg/d or 10 mg/d	C	Administer with caution with anticonvulsants because may lower seizure threshold; prolongs QT interval, so avoid use with phenothiazines, antidysrhythmics, tricyclic antidepressants; *increase effects of CNS depressants*	55 h	UK	UK	6–8 h	UK
Pipecuronium bromide (Arduan) *Skeletal muscle relaxant*	A: IV: 0.15 mg/kg push over 5–15 sec; may follow with 0.1 mg/kg C 2–12 y: IV: 0.2 mg/kg push over 5–15 sec	C	Similar to atracurium besylate	2–3 h	32%	1–2 min	5 min	20–60 min

Piperazine citrate (Antepar) *Anthelmintic drug*	*Roundworm:* A: PO: 3.5 g/d × 2 d C: PO: 75 mg/kg/d × 2 d; max: 3.5 g/d *Pinworm:* A&C: 65 mg/kg/d × 7 d; max: 2.5 g/d	B	*Increase* EPS with phenothiazines	UK	UK	UK	UK
Praziquantel (Biltricide) *Anthelmintic drug*	*Tapeworms:* A&C: PO: 10–20 mg/kg single dose *Blood flukes:* A&C: PO: 20 mg/kg t.i.d. × 1 d *Liver, lung, and intestinal flukes:* A&C: PO: 25 mg/kg t.i.d. × 1–2 d	B	None significant reported	0.8–1.5 h	UK	UK	1–3 h	UK
Pyrantel pamoate (Antiminth) *Anthelmintic drug*	A&C: 11 mg/kg single dose; repeat in 2 wk if necessary; max 1 g	C	*Decrease* effect with piperazine	1–2 h	UK	UK	1–3 h	UK
Pyrazinamide (Tebrazid) *Antitubercular agent*	A: PO: 20–35 mg/kg/d in 3–4 divided doses; max: 3 g/d	C	None significant reported	9.5 h	10–20%	UK	2 h	UK
Rimexolone (Vexol) *Corticosteroid*	*Anterior uveitis:* A: susp 1%: 1–2 gtt in sac qh while awake for 1 wk; then 1 gt q2h while awake for 2nd wk; taper until healed *Postoperative:* A: 1–2 gtt	C	None significant reported	NA	NA	UK	UK	UK

continued

Additional FDA Approved Drugs—Continued

Generic (Brand)	Route and Dosage	Preg Cat	Interaction	t1/2	PB	Onset	Peak	Duration
Ritonavir (Norvir) *Antiviral agent (HIV)*	A: PO: Initially: 300 mg/d; may increase dose 100 mg per d; maint: 600 mg q12h	B	*Increase* effects with clarithromycin, fluconazole, fluoxetine; *decrease* effects of zidovudine (AZT); *increase* effects of meperidine, propoxyphene, flecainide	UK	95%	UK	2 h	UK
Saquinavir mesylate *Antiviral agent (HIV)*	A: PO: 600 mg q8h; reduce dose if given with AZT	B	Similar to indinavir sulfate	UK	98%	UK	UK	7 h
Stavudine (d4T) (Zerit) *Antiviral agent (HIV)*	A >60 kg: PO: 40 mg q12h; <60 kg: PO: 30 mg q12h; Cl_{cr} 25–50 mL/min: 15–20 mg q12h	C	None significant reported	1–1.6 h	<25%	UK	1 h	UK
Sulfacetamide sodium (Bleph-10, Liquifilm Ophthalmic, Cetimide Ophthalmic) *Antiinfective, ophthalmic*	*Corneal ulcers, trachoma, chlamydial infections, conjunctivitis:* A&C: Sol 10, 15, 30%: 1–3 gtt in sac q2–3h; taper as condition improves Oint 10%: 0.5–1 inch q6h and h.s.	UK	*Decrease* effects with PABP-based local anesthetics; drug precipitated with silver preparations	UK	UK	UK	UK	UK
Thiabendazole (Mintezol, Minzolum) *Anthelmintic drug*	*Threadworm, roundworm:* A&C: PO: 25 mg/kg b.i.d. for 2 d; max: 3 g/d	C	May *increase* theophylline level	UK	UK	UK	1–2 h	UK

Drug	Dosage		Contraindications / Interactions					
Tobramycin (Nebcin, Tobrex) *Antiinfective, ophthalmic*	Oint 0.3%: 1 cm b.i.d./t.i.d. Sol 0.3%: 1–2 gtt q4h *For severe infections:* Oint: q3–4 h Sol: 2 gtt q30–60 min until improvement, then decrease frequency	D	None significant reported	NA	NA	Rapid	1–1.5 h	8 h
Tramadol HCl (Ultram) *Analgesic*	A: PO: 50–100 mg q4–6h PRN; max: 400 mg/d Elderly >75 y: max: 300 mg/d *Hepatic dysfunction:* 50 mg q12 h *Renal dysfunction:* Cl$_{cr}$ <30 mL/min: 50–100 mg q12h	C	*Increased* effect with CNS depressants; *increased* risk of seizures with MAOIs; *decreased* effect with carbamazepine	UK	UK	UK	Serum 2 h	UK
Triamcinolone acetonide (Azmacort, Trilog) *Corticosteroid*	A: Inhal: 2 inhal t.i.d./q.i.d.; max: 16 inhal/d C 6–12 y: Inhal: 1–2 inhal t.i.d./q.i.d.; max: 12 sprays /d	C	Similar to prednisone	2–5 h	65–90%	1 h	1–2 h	UK
Tubocurarine Cl *Skeletal muscle relaxant*	A: IV: 6–9 mg; may follow with 3–4.5 mg	C	May *increase* neuromuscular blockade with aminoglycosides, clindamycin, antidysryhthmics, diuretics	1–3 h	50%	Immediate	2–5 min	30 min
Valacyclovir HCl (Valtrex) *Antiviral agent (HSV 1, HSV 2, herpes zoster)*	*Herpes zoster:* A: PO: 1 g t.i.d. × 7 d in 3 divided doses *Recurrent genital herpes:* A: PO: 500 mg b.i.d. × 5 d	B	*Decrease* effects with cimetidine, probenecid	2.5–3.5 h	13–18%	UK	3 h	UK

INDEX

Note: Page numbers followed by the letter t refer to tables.

Abbokinase (urokinase), 321t
acarbose, 484t
Accupril (quinapril HCl), 309t
acebutolol HCl, 96t, 280t, 296t
acetaminophen, 34, 35
  nursing process, 35
  prototype, 34
acetazolamide, 56t, 289t, 377t
acetohexamide, 414
acetophenazine maleate, 484t
acetylcholine Cl, 375t
acetylcysteine, 484t
Achromycin (tetracycline), 166, 382t, 384t
Acon, 2
ACTH, 388, 389, 391
Acthar (corticotropin), 388, 389
Acthar gel (corticotropin repository), 388, 391t
Actidil (triprolidine HCl), 247t
Actifed (pseudoephedrine), 246t, 253t
Actimmune (interferon gamma-1b), 238t
actinomycin (dactinomycin), 227t
activated charcoal, 454t
Acular ophth (ketorolac), 383t
Acutrim (phenylpropanolamine HCl), 20t
acyclovir sodium, 194, 195
  nursing process, 194, 195
  prototype, 194
Adalat (nifedipine), 275t
Adenocard (adenosine), 281t, 446t
adenosine, 281t, 446t
Adipex-P (phentermine HCl), 20t
Adipost (phendimetrazine tartrate), 19t
adrenal hormone replacement, 404–409
Adrenalin (epinephrine), 86–88, 446t
adrenergic agonists, 86–93
  nursing process, 87, 88
  prototype, 86

adrenergic blockers, 94–97
  nursing process, 95
  prototype, 94
adrenocorticotropic hormone replacement, 388, 389, 391
Adriamycin (doxorubicin), 227t
Adrucil (fluorouracil), 222
Advil (ibuprofen), 36t, 132, 134
Aerosporin (polymyxin B), 381t
Afrin (oxymetazoline HCl), 252t
agonist-antagonist narcotics, 44–47
AK-Dex ophthalmic (dexamethasone), 383t
AK-Dilate (phenylephrine HCl), 380t
Akineton (biperiden lactate), 111t, 114t
Albalon (naphazoline HCl), 252t
albuterol, 89t, 256t
Aldactazide (spironolactone and hydrochlorothiazide), 292t
Aldactone (spironolactone), 292t
aldesleukin, 229t, 484t
Aldomet (methyldopa), 298t
Alferon N (interferon alfa-n3), 238t
Alka-Seltzer, 32
Alkeran (melphalan), 218t
alkylating drugs, 216–220
  nursing process, 216, 217
  prototype, 216
Allerdryl (diphenhydramine HCl), 242, 243
Allerest (naphazoline HCl), 252t
Alloprin (allopurinol), 144
allopurinol, 144, 145
  nursing process, 145
  prototype, 144
Alpha-adrenergic blockers, 300–302
alprazolam, 74t
Altace (ramipril), 309t
Alteplase (tissue-type plasminogen activator), 320t
ALternaGEL (aluminum hydroxide), 358, 359

499

Index

altretamine, 219t
Alu-Tab (aluminum hydroxide), 358, 359
Aludrox, 361t
aluminum carbonate, 360t
aluminum hydroxide, 358, 359
  nursing process, 359
  prototype, 358
Alupent (metaproterenol), 90t, 254, 255
Alurate (aprobarbital), 26t
amantadine HCl, 118, 196t
ambenonium Cl, 102t, 122t
Ambien (zolpidem tartrate), 31t
Amen (medroxyprogesterone acetate), 431t
Amersol (ibuprofen), 132
Amicar (aminocaproic acid), 321t
amifostine, 484t
amikacin sulfate, 172t
Amikin (amikacin sulfate), 172t
amiloride HCl, 292t
aminocaproic acid, 321t
aminoglutethimide, 229t
aminoglycosides, 170–173
  nursing process, 170, 171
  prototype, 170
aminophylline, 263t
aminosalicylate sodium, 187t
amiodarone HCl, 281t
amitriptyline HCl, 78t
amlodipine besylate, 273t, 484t
amobarbital sodium, 26t, 52t
amoxapine, 76, 77
  nursing process, 77
  prototype, 76
amoxicillin trihydrate, 148, 149
  nursing process, 149
  prototype, 148
amoxicillin-clavulanate, 148, 149
Amoxil (amoxicillin trihydrate), 148
amphetamine sulfate, 18t
Amphojel (aluminum hydroxide), 358, 359
amphotericin B, 190t
ampicillin, 151t
ampicillin-sulbactam, 151t
amrinone lactate, 268t
amyl nitrite, 272t
Amytal sodium (amobarbital sodium), 26t, 52tt
Anafranil (clomipramine HCl), 78t
analgesics, 32–37
Anaspaz (hyoscyamine sulfate), 108t
anastrozole, 485t
Anavar (oxandrolone), 439t
Ancef (cefazolin sodium), 158t

Ancobon (flucytosine), 191t
Andro-Cyp 100 (testosterone), 434
androgens, 434–439
  nursing process, 435, 436
  prototype, 434
Android (methyltestosterone), 439t
Androlone-D (nandrolone decanoate), 438t
Anectine Cl (succinylcholine Cl), 129t
angiotensin antagonists, 306–309
anistreplase, 320t
Anorex (phendimetrazine tartrate), 19t
Ansaid (flurbiprofen sodium), 137t
antacids, 358–361
  nursing process, 358, 359
  prototype, 358
Antepar (piperazine citrate), 494t
antianginals, 270–275
  nursing process, 271
  prototype, 270
antibacterials, 148–183
anticholinergics, 104–111
  nursing process, 105, 106
  prototype, 104
anticoagulants, 312–315
  nursing process, 313, 314
  prototype, 312
anticonvulsants, 50, 57
antidepressants, 76–81
antidiabetics, 410–417
  insulin, 410–413
    nursing process, 410, 411
    prototype, 410
  sulfonylurea, 414–417
    nursing process, 414, 415
    prototype, 414
antidiarrheals, 344–349
  nursing process, 344, 345
  prototype, 344
antidysrhythmics, 276–281, 444
  nursing process, 277
  prototype, 276
antiemetics, 334–339
  cannabinoid, 337t
  motion sickness, 339t
  phenothiazine, 334–336
    nursing process, 335
    prototype, 334
antifungals, 188–191
antigout agents, 144–146
  nursing process, 145
  prototype, 144
antihistamines, 242–244
  nursing process, 242
  prototype, 242

Index

antihypertensives, 294–310
antiinfectives, 148–201
  topical, 198–201
antiinflammatory agents, 132–142
antilipemics, 322–327
  nursing process, 323, 324
  prototype, 322
antimalarials, 192t, 193t
antimanics, 82–84
antimetabolites, 222–224
  nursing process, 223
  prototype, 222
Antiminth (pyrantel pamoate), 494t
antineoplastics, 216–231
antipsychotics, 60–71
  nonphenothiazine, 66–71
  phenothiazine, 60–65
Antispas (dicyclomine HCl), 107t
antitubercular agents, 184–187
Anti-Tuss (guaifenesin), 251t
antitussives, 248–251
  nursing process, 249
  prototype, 248
antiulcer drugs, 358–370
  histamine$_2$ blocker, 364–366
    nursing process, 365
    prototype, 364
  pepsin inhibitor, 368–370
    nursing process, 369
    prototype, 368
Antivert (meclizine HCl), 339t
antivirals, 194–197
Antrizine (meclizine HCl), 339t
Anturane (sulfinpyrazone), 146t, 317t
anxiolytics, 72–75
Aparkane (trihexyphenidyl), 112
Aphen (trihexyphenidyl HCl), 112t
Apo-Amoxi (amoxicillin trihydrate), 148
Apo-Bisacodyl (bisacodyl), 350, 351
Apo-Captopril (captopril), 306
Apo-Diazepam (diazepam), 72, 73
Apo-Erythro-S or Base (erythromycin), 162
Apo-Flurazepam (flurazepam HCl), 28, 29
Apo-Hydro (hydrochlorothiazide), 282
Apo-Metoprolol (metoprolol tartrate), 294
Apo-Nitrofurantoin (nitrofurantoin), 204, 205
Apo-Perphenazine (perphenazine), 334, 335
Apo-Prednisone (prednisone), 404
Apo-Propranolol (propranolol HCl), 94

apomorphine, 342t
apresoline HCl, 304t
aprobarbital, 26t
APSAC (anistreplase), 320t
AquaMEPHYTON (vitamin K$_1$), 317t
Aquasol A, 2
Aquatag (benzthiazide), 284t
Aquatensen (methyclothiazide), 285t
Aralen HCl (chloroquine HCl), 192t
Arduan (pipecuronium bromide), 494t
Arimidex (anastrozole), 485t
Aristocort (triamcinolone), 409t
Arlidin (nylidrin HCl), 330t
Armour Thyroid (thyroid), 397t
Arrestin (trimethobenzamide), 338t
Artane (trihexyphenidyl HCl), 111t, 112, 113
ASA (aspirin), 32, 33, 135t
ascorbic acid, 5t
Asendin (amoxapine), 76, 77
  nursing process, 77
  prototype, 76
asparaginase, 230t
aspirin, 32, 33, 135t, 316t
  nursing process, 33
  prototype, 32
astemizole, 247t
Astrin (aspirin), 32, 33
Atabrine HCl (quinacrine HCl), 193t
Atarax (hydroxyzine HCl), 74t, 244t
Atasol (acetaminophen), 34, 35
atenolol, 96t, 273t, 296t
Ativan (lorazepam), 30t, 54t, 75t
atovaquone, 191t
atracurium besylate, 128t
Atromid-S (clofibrate), 325t
Atropair (atropine), 104
atropine sulfate, 104–106, 378t, 446t
  nursing process, 105, 106
  prototype, 104
Atropisol, 104
Atrovent (ipratropium bromide), 258t
Augmentin (amoxicillin-clavulanate), 148
auranofin, 140–142
  nursing process, 141, 142
  prototype, 140
aurothioglucose, 143t
Aventyl (nortriptyline HCl), 79t
Axid (nizatidine), 366t
Azactam (aztreonam), 177t, 208t
Azaline (sulfasalazine), 182t
azatadine maleate, 246t
azithromycin, 164t

501

Index

Azmacort (triamcinolone acetonide), 496t
aztreonam, 177t, 208t
Azulfidine (sulfasalazine), 182t

bacampicillin HCl, 151t
Bacarate (phendimetrazine tartrate), 19t
bacitracin, 183t, 381t
Bacitrin (bacitracin), 183t
baclofen, 127t
Bactocill (oxacillin), 153t
Bactrim (trimethoprim-sulfamethoxazole), 178–180. See *Septra (sulfamethoxazole-trimethoprim)*.
Bactroban (mupirocin), 154t
Balminil DM (dextromethorphan hydrobromide) 248, 249
Banflex (orphenadrine HCl), 115t
barbiturates, 22–26, 52t, 53t
  nursing process, 23, 24
Basaljel (aluminum carbonate), 360t
Bayer (aspirin), 32, 33
beclomethasone, 407t
beclomethasone dipropionate, nasal spray, 485t
Beclovent (beclomethasone dipropionate), 485t
belladonna tincture, 362t
Benadryl (diphenhydramine HCl), 242, 243, 458t
benazepril HCl, 308t
bendroflumethiazide, 284t
Benemid (probenecid), 146t
Bentyl (dicyclomine HCl), 107t
Benylin (dextromethorphan hydrobromide), 250t
Benylin DM (dextromethorphan hydrobromide), 248, 248t, 249
Benzac (benzoyl peroxide), 200t
Benzodiazepines, 28–31, 72
  nursing process, 29, 30
  prototype, 28
benzonatate, 250t
benzoyl peroxide, 200t
benzphetamine HCl, 19t
benzquinamide HCl, 337t
benzthiazide, 284t
benztropine mesylate, 110t, 114t
bepridil HCl, 274t
beta blockers, 294–297
Betagan liquifilm (levobunolol HCl), 376t
Betaloc (metoprolol tartrate), 294

betamethasone, 407t
Betapen-VK (penicillin V potassium), 151t
Betaseron (interferon beta-1b), 238t
betaxolol HCl, 296t, 376t
bethanechol Cl, 98–100, 212t
  nursing process, 99, 100
  prototype, 98
Betoptic (betaxolol HCl), 376t
Biaxin (clarithromycin), 164t
bicalutamide, 485t
Bicillin (penicillin G benzathine), 150t
BiCNU, 219t
Biltricide (praziquantel), 494t
biologic response modifiers, 232–238
  nursing process, 233, 234
  prototype, 232
biotin, 4t
biperiden lactate, 111t, 114t
bisacodyl, 350, 351
  nursing process, 351
  prototype, 350
bishydroxycoumarin (dicumarol), 315t
bismuth salts, 347t
bisoprolol fumarate, 296t
bitolterol mesylate, 256t
Blenoxane (bleomycin sulfate), 224t
bleomycin sulfate, 226t
Blocadren (timolol maleate), 93t, 297t
body weight (calculations), xxi
Bonine (meclizine HCl), 339t
boric acid, 384t
Brethaire (terbutaline sulfate), 93t, 258t, 423t
Brethine (terbutaline sulfate), 93t, 258t, 423t
bretylium tosylate, 281t, 446t
Bretylol (bretylium tosylate), 281t, 446t
BRMs, 232–238
broad-spectrum penicillins, 148, 149, 151
  nursing process, 148, 149
  prototype, 148
bromocriptine mesylate, 119t, 442t
Bromphen (brompheniramine maleate), 246t
brompheniramine maleate, 246t
bronchodilators, 254–263
Bronkaid Mist (epinephrine), 256t
Bronkephrine (ethylnorepinephrine HCl), 258t
Bronkosol (isoetharine HCl), 90t, 257t

Index

Bucladin-S (buclizine HCl), 339t
buclizine HCl, 339t
bulk-forming laxatives, 354–357
bumetanide, 288t
Bumex (bumetanide), 288t
Buprenex (buprenorphine HCl), 46t
buprenorphine HCl, 46t
bupropion HCl, 80t
burn agents, 198, 199
BuSpar (buspirone HCl), 75t
busulfan, 219t
butabarbital sodium (Butisol Sodium), 26t
Butazolidin (phenylbutazone), 37t
Butisol sodium (butabarbital sodium), 26t
butorphanol tartrate, 46t

C.E.S. (conjugated estrogens), 428–430
caffeine, 20t
Calan (verapamil HCl), 275t, 280t, 310t, 447t
calcifediol, 402t
Calciferol, 5t
Calcimar (calcitonin [salmon]), 403t
calcitonin (salmon), 403t
calcitonin (human), 403t
calcitriol, 400, 402t
calcium, 12–14
 nursing process, 13, 14
 prototype, 12
calcium carbonate, 12, 360t
calcium chloride, 12
calcium lactate, 12
calcium polycarbophil, 356t
calculations (drug), xxi
Calderol (calcifediol), 402t
Calm-X (dimenhydrinate), 339t
Caltrate, 12
Camalox, 361t
Camphorated opium tincture, 346t
Canadian drug names, 465–477
 Canadian brand names to generic names, 471–477
 generic drugs to Canadian brand names, 465–469
Cantil (mepenzolate bromide), 109t
Capastat Sulfate (capreomycin sulfate), 485t
Capoten (captopril), 306, 307
captopril, 306, 307
 nursing process, 306, 307
 prototype, 306
capreomycin sulfate, 485t

Carafate (sucralfate), 368
carbachol, 101t, 375t
carbamazepine (Tegretol), 55t
carbamide peroxide, 384t
carbenicillin disodium, 153t
carbidopa-levodopa, 116, 117
 nursing process, 117
 prototype, 116
carbinoxamine/pseudoephedrine, 245t
Carbiset (carbinoxamine), 245t
Carbodec (carbinoxamine), 245t
Carbolith (lithium carbonate), 82–84
carboplatin, 219t
carboprost tromethamine, 427t
Carcholin (carbachol), 101t
Cardene SR (nicardipine HCl), 274t
cardiac glycosides, 266–268
 nursing process, 266, 267
 prototype, 266
cardiotonics, 266–268
Cardizem (diltiazem HCl), 274t, 309t
Cardura (doxazosin mesylate), 302t
carisoprodol, 124, 125
 nursing process, 125
 prototype, 124
carmustine, 219t
carteolol HCl, 296t
Cartrol (carteolol HCl), 296t
carvedilol, 485t
cascara sagrada, 353t
Casodex (bicalutamide), 485t
castor oil, 353t
Cataflam (diclofenac sodium), 383t
Catapres (clonidine HCl), 298t
Ceclor (cefaclor), 156, 157, 385t
Cedilanid-D (deslanoside), 268t
CeeNu (lomustine), 219t
cefaclor, 156, 157, 385t
 nursing process, 156, 157
 prototype, 156
cefadroxil, 158t
Cefadyl (cephapirin), 159t
cefamandole, 159t
cefazolin sodium, 158t
cefixime, 161t
Cefizox (ceftizoxime), 161t
cefmetazole sodium, 159t
Cefobid (cefoperazone), 161t
cefonicid sodium, 159t
cefoperazone, 161t
ceforanide, 159t
ceforozil monohydrate, 160t
Cefotan (cefotetan), 161t
cefotaxime, 161t
cefotetan, 161t

503

Index

cefoxitin sodium, 160t
cefpodoxime, 160t
ceftazidime, 161t
Ceftin (cefuroxime), 160t
ceftizoxime, 161t
ceftriaxone, 161t
cefuroxime, 160t
Cefzil (cefprozil), 160t
Celestone (betamethasone), 407t
Celontin (methsuximide), 55t
central nervous system stimulants, 16–21
   nursing process, 17
Centrax (prazepam), 75t
cephalexin, 158t
cephalosporins, 156–161
   first generation, 158t
   second generation, 159t, 160t
   third generation, 161t
cephapirin, 159t
cephradine, 159t
Cephulac (lactulose), 352t
Cerubidine (daunorubicin HCl), 227t
Cerumenex, 384t
Cesamet (nabilone), 337t
cetirizine, 247t
Charcoaid (charcoal), 342t
charcoal, 342t
CharcoCaps (charcoal), 342t
Cheracol (guaifenesin and codeine), 250t
Chibroxin (norfloxacin), 381t
chloral hydrate, 27t
chlorambucil, 218t
chloramphenicol, 177t
   ophth, 381t
   optic, 384t
chlordiazepoxide HCl, 74t
Chloromycetin (chloramphenicol), 177t
   ophth, 381t
chloroquine HCl, 192t
chlorothiazide, 284t
chlorotrianisene, 431t
chlorphenesin carbamate, 127t
chlorpheniramine maleate, 244t
Chlorpromanyl (chlorpromazine), 60, 61
chlorpromazine, 60–63
   nursing process, 61–63
   prototype, 60, 61
chlorpropamide, 417t
chlorprothixene HCl, 70t
chlorthalidone, 285t
Chlor-Trimeton (chlorpheniramine maleate), 244t
chlorzoxazone, 127t

Cholac (lactulose), 352t
Choledyl (oxtriphylline), 263t
cholestyramine resin, 325t
Choloxin (dextrothyroxine sodium), 325t
Chorex (human chorionic gonadotropin), 442t
Cibacalcin (calcitonin [human]), 403t
cimetidine, 366t
Cinobac (cinoxacin), 176t, 206t
cinoxacin, 176t, 206t
Cipro (ciprofloxacin), 174, 207t, 381t
ciprofloxacin, 174, 175, 207t, 381t, 485t
   nursing process, 174, 175
   ophth, 381t
   prototype, 174
cisapride, 486t
cisplatin, 219t
citrate of magnesia (magnesium citrate), 490t
Citroma (magnesium citrate), 352t
Citrucel (methylcellulose), 356t
Clabulin (amoxicillin-clavulanate), 148t
cladribine, 224t
Claforan (cefotaxime), 161t
clarithromycin, 164t
   otic, 486t
Claritin (loratadine), 247t
clemastine fumarate, 245t
Cleocin (clindamycin), 165t
clidinium bromide, 108t
clidinium bromide and chlordiazepoxide HCl, 362t
clindamycin HCl, 165t
clindamycin palmitate, 165t
Clinoril (sulindac), 136t
clofazimine, 446t
clofibrate, 325t
Clomid (clomiphene citrate), 440t
clomiphene citrate, 440t
clomipramine HCl, 78t
clonazepam (Klonopin), 53t
clonidine HCl, 298t
clorazepate dipotassium, 53t, 74t
cloxacillin, 152t
clozapine, 71t
Clozaril, 71t
CNS stimulants, 16–21
Co-trimoxazole (trimethoprim-sulfamethoxazole), 178, 180. See also *Septra (sulfamethoxazole-trimethoprim)*.
   nursing process, 179, 180
   prototype, 178

Index

cobalamin, 4t
codeine sulfate and phosphate, 42t, 250t
Cogentin (benztropine mesylate), 110t
Cognex (tacrine HCl), 101t
Colace (docusate sodium), 357t
colchicine, 146t
Colestid (colestipol HCl), 326t
colestipol HCl, 326t
colistimethate sodium, 183t
colistin sulfate, 183t, 348t
Cologel (methylcellulose), 356t
Colsalide (colchicine), 146t
Coly-Mycin M (colistimethate sodium), 183t
Coly-Mycin S (colistin sulfate), 183t, 348t
Colyte (polyethylene glycol), 357t
Compazine (prochlorperazine maleate), 64t, 336t
conjugated estrogens, 428
Constilac (lactulose), 352t
Contac (phenylpropanolamine HCl), 92t
contact laxatives, 350–353
Control (phenylpropanolamine HCl), 20t
conversion tables, xxi
Cordarone (amiodarone HCl), 281t
Coreg (carvedilol), 485t
Corgard (nadolol), 96t, 297t
Correctol (phenolphthalein), 353t
Cortef (hydrocortisone), 408t
Corticotropin, 388, 389
 prototype, 388
 repository, 390t
cortisone acetate, 408t
Cortistan (cortisone acetate), 408t
Cortone Acetate (cortisone acetate), 408t
Cortrophin-Zinc (corticotropin), 388
Cortrosyn (cosyntropin), 391t
Corvert (ibutilide fumarate), 489t
Cosmegen (dactinomycin), 227t
cosyntropin, 391t
Coumadin (warfarin sodium), 312
Cozaar (losartan potassium), 489t
cromolyn sodium, 247t
Crysticillin (penicillin G procaine), 150t
Crystodigin (digitoxin), 268t
Curretab (medroxyprogesterone acetate), 431t
cyclacillin, 151t
cyclandelate, 330t
Cyclapen (cyclacillin), 151t
cyclizine HCl, 339t

cyclobenzaprine HCl, 127t
Cyclogyl (cyclopentolate HCl), 107t, 379t
cyclopentolate HCl, 107t, 379t
cyclophosphamide, 216, 217
 nursing process, 216, 217
 prototype, 216
cycloserine, 486t
Cyclospasmol (cyclandelate), 330t
Cycrin (medroxyprogesterone acetate), 431t
Cylert (pemoline), 18t
cyproheptadine HCl, 246t
Cystospaz (hyoscyamine sulfate), 108t
Cytadren (aminoglutethimide), 229t
cytarabine HCl, 224t
Cytomel (liothyronine sodium), 397t
Cytosar-U (cytarabine HCl), 224t
Cytotec (misoprostol), 370t
Cytovene (ganciclovir sodium), 197t
Cytoxan (cyclophosphamide), 216

dacarbazine, 220t
dactinomycin, 227t
Dalgan (dezocine), 46t
Dalmane (flurazepam HCl), 28–30
dalteparin sodium, 316t
danazol, 437t
Danocrine (danazol), 437t
Dantrium (dantrolene sodium), 130t
dantrolene sodium, 130t
dapiprazole HCl, 487t
Daranide (dichlorphenamide), 289t, 377t
Daraprim (pyrimethamine), 193t
Darbid (isopropamide iodide), 109t
Daricon (oxyphencyclimine HCl), 109t
Darvon (propoxyphene HCl), 43t
Darvon-N (propoxyphene napsylate), 43t
Datril (acetaminophen), 34, 35
daunorubicin HCl, 227t
Daypro (oxaprozin), 138t
DDAVP (desmopressin acetate), 391t
Debrox (carbamide peroxide), 384t
Deca-Durabolin (nandrolone decanoate), 438t
Decadron (dexamethasone), 408t
Declomycin (demeclocycline HCl), 168t
Delatestryl (testosterone), 437t
Delaxin (methocarbamol), 128t
Delta-Cortef (prednisolone), 409t

505

Index

Deltasone (prednisone), 404
Demadex (torsemide), 288t
demecarium bromide, 101t, 376t
demeclocycline HCl, 168t
Demerol HCl (meperidine HCl), 40, 41
  nursing process, 41
  prototype, 40
deodorized opium tincture, 346t
Depakene (valproic acid), 56t
depAndrogyn (testosterone), 434
Depo-Estradiol Cypionate (estradiol cypionate), 431t
Depo-Medrol (methylprednisolone), 408t
Depo-Provera (medroxyprogesterone acetate), 431t
DEPO-Testosterone (testosterone), 434, 437t
Depotest 100 (testosterone), 434, 437t
Dervoid (bethanechol Cl), 98
desipramine HCl, 78t
deslanoside, 268t
desmopressin acetate, 391t
Desoxyn (methamphetamine HCl), 18t
Desquam (benzoyl peroxide), 200t
Desyrel (trazodone HCl), 81t
Detensol (propranolol HCl), 94
dexamethasone, 383t, 408t
Dexatrim (phenylpropanolamine HCl), 20t
Dexchlor (dexchlorpheniramine maleate), 246t
dexchlorpheniramine maleate, 246t
Dexedrine (dextroamphetamine sulfate), 18t, 19t
dextroamphetamine sulfate, 18t, 19t
dexfenfluramine, 487t
dextromethorphan hydrobromide, 248, 249
  nursing process, 249
  prototype, 248
Dextrose 50%, 458t
dextrothyroxine sodium, 325t
dezocine, 46t
DHT Intensol (dihydrotachysterol), 487t
DiaBeta (glyburide nonmicronized), 417t
Diabinese (chlorpropamide), 417t
Diachlor (chlorothiazide), 284t
Dialose (docusate potassium), 356t
Diamox (acetazolamide), 56t, 289t
Diamox Sequels (acetazolamide), 377t

Diapid (lypressin), 391t
Diazemuls (diazepam), 72, 73
diazepam (Valium), 54t, 72, 73, 126t
diazoxide, 462t
Dibenzyline (phenoxybenzamine HCl), 302t
Dicarbosil (calcium carbonate), 360t
dichlorphenamide, 289t, 377t
diclofenac sodium, 139t, 383t
dicloxacillin, 152t
dicumarol (bishydroxycoumarin), 315t
dicyclomine HCl, 107t
didanosine, 196t
Didrex (benzphetamine HCl), 19t
Didronel (etidronate), 403t
dienestrol, 431t
diethylcarbamazine citrate, 487t
diethylpropion HCl, 19t
diethylstilbestrol, 431t
difenoxin and atropine, 348t
Diflucan (fluconazole), 190t
diflunisal, 37t, 135t
Di-Gel, 361t
digitoxin, 268t
digoxin, 266, 267
  nursing process, 266, 267
  prototype, 266
dihydrotachysterol, 487t
dihydroxyaluminum sodium carbonate, 360t
Dilantin (phenytoin), 50, 51, 279t
  nursing process, 51
  prototype, 50
Dilaudid (hydromorphone HCl), 42t
Dilor (dyphylline), 263t
diltiazem, emergency, 487t
diltiazem HCl, 274t, 309t
Dimelor (acetohexamide), 414
dimenhydrinate, 339t
dimensional analysis, xxi
Dimetabs (dimenhydrinate), 339t
Dimetane (brompheniramine), 246t
Dimetapp (phenylpropanolamine HCl), 92t
dimethyl sulfoxide, 213t
dinoprostone cervical gel, 427t
diphenhydramine HCl, 242, 243, 458t
  nursing process, 243
  prototype, 242
diphenidol HCl, 337t
diphenoxylate with atropine, 344, 345, 346t
  nursing process, 345
  prototype, 344
dipivefrin HCl, 379t

dipyridamole, 316t
dirithromycin, 487t
Disipal (orphenadrine HCl), 115t
disopyramide phosphate, 278t
Di-Spaz (dicyclomine HCl), 107t
Ditropan (oxybutynin Cl), 213t
Diucardin (hydroflumethiazide), 284t
diuretics, 282–293
  loop, 286–288
    nursing process, 287
    prototype, 286
  potassium-sparing, 290–293
    nursing process, 291
    prototype, 290
  thiazide, 282–285
    nursing process, 283
    prototype, 282
Diuril (chlorothiazide), 284t
DMSO (dimethyl sulfoxide), 213t
Doan's Pills (magnesium salicylate), 490t
dobutamine HCl, 89t, 458t
docusate calcium, 356t
docusate sodium, 357t
docusate potassium, 356t
Dolobid (diflunisal), 37t, 135t
Domeboro, otic, 384t
Donnagel, 349t
Donnagel-PG, 349t
dopamine HCl, 89t, 456
  nursing process, 457
  prototype, 456
dopaminergics, 116–119
Dopar (levodopa), 118t
Dopram (doxapram HCl), 21t
Doral (quazepam), 30t
Doriden (glutethimide), 31t
dorzolamide HCl, 377t
Dospan (diethylpropion HCl), 19t
doxacurium Cl, 128t
doxapram HCl, 21t
doxazosin mesylate, 302t
doxepin HCl, 78t
doxorubicin, 227t
doxycycline hyclate, 168t
Dramamine (dimenhydrinate), 229t
Drisdol Drops, 403t
Dristan (phenylephrine HCl), 92t
dronabinol, 337t
droperidol, 70t, 337t
drug calculations, xxi
DTIC (dacarbazine), 220t
Dulcolax (bisacodyl), 350, 351
Durabolin (nandrolone phenpropionate), 438t
Duragesic (fentanyl), 47t

Duramorph (morphine sulfate), 38, 39
Duraquin (quinidine sulfate), 278t
Duratest 100 (testosterone), 434, 437t
Duricef (cefadroxil), 158t
Duvoid (bethanechol Cl), 212t
Dyazide (triamterene and hydrochlorothiazide), 293t
Dyline (dyphylline), 263t
Dymelor (acetohexamide), 414
Dynabac (dirithromycin), 487t
DynaCirc (isradipine), 274t, 310t
Dynapen (dicloxacillin), 152t
dyphylline, 263t
Dyrenium (triamterene), 290

echothiophate iodide, 101t, 375t
Ecotrin, 32, 33
Ectasule (ephedrine sulfate), 252t
Edecrin (ethacrynic acid), 288t
edrophonium Cl, 102t, 122t
Efedrin (ephedrine sulfate), 90t
Efedron (ephedrine HCl), 90t
Effexor (venlafaxine), 81t
Efidac (pseudoephedrine HCl), 253t
Elavil (amitriptyline HCl), 78t
Eldepryl (selegiline HCl), 119t
electrolyte(s), 8–14
  calcium as, 12–14
  potassium as, 8–11
  magnesium as, 490t
Elixophyllin-KI (theophylline), 260
Elspar (asparaginase), 230t
Eltroxin (levothyroxine), 394
Emcyt (estramustine), 218t, 487t
emergency drugs, 444–462
emetics, 340–342
  nursing process, 340, 341
  prototype, 340
Eminase (anistreplase), 320t
Empirin, 32, 33
Emulsoil (castor oil), 353t
E-Mycin (erythromycin) (optic), 162, 386t
enalapril maleate, 308t
encainide HCl, 279t
Endep (amitriptyline HCl), 78t
endocrine agents, 387–417
Enduron (methyclothiazide), 285t
Enkaid (encainide HCl), 279t
Enovil (amitriptyline HCl), 78t
enoxacin, 176t, 209t
enoxaparin sodium, 315t
Entrophen (aspirin), 32, 33

Index

Enulose (lactulose), 352t
ephedrine sulfate, 90t, 252t, 256t
Epifrin (epinephrine HCl), 379t
Epinal (epinephrine borate), 39t
epinephrine, 86–88, 256t, 379t, 446t, 459t
   nursing process, 86–88
   prototype, 86
epinephrine borate, 379t
Epivir (lamivudine), 489t
epoetin alfa, 232
Epogen (erythropoietin), 232
Eppy/N (epinephrine borate), 379t
Epsom salts (magnesium sulfate), 353t
Equanil (meprobamate), 126t
ergocalciferol, 403t
ergoloid mesylate, 331t
ergonovine maleate, 426t
Ergotrate (ergonovine maleate), 426t
Erythrocin (erythromycin), 162
Erythrocin (IV) (erythromycin lactobionate), 162
Erythromid (erythromycin), 162
erythromycin, 162, 163, 381t, 386t
   nursing process, 163
   ophth, 381t, 386t
   prototype, 162
erythromycin lactobionate, 162, 163
erythropoietin (EPO), 232–234
   nursing process, 233, 234
   prototype, 232
Eserine Salicylate (physostigmine), 103t
Esidrix (hydrochlorothiazide), 282
Eskalith (lithium carbonate), 82
estazolam, 30t
esterified estrogens, 431t
Estrace (estradiol), 431t
Estraderm (estradiol), 431t
estradiol, 431t
estradiol cypionate, 431
Estradurin (polyestradiol phosphate), 231t
estramustine phosphate sodium, 218t, 487t
Estratab (esterified estrogens), 431t
estrogen replacements, 428–430
   nursing process, 428–430
   prototype, 428
estrogens and progestins, 431, 432
estrone, 431t
estropipate sulfate, 431t
ethacrynic acid, 288t
ethambutol HCl, 187t
ethchlorvynol, 25t
ethionamide, 487t

Ethmozine (moricizine HCl), 492t
ethopropazine HCl, 115t
ethosuximide, 55t
ethotoin, 54t
ethylnorepinephrine HCl, 258t
Ethyol (amifostine), 484t
etidronate, 403t
etodolac, 139t
etoposide, 226t
etretinate, 201t
Eulexin (flutamide), 230t
Euthroid (liotrix), 397t
Evac-Q-Mag (magnesium citrate), 352t
Everone (testosterone), 434, 437t
Ex-Lax (phenolphthalein), 353t

famciclovir, 197t
famotidine, 366t
Famvir (famciclovir), 197t
Fastin (phentermine HCl), 20t
feces, drugs causing discoloration of, xxv
Feen-A-Mint (phenolphthalein), 353t
felbamate, 488t
Felbatol (felbamate), 488t
Feldene (piroxicam), 139t
felodipine, 309t
fenfluramine HCl, 19t
fenofibrate, 326t
fenoprofen calcium, 137t
fentanyl, 47t
Feosol, 6
Feostat, 6
Fer-Iron, 6
Feosol, 6
Fergon, 6
ferrous fumarate, 6
ferrous gluconate, 6
ferrous sulfate, 6
Fetinic, 6
Fiberall (calcium polycarbophil), 356t
FiberCon (calcium polycarbophil), 356t
filgrastim, 234, 235
   nursing process, 235
Flagyl (metronidazole HCl), 491t
flavoxate HCl, 213t
flecainide, 278t
Fleet Enema, 353t
Fleet Phospho-Soda (sodium biphosphate), 353t
Flexeril (cyclobenzaprine HCl), 127t
Flexon (orphenadrine citrate), 128t
Florinef Acetate (fludrocortisone acetate), 408t

Index

Floropryl (isoflurophate), 101t, 376t
Floxin (ofloxacin), 177t
floxuridine, 224t
fluconazole, 190t
flucytosine, 191t
Fludara (fludarabine), 225t
fludarabine, 225t
fludrocortisone acetate, 408t
Flumadine (rimantadine HCl), 196t
flunisolide, 252t
fluorometholone, 488t
fluoroquinolone, ciprofloxacin as, 174
fluorouracil, 222, 223
  nursing process, 222, 223
  prototype, 222
fluoxetine HCl, 80t
fluoxymesterone, 438t
fluphenazine HCl, 64t
flurazepam HCl, 28–30
  nursing process, 29, 30
  prototype, 28
FML liquifilm (fluorometholone), 488t
folic acid, 5t
Follutein (human chorionic gonadotropin), 442t
Fortaz (ceftazidime), 161t
fosinopril, 308t
Fragmin (dalteparin sodium), 316t
Freezone (salicylic acid), 200t
5-FU (fluorouracil), 222
FUDR (floxuridine), 224t
Fulvicin (griseofulvin microsize), 489t
Fumerin, 6
Fumide (furosemide), 286
Fungizone (amphotericin B), 190t
Furacin (nitrofurazone), 200t
Furadantin (nitrofurantoin), 204, 205
Furalan (nitrofurantoin), 204, 205
Furan (nitrofurantoin), 204, 205
furazolidone, 348t
Furomide (furosemide), 286
furosemide, 286, 287
  nursing process, 286, 287
  prototype, 286
Furoxone (furazolidine), 348t

gabapentin (Neurontin), 56t
ganciclovir sodium, 197t
Gantanol (sulfamethoxazole), 182t
Gantrisin (sulfisoxazole), 181t
Garamycin (gentamicin sulfate), 170t, 381t
Gaviscon (magnesium trisilicate), 361t
Gelusil-I, 361t
Gelusil-II, 361t
Gelusil-M, 361t
gemfibrozil, 326t
gentamicin sulfate, 170t, 171, 381t
  nursing process, 170, 171
  ophth, 381t
  prototype, 170
Geocillin (carbenicillin disodium), 153t
Geopen (carbenicillin disodium), 153t
Geref (sermorelin acetate), 390t
Gesterol 50 (progesterone), 231t
Glaucon (epinephrine HCl), 379t
glipizide, 417t
glucagon, 459t
glucocorticoids, 404–409
  nursing process, 405, 406
  prototype, 404
Glucophage (metformin HCl), 491t
Glucotrol (glipizide), 417t
Glukor (human chorionic gonadotropin), 442t
glutethimide, 31t
glyburide micronized, 417t
glyburide nonmicronized, 417t
glycerin, 378t
glycopyrrolate, 108t, 362t
Glycotuss, 251t
Glynase (glyburide micronized), 417t
Glyrol (glycerin), 378t
gold preparations, 140–143
  nursing process, 141, 142
  prototype, 140
gold sodium thiomalate, 143t
GoLYTELY (polyethylene glycol), 357t
gonadorelin acetate, 442t
Gonic (human chorionic gonadotropin), 442t
goserelin acetate, 230t
gout drugs, 146t
granisetron, 338t
granulocyte colony-stimulating factor, 234, 235
granulocyte-macrophage colony-stimulating factor, 236
Grifulvin V (griseofulvin microsize), 489t
Grisactin (griseofulvin microsize), 489t
griseofulvin microsize, 489t
guaifenesin, 251t
guaifenesin and codeine, 250t
guaifenesin and dextromethorphan, 251t

509

Index

guanabenz acetate, 298t
guanadrel sulfate, 303t
guanethidine monosulfate, 303t
guanfacine HCl, 298t

halazepam, 75t
Halcion (triazolam), 31t
Haldol (haloperidol), 66–68
  nursing process, 67, 68
  prototype, 66
Haldrone (paramethasone acetate), 409t
haloperidol, 66–68
Halotestin (fluoxymesterone), 438t
HCTZ (hydrochlorothiazide), 282
Hemabate (carboprost tromethamine), 427t
heparin sodium, 315t
Herplex Liquifilm, 383t
Hetrazan (diethylcarbamazine), 487t
Hexalen (altretamine), 219t
Hexaphen (trihexyphenidyl HCl), 112
Hiprex (methenamine hippurate), 207t
Hismanal (astemizole), 247t
Histaject (brompheniramine maleate), 246t
Histerone (testosterone), 434, 435, 436t
Hivid (zalcitabine), 197t
Homatropine, 107t
homatropine hydrobromide, 380t
human chorionic gonadotropin (hCG), 442t
human menopausal gonadotropin, 442t
Humatrope (somatropin), 390t
Humorsol (demecarium bromide), 101t, 376t
Humulin L insulin, 413t
Humulin N insulin, 413t
Humulin R insulin, 412t
Hycodan (hydrocodone), 250t
hydantoin, 50, 51, 54t
Hydeltrasol (prednisolone), 409t
Hydergine (ergoloid mesylate), 331t
hydralazine HCL, 304t
Hydrea (hydroxyurea), 225t
Hydrex (benzthiazide), 284t
hydrochlorothiazide, 282, 283
  nursing process, 283
  prototype, 282
hydrocodone, 250t
hydrocortisone, 408t

Hydrocortone (hydrocortisone), 408t
HydroDIURIL (hydrochlorothiazide), 282
hydroflumethiazide, 284t
hydromorphone HCl, 42t
Hydromox (quinethazone), 285t
hydroxychloroquine sulfate, 192t
hydroxyurea, 225t
hydroxyzine HCl, 74t, 244t
Hygroton (chlorthalidone), 285t
Hylorel (guanadrel sulfate), 303t
hyoscyamine sulfate, 108t
Hyperstat (diazoxide), 304t, 462t
hypnotics, 22–31
Hytakerol (dihydrotachysterol), 487t
Hytrin (terazosin HCl), 302t

ibuprofen, 36t, 132–134
  nursing process, 133–134
  prototype, 132
ibutilide fumarate, 489t
Idamycin (idarubicin), 227t
idarubicin, 227t
idoxuridine, 382t
IDU (idoxuridine), 382t
Ifex (ifosfamide), 218t
ifosfamide, 218t
Ilosone (erythromycin estolate), 164t
Ilotycin (erythromycin), 164t, 381t
Imdur (isosorbide mononitrate), 272t
iminostilbenes, 54t
imipenem, 177t, 209t
imipenem-cilastatin, 177t
imipramine HCl, 79t
Imitrex (sumatriptan succinate), 21t
Imodium (loperamide HCl), 347t
Inapsine (droperidol), 70t, 337t
indapamide, 285t
Inderal (propranolol HCl), 273t, 297t
  nursing process, 95
  prototype, 94
indinavir sulfate, 489t
Indocin (indomethacin), 136t
indomethacin, 136t
INH (isoniazid), 184–186
  nursing process, 185–186
  prototype, 184
Inocor (amrinone lactate), 268t
insulins, 410–413
Intal (cromolyn sodium), 247t
interferons, 238t
interleukin-2 (aldesleukin), 229t, 484t
intravenous (IV) flow rates, xxiii
Intron-A (interferon alfa-2b), 238t

Index

Intropin (dopamine HCl), 89t
  nursing process, 457
  prototype, 456
iodinated glycerol, 251t
iodine: strong iodine solution, 398t
Iophen (iodinated glycerol), 251t
ipecac syrup, 454t
  nursing process, 341
  prototype, 340
ipratropium bromide, 257t
iron, 6, 7
  nursing process, 7
  prototype, 6
Ismelin sulfate, 303t
Ismotic (isosorbide), 378t
isocarboxazid, 81t
isoetharine HCl, 90t, 257t
isoflurophate, 101t, 376t
isoniazid, 184–186
  nursing process, 185, 186
  prototype, 184
isopropamide iodide, 109t
isoproterenol HCl, 90, 257t
Isoptin (verapamil HCl), 275t, 447t
Isoptin SR (verapamil HCl), 310t
Isopto Atropine (atropine sulfate), 379t
Isopto Carpine (pilocarpine), 372–374
  nursing process, 373, 374
  prototype, 372
Isopto Eserine (physostigmine salicylate), 375t
Isopto Homatropine (homatropine), 107, 380t
Isopto Hyoscine (scopolamine hydrobromide), 380t
Isordil (isosorbide dinitrate), 272t
isosorbide dinitrate, 272t, 378t
isosorbide mononitrate, 72t
Isotamine (isoniazid), 184
isoxsuprine HCl, 328, 329
  nursing process, 329
  prototype, 328
isradipine, 274t, 310t
Isuprel (isoproterenol HCl), 90t, 257t
itraconazole, 190t

Kabikinase (streptokinase), 318, 319
Kalcinate (calcium gluconate), 12
kanamycin sulfate, 172t
Kantrex (kanamycin sulfate), 172t
Kaochlor (potassium chloride), 12
kaolin-pectin, 347t
Kaon-Cl (potassium chloride), 12

Kaopectate (kaolin-pectin), 347t
Karasil (psyllium hydrophilic muciloid), 354, 355
Kay Ciel (potassium chloride), 12
K-Dur (potassium chloride), 12
Keflex (cephalexin), 158t
Kefzol (cefazolin sodium), 158t
Kemadrin (procyclidine HCl), 11t, 115t
Kenacort (triamcinolone), 409t
Kenalog (triamcinolone), 409t
Kerlone (betaxolol HCl), 296t
Kestrone 5 (estrone), 431t
ketoconazole, 191t
ketoprofen, 36t, 138t
ketorolac, 139t, 383t
Klonopin (clonazepam), 53t
Kloromin (chlorpheniramine maleate), 244t
Konakion (phytonadione), 317t
Kytril (granisetron), 338t

labetalol HCl, 305t
Lactinex *(Lactobacillus),* 348t
Lactobacillus acidophilus, 348t
Lactobacillus bulgaricus, 348t
lactulose, 352t
Lamictal (lamotrigine), 57t
Lamisil (terbinafine HCl), 191t
lamivudine, 489t
lamotrigine, 57t
Lamprene (clofazimine), 486t
Lanoxin (digoxin), 266, 267
  nursing process, 267
  prototype, 266
lansoprazole, 370t
Lariam (mefloquine HCl), 193t
Lasix (furosemide), 286, 287
laxatives, 350–357
  bulk-forming, 356t
  contact, 353t
  emollient, 356t
  evacuant, 357t
  osmotic, 352t
Lente insulin, 413t
Lescol (fluvastatin), 326t
Leukeran (chlorambucil), 218t
Leukine (sargramostim), 233, 235–237
leuprolide acetate, 489t
Leustatin (cladribine), 224t
levarterenol (norepinephrine bitartrate), 91t
Levatol (penbutolol sulfate), 297t

511

Index

Levo-Dromoran (levorphanol tartrate), 42t
levobunolol HCl, 376t
levomethadyl acetate HCl, 43t
Levophed (norepinephrine bitartrate), 91t, 459t
Levoprome (methotrimeprazine), 37t
levorphanol tartrate, 42t
Levothroid (levothyroxine sodium), 394–396
levothyroxine sodium 394–396
  nursing process, 395, 396
  prototype, 394
Levsin (hyoscyamine sulfate), 108t
Librax, 362t
Librium (chlordiazepoxide HCl), 74t
lidocaine HCl, 444, 445
  nursing process, 445
  prototype, 444
lincomycin, 165t
Lincorex (lincomycin), 165t
lincosamides, 165t
Lioresal (baclofen), 127t
liothyronine sodium, 397t
liotrix, 397t
Lipidil (fenofibrate), 326t
Lipo-Hepin (heparin sodium), 315t
Liquifilm (idoxuridine), 383t
lisinopril, 308t
Lithane (lithium carbonate), 82–84
lithium carbonate, 81t, 82–84
  nursing process, 83, 84
  prototype, 82
lithium citrate, 81t
Lithizine (lithium carbonate), 82–84
Lithobid (lithium carbonate), 82–84
Lodine (etodolac), 139t
lomefloxacin HCl, 176t
Lomotil (diphenoxylate with atropine), 346t
  nursing process, 345
  prototype, 344
lomustine, 219t
Loniten (minoxidil), 305t
loperamide HCl, 347t
Lopid (gemfibrozil), 326t
Lopressor (metoprolol tartrate), 96t, 273t, 294t, 295t
Lorabid (loracarbef), 160t
loracarbef, 160t, 385t
loratadine, 247t
lorazepam, 30t, 54t, 75t, 338t
Lorelco (probucol), 327t
losartan potassium, 489t
Lotensin (benazepril HCl), 308t

Lotrel (amlodipine besylate), 484t
lovastatin, 322–324
  nursing process, 323, 324
  prototype, 322
Lovenox (enoxaparin sodium), 315t
Lowsium (magaldrate with simethicone), 361t
loxapine, 70t
Loxitane (loxapine), 70t
Lozol (indapamide), 285t
Ludiomil (maprotiline HCl), 80t
Lufyllin (dyphylline), 263t
Lugol solution (strong iodine solution), 398t
Luminal (phenobarbital) 52t
Lupron (leuprolide acetate), 489t
Lutrepulse (gonadorelin acetate), 442t
lypressin, 391t
Lysodren (mitotane), 230t

Maalox (magnesium hydroxide and aluminum hydroxide), 361t
Maalox Plus, 361t
Macrodantin (nitrofurantoin), 204, 205
macrolides, 162–164
  nursing process, 163
  prototype, 162
mafenide acetate, 198, 199
  nursing process, 199
  prototype, 198
Mag-Ox 400 (magnesium oxide), 490t
magaldrate, 361t
magnesium citrate, 352t, 490t
magnesium hydroxide, 352t, 490t
magnesium hydroxide–aluminum hydroxide, 361t
magnesium hydroxide–aluminum hydroxide–calcium carbonate, 361t
magnesium hydroxide–aluminum hydroxide–simethicone, 361t
magnesium oxide, 352t, 490t
magnesium salicylate, 490t
magnesium sulfate, 57t, 353t, 423t, 490t
magnesium trisilicate, 361t
Malogen (testosterone), 434–436
Mandelamine (methenamine), 206t
Mandol (cefamandole), 159t
mannitol, 288t
  nursing process, 449
  prototype, 448

Index

Maolate (chlorphenesin), 127t
Maox (magnesium oxide), 352t, 490t
maprotiline HCl, 80t
Marbaxin (methcarbamol), 128t
Marezine (cyclizine HCl), 339t
Maridex ophthalmic (dexamethasone), 383t
Marinol (dronabinol), 337t
Marplan (isocarboxazid), 81t
Matulane (procarbazine HCl), 220t
Maxair (pirbuterol acetate), 257t
Maxaquin (lomefloxacin HCl), 176t
Maxzide (triamterene and hydrochlorothiazide), 293t
Mazanor (mazindol), 19t
mazindol, 19t
Mebaral (mephobarbital), 52t
mebendazole, 491t
mechlorethamine HCl, 218t
Meclan (meclocycline), 201t
meclizine HCl, 339t
meclocycline, 201t
meclofenamate, 138t
Meclomen (meclofenamate), 138t
Medication use in community settings, 481
Medipren (ibuprofen), 36t, 132–134
Medrol (methylprednisolone), 408t
medroxyprogesterone acetate, 431t
medrysone, 383t
mefenamic acid, 139t
mefloquine HCl, 193t
Mega-Cal (potassium chloride), 12
Megace (megestrol acetate), 432t
megestrol acetate, 231t, 432t
Mellaril (thioridazine HCl), 65t
melphalan, 218t
Menest (esterified estrogens), 431t
menadiol sodium diphosphate, 317t
menotropins, 442t
Mentane (velnacrine), 101t
mepenzolate bromide, 109t
meperidine HCl, 40, 41
  nursing process, 41
  prototype, 40
mephentermine sulfate, 491t
mephenytoin, 54t
mephobarbital, 52t
Mephyton (phytonadione), 317t
meprobamate, 75t, 126t
Mepron (atovaquone), 191t
6-mercaptopurine, 225t
Mesantoin (mephenytoin), 54t
mesoridazine besylate, 65t
Mestinon (pyridostigmine bromide), 103t, 120t, 121t

Metahydrin (trichlormethiazide), 285t
Metamucil (psyllium hydrophilic mucilloid), 354, 355
  nursing process, 355
  prototype, 354
Metaprel (metaproterenol sulfate), 91t, 254, 255
  nursing process, 255
  prototype, 254
metaproterenol sulfate, 91t, 254, 255
metformin HCl, 491t
methamphetamine HCl (Desoxyn), 18t
methazolamide, 289t, 377t
methdilazine HCl, 247t
methenamine mandelate, 206t
methenamine hippurate, 207t
Methergine (methylergonovine maleate), 426t
methicillin, 152t
methimazole, 398t
methocarbamol, 128t
methotrexate, 224t
methotrimeprazine HCl, 36t
methoxsalen, 201t
methsuximide, 55t
methyclothiazide, 285t
methylcellulose, 356t
methyldopa, 298t
methylene blue, 209t
methylergonovine maleate, 426t
methylphenidate HCl, 16, 17
  nursing process, 17
  prototype, 16
methylprednisolone, 408t, 450t
methyltestosterone, 438t
methylxanthines, 20, 21
methyprylon, 31t
methysergide maleate, 491t
Meticorten (prednisone), 404–406
metoclopramide monohydrochloride monohydrate, 338t
metolazone, 285t
metoprolol tartrate, 96t, 273t, 294, 295
  nursing process, 295
  prototype, 294
Metrodin (urofollitropin), 442t
MetroGel (metronidazole HCl), 491t
metronidazole HCl, 491t
Mevacor (lovastatin), 322–324
mexiletine HCl, 279t
Mexitil (mexiletine HCl), 279t
Mezlin (mezlocillin), 153t
Miacalcin (calcitonin nasal spray), 491t

513

Index

Micatin (miconazole nitrate), 191t
miconazole nitrate, 191t
Micro-K (potassium chloride), 12
Micronase (glyburide nonmicronized), 417t
Microsulfon (sulfadiazine), 181t
Midamor (amiloride HCl), 292t
midazolam HCl, 492t
milk of magnesia (magnesium hydroxide), 352t, 490t
Milontin (phensuximide), 55t
Milophene (clomiphene citrate), 440, 441
  nursing process, 441
  prototype, 440
Milprem-400 (conjugated estrogens), 428–430
  nursing process, 429, 430
  prototype, 428
milrinone lactate, 268t
Miltown (meprobamate), 75t, 126t
mineral oil, 357t
minerals, 6, 7
Minipress (prazosin HCl), 97t, 300, 301
Minocin (minocycline HCl), 168t
minocycline HCl, 168t
Minodyl (minoxidil), 305t
minoxidil, 305t
Mintezol (thiabendazole), 496t
Minzolum (thiabendazole), 496t
Miochol (acetylcholine Cl), 375t
Miostat (carbachol), 101t, 375t
miotics, 372–376
misoprostol, 370t
Mithracin (plicamycin), 228t
mithramycin (plicamycin), 228t
mitomycin, 227t
mitotane, 230t
mitoxantrone, 231t
Mitrolan (calcium polycarbophil), 356t
Mivacron (mivacurium Cl), 492t
mivacurium Cl, 492t
Moban (molindone HCl), 71t
Moduretic (amiloride HCl and hydrochlorothiazide), 293t
moexipril HCl, 492t
molindone HCl, 71t
Monistat (miconazole nitrate), 191t
monoamine oxidase (MAO) inhibitors, 81t
Monocid (cefonocid sodium), 159t
Monopril (fosinopril), 308t
More-Dophilus (Bacid plus carboxymethylcellulose), 348t
moricizine HCl, 492t

morphine sulfate, 38, 39, 446t
  nursing process, 39
  prototype, 38
Motofen (difenoxin and atropine), 348t
Motrin (ibuprofen), 36t, 132–134
  nursing process, 133, 134
  prototype, 132
moxalactam disodium, 161t
Moxam (moxalactam disodium), 161t
MS Contin (morphine sulfate), 38, 39
Mucomyst (acetylcysteine), 484t
mupirocin, 154t
muscle relaxants, 124–130
Mustargen (mechlorethamine HCl), 218t
Mutamycin (mitomycin), 227t
Myambutol (ethambutol HCl), 187t
myasthenia gravis agents, 120–123
Mycifradin (neomycin sulfate), 172t
Mycobutin (rifabutin), 187t
Mycostatin (nystatin), 188, 189
Mydriacyl ophthalmic (tropicamide), 107t, 380t
Myidyl (triprolidine HCl), 247t
Mylanta (magnesium hydroxide, aluminum hydroxide, simethicone), 361t
Mylanta III, 361t
Myleran (busulfan), 219t
Myochrysine (gold sodium thiomalate), 143t
Mysoline (primidone), 53t
Mytelase (ambenonium chloride), 102t, 122t

nabilone, 337t
nabumetone, 493t
nadolol, 96t, 297t
Nafcil (nafcillin), 152t
nafcillin, 152t
nalbuphine HCl, 46t
Nalfon (fenoprofen calcium), 137t
nalidixic acid, 176t, 207t
naloxone HCl, 47t, 452, 453
  nursing process, 453
  prototype, 452
nandrolone decanoate, 438t
nandrolone phenpropionate, 438t
Napamide (disopyramide phosphate), 278t
naphazoline HCl, 252t
Naprosyn (naproxen), 138t
naproxen, 138t

Index

Naqua (trichlormethiazide), 285t
Narcan (naloxone HCl), 452, 453
  nursing process, 453
  prototype, 452
narcotic antitussives, 250t
narcotics, 38–47
  nursing process, 39, 41
  prototype, 38, 40
Nardil (phenelzine sulfate), 81t
Nasahist B (brompheniramine maleate), 246t
Nasalide (flunisolide), 252t
Natacyn ophthalmic (natamycin), 382t
natamycin, 382t
Naturacil (psyllium hydrophilic mucilloid), 354, 355
  nursing process, 355
  prototype, 354
Naturetin (bendroflumethiazide), 284t
Navane (thiothixene HCl), 65t, 70t
Navelbine (vinorelbine), 228t
Nebcin (tobramycin sulfate), 173t
nefazodone HCl, 493t
NegGram (nalidixic acid), 176t, 207t
Nembutal sodium (pentobarbital sodium), 22–24
  nursing process, 23, 24
  prototype, 22
Neo-Synephrine (oxymetazoline HCl), 92t
Neo-Synephrine (phenylephrine HCl), 252t
Neoloid (castor oil), 353t
neomycin sulfate, 172t, 381t
neostigmine bromide, 103t, 123t
neostigmine methylsulfate, 103t, 123t
Neptazane (methazolamide), 289t, 377t
netilmicin, 173t
Netromycin (netilmicin), 173t
Neupogen (filgrastim), 234, 235
Neurontin (gabapentin), 56t
NeuTrexin (trimetrexate glucuronate), 229t
niacin (nicotinic acid), 5t, 326t
nicardipine HCl, 275t
Niclocide (niclosamide), 493t
niclosamide, 493t
nicotinic acid (niacin), 5t, 326t
nicotinyl alcohol, 331t
nifedipine, 275t, 310t
Nipent (pentostatin), 226t
Nipride, 305t, 460, 461
  nursing process, 461
  prototype, 460

nisoldipine, 493t
Nitro-Bid (nitroglycerin), 270, 271
nitrofurantoin, 204, 205
  nursing process, 205
  prototype, 204
nitrofurazone, 200t
nitrogen mustards, 218t
nitroglycerin, 270, 271, 447t
  nursing process, 271
  prototype, 270
Nitrol (nitroglycerin), 270
Nitropress, 305t
nitrosoureas, 219t
Nitrostat (nitroglycerin), 270, 271, 447t
nizatidine, 366t
Nizoral (ketoconazole), 190t
No Doz (caffeine), 20t
Noctec (chloral hydrate), 27t
Nodostine (nystatin), 188
Noludar (methyprylon), 31t
Nolvadex (tamoxifen), 231t
nonnarcotic antitussives, 250t, 251t
nonsteroidal antiinflammatory drugs (NSAIDs), 36t, 37t, 132–139
nonsteroidal estrogens, 431t
Norcuron (vecuronium), 129t
norepinephrine bitartrate, 91t, 459t
norethindrone, 432t
Norflex (orphenadrine HCl/citrate), 115t, 128t
norfloxacin, 177t, 208t, 381t
Norlutin (norethindrone), 432t
Noroxin (norfloxacin), 176t, 208t
Norpace (disopyramide phosphate), 278t
Norpramin (desipramine HCl), 78t
nortriptyline HCl, 79t
Norvasc (amlodipine), 273t
Norvir (ritonavir), 496t
Norzine (thiethylperazine maleate), 336t
Novafed (pseudoephedrine), 253t
Novantrone (mitoxantrone), 231t
Novasen (aspirin), 32, 33
Novocolchine (colchicine), 146t
Novodipam (diazepam), 72, 73
Novodoxylin (digoxin), 266
Novoflupam (flurazepam HCl), 28, 29
Novopentobarb (pentobarbital sodium), 22–24
Novopranol (propranolol HCl), 94
Novorythro (erythromycin), 162
Novotetra (tetracycline), 166
NPH insulin, 410, 411
  nursing process, 411
  prototype, 410

515

Index

NSAIDs, 36t, 37t, 132–139
NTG (nitroglycerin), 270, 271
Nubain (nalbuphine HCl), 46t
Numorphan (oxymorphone HCl), 43t
Nuprin (ibuprofen), 36t, 132t
Nuromax (doxacurium Cl), 128t
Nydrazid (isoniazid), 184–186
   nursing process, 185, 186
   prototype, 184
nylidrin HCl, 330t
Nysderm (nystatin), 188
nystatin, 188, 189
   nursing process, 189
   prototype, 188

octreotide acetate, 349t
Ocufen (flurbiprofen sodium), 137t, 383t
Ocusert Pilo-20 and Pilo-40 (pilocarpine), 372–374
ofloxacin, 177t, 493t
Ogen (estropipate sulfate), 431t
omeprazole, 370t
Omnipen (ampicillin), 151t
Oncovin (vincristine sulfate), 228t
ondansetron HCl, 338t
ophthalmic agents, 37–383
opiates, 346t, 347t
Optimine (azatadine maleate), 246t
Oral contraceptives, 432, 433
Oraminic II (brompheniramine maleate), 246t
Orap (pimozide), 70t
Orasone (prednisone), 404–406
Oratrol (dichlorphenamide), 289t
Oretic (hydrochlorothiazide), 282, 283
Oreton-Methyl (methyltestosterone), 438t
Orinase (tolbutamide), 416t
Orlaam (levomethadyl acetate HCl), 43t
Ornex DM (dextromethorphan hydrobromide), 248, 249
orphenadrine, 115t, 128t
Ortho-Est (estropipate sulfate), 431t
Orudis (ketoprofen), 36t, 138t
Os-Cal (calcium carbonate), 12
Osmitrol (mannitol), 448, 449
   nursing process, 449
   prototype, 448
otic agents, 384–386
Otic Domeboro (acetic acid and aluminum acetate), 384t

Otrivin (xylometazoline HCl), 253t
ovulation stimulants, 440–442
oxacillin, 153t
oxamniquine, 493t
Oxandrin (oxandrolone), 439t
oxandrolone, 439t
oxaprozin, 138t
oxazepam, 75t
oxazolidones, 55t
Oxsoralen-Ultra (methoxsalen), 201t
oxtriphylline, 263t
oxybutynin Cl, 213t
oxycodone HCl, 42t
oxymetazoline HCl, 92t, 252t
oxymetholone, 439t
oxymorphone HCl, 43t
oxyphencyclimine HCl, 109t
oxytetracycline HCl, 168t
oxytocin nasal solution, 493t
oxytocin, 424–427, 427t
   nursing process, 425
   prototype, 424

P.A.S. sodium (aminosalicylate sodium), 187t
paclitaxel, 226t
Pamine (methscopolamine bromide), 109t
Pan-heparin (heparin sodium) 315t
Panadol (acetaminophen), 34, 35
Panasol-S (prednisone), 404–406
pancuronium bromide, 129t
Panmycin (tetracycline), 166, 167
pantothenic acid, 5t
Panwarfin (warfarin sodium), 310t
papaverine, 331t
Paradione (paramethadione), 55t
Paraflex (chlorzoxazone), 127t
Parafon Forte (chlorzoxazone), 127t
Paral (paraldehyde), 27t
paraldehyde, 27t
paramethadione, 55t
paramethasone acetate, 409t
Paraplatin (carboplatin), 219t
parathyroid hormone, 400–403
Paregoric (camphorated opium tincture), 346t
Parepectolin, 349t
Parlodel (bromocriptine mesylate), 119t, 442t
Parnate (tranylcypromine sulfate), 81t
paromomycin, 173t
paroxetine HCl, 80t
Parsidol (ethopropazine HCl), 115t

Index

Pathilon (tridihexethyl chloride), 362t
Pavabid, 331t
Pavulon (pancuronium bromide), 129t
Paxil (paroxetine HCl), 80t
Paxipam (halazepam), 5t
PediaCare I (dextromethorphan hydrobromide), 248, 249
PediaCare (pseudoephedrine HCl), 92t
Pediamycin (erythromycin ethylsuccinate), 164t
Peganone (ethotoin), 54t
Pelamine (tripelennamine HCl), 245t
pemoline (Cylert), 18t
penbutolol sulfate, 297t
Penetrex (enoxacin), 176t, 209t
penicillin G benzathine, 150t
penicillin G procaine, 150t
penicillin G sodium/potassium, 150t
penicillins, 148–154, 386t
pentaerythritol tetranitrate, 272t
pentazocine lactate, 44, 45
  nursing process, 45
  prototype, 44
Pentids (penicillin), 150t, 386t
pentobarbital sodium, 22–24
  nursing process, 23, 24
  prototype, 22
pentostatin, 226t
pentoxifylline, 331t
Pen-V (penicillin), 386t
Pepcid AC (OTC), 366t
Pepcid (famotidine), 366t
peptides, 183t
Pepto-Bismol (bismuth salts), 347t
Percocet (oxycodone HCl), 42t
Percodan (oxycodone terephthalate), 42t
pergolide mesylate, 119t
Pergonal (human menopausal gonadotropin), 442t
Periactin (cyproheptadine HCl), 246t
Peri-Colace (docusate sodium with casanthranol), 357t
Peridol (haloperidol), 66–68
Peritrate (pentaerythritol), 272t
Permax (pergolide mesylate), 119t
perphenazine, 64t, 334, 335
  nursing process, 335
  prototype, 334
Persa-Gel (benzoyl peroxide), 200t
Persantine (dipyridamole), 316t
Pertofrane (desipramine HCl), 78t
Pethadol (meperidine HCl), 40, 41

Pethidine HCl (meperidine HCl), 40, 41
Pfizerpen (penicillin G sodium/potassium), 150t
phenacemide, 494t
Phenazo (phenazopyridine), 210, 211
phenazopyridine, 210, 211
  nursing process, 211
  prototype, 210
phendimetrazine tartrate, 19t
phenelzine sulfate, 81t
Phenergan (promethazine HCl), 244t, 338t
Phenetron (chlorpheniramine maleate), 244t
phenmetrazine HCl, 20t
phenobarbital, 52t
phenolphthalein, 353t
phenothiazine antiemetics, 334–336
phenothiazine antihistamines, 244t
phenoxybenzamine HCl, 302t
phensuximide, 55t
phentermine HCl, 20t
phentolamine mesylate, 97t, 302t
Phenurone (phenacemide), 494t
phenylephrine HCl, 92t
phenylpropanolamine HCl, 20t, 92t, 253t
phenytoin, 50, 51, 279t
  nursing process, 51
  prototype, 50
Phospholine Iodide (echothiophate iodide), 101t, 375t
physostigmine salicylate, 103t, 120, 121, 375t
  nursing process, 121
  prototype, 120
phytonadione, 317t
Pilocar (pilocarpine HCl), 101t
pilocarpine HCl, 101t, 372–374
  nursing process, 373, 374
  prototype, 372
Pilopine HS (pilocarpine HCl), 101t, 372–374
pimozide, 70t, 494t
pindolol, 97t, 297t
pipecuronium bromide, 494t
piperacillin, 154t
piperacillin–tazobactam sodium, 154t
piperazine citrate, 495t
pipobroman, 220t
Pipracil (piperacillin), 154t
pirbuterol acetate, 257t
piroxicam, 139t
Pitocin (oxytocin), 424, 425, 427t
Pitressin (vasopressin), 392t

Index

Pitressin Tannate (vasopressin tannate), 392t
pituitary hormones, 388–39
Placidyl (ethchlorvynol), 25t
Plaquenil Sulfate (hydroxychloroquine sulfate), 192t
Platinol (cisplatin), 219t
Plendil (felodipine), 309t
plicamycin, 228t
PMB (conjugated estrogens), 428–430
  nursing process, 429, 430
  prototype, 428
PMS Theophylline (theophylline), 261, 262
PMS Isoniazid (isoniazid), 184
Poladex (dexchlorpheniramine maleate), 246t
Polaramine (dexchlorpheniramine maleate), 246t
Polargen (dexchlorpheniramine maleate), 246t
Polycillin (ampicillin), 151t, 385t
polyestradiol phosphate, 231t
polyethylene glycol, 357t
polygalactorate, 278t
polymyxin B sulfate, 183t, 209t, 381t, 384t
polymyxin E (colistin), 183t
polythiazide, 285t
Pondimin (fenfluramine HCl), 19t
Ponstel (mefenamic acid), 139t
potassium, 8–11
potassium chloride, 8–10
  nursing process, 9, 10
  prototype, 8
potassium iodide, 251t
potassium iodine solution, 398t
Pravachol (pravastatin), 326t
prazepam, 75t
praziquantel, 495t
prazosin HCl, 9t, 300, 301
  nursing process, 301
  prototype, 300
Precef (ceforanide), 159t
Precose (acarbose), 484t
Pred Forte ophthalmic (prednisolone acetate), 383t
Pred Mild ophthalmic (prednisolone acetate), 383t
prednisolone, 409t
prednisolone acetate, 383t
prednisolone sodium phosphate, 383t
prednisone, 404–406
  nursing process, 405, 406
  prototype, 404
Preludin (phenmetrazine HCl), 20t

Premarin (conjugated estrogens), 428–430
  nursing process, 429, 430
  prototype, 428
Prepidil gel (dinoprostone gel), 427t
Prevacid (lansoprazole), 370t
Preznyl (human chorionic gonadotropin), 442t
Prilosec (omeprazole), 370t
Primacor (milrinone lactate), 268t
primaquine phosphate, 193t
Primatene Mist (epinephrine), 256t
Primaxin (imipenem), 209t
Primaxin (imipenem-cilastatin), 177t
primidone, 53t
Prinivil (lisinopril), 308t
Priscoline HCl (tolazoline), 97t, 302t, 330t
Pro-Banthine (propantheline), 109t, 213t, 362t
probenecid, 146t
probucol, 327t
procainamide HCl, 276, 277, 447t
  nursing process, 277
  prototype, 276
Procan (procainamide HCl), 276, 277
procarbazine HCl, 220t
Procardia (nifedipine), 275t, 310t
prochlorperazine maleate, 64t, 336t
procyclidine HCl, 111t, 115t
Procytox (cyclophosphamide), 216
Profasi HP (human chorionic gonadotropin), 442t
Profenal (suprofen), 383t
Progestaject (progesterone), 231t
Progestasert (progesterone), 231t
progesterone, 231t, 431t
progestins, 431t
progestins and estrogens, 431, 432
Proglycem (diazoxide), 304t
Prokine (sargramostim), 233, 235–257
Prolamine (phenylpropanolamine HCl), 20t
Prolixin (fluphenazine HCl), 64t
Proloid (thyroglobulin), 397t
proloprim (trimethoprim), 206t
promazine HCl, 64t
Prometh (promethazine HCl), 244t
promethazine HCl, 244t, 338t
promethazine with dextromethorphan, 251t
Pronestyl (procainamide HCl), 276, 277, 447t
propafenone HCl, 281t
propantheline bromide, 109t, 213t, 362t

Propine (dipivefrin HCl), 379t
propoxyphene HCl, 43t
propoxyphene napsylate, 43t
propranolol HCl, 94, 95, 97t, 273t, 280t, 297t
  nursing process, 95
  prototype, 94
Propulsid (cisapride), 486t
propylamine derivatives, 246t
Prorex (promethazine), 244t
ProSom (estazolam), 30t
Prostaphlin (oxacillin), 153t
Prostigmin (neostigmine bromide), 103t, 123t
protamine sulfate, 317t
Protostat (metronidazole HCl), 491t
protriptyline HCl, 79t
Protropin (somatrem), 390t
provastatin sodium, 326t
Proventil (albuterol), 89t, 256t
Provera (medroxyprogesterone acetate), 431t
proxetil (cefpodoxime), 160t
Prozac (fluoxetine HCl), 80t
pseudoephedrine HCl, 92t, 253t
psyllium hydrophilic mucilloid, 354, 355
  nursing process, 355
  prototype, 354
PTU (propylthiouracil), 398t
Pulmophylline (theophylline), 261, 262
Purge (castor oil), 353t
Purinethol (6-mercaptopurine), 225t
Purinol (allopurinol), 144
pyrantel pamoate, 495t
pyrazinamide, 495t
Pyridium (phenazopyridine), 211, 212
pyridostigmine bromide, 103t, 120, 121
  nursing process, 121
  prototype, 120
pyridoxine, 4t
pyrimethamine, 193t
Pyronium (phenazopyridine), 210, 211
PZI (protamine zinc insulin), 413t

Quarzan (clidinium bromide), 108t
quazepam, 30t
Quelicin (succinylcholine), 129t
Questran (cholestyramine resin), 325t
Quibron (theophylline), 260–262
Quin-260 (quinine sulfate), 193t
quinacrine HCl, 193t
quinapril HCl, 309t
quinestrol, 431t
quinethazone, 285t
Quinidex (quinidine sulfate), 278t
quinidine sulfate, 278t
quinine sulfate, 193t
quinolones, 174, 175, 176t, 177t, 206t–208t
  nursing process, 175
  prototype, 174
Quiphile (quinine sulfate), 193t

ramipril, 309
ranitidine, 364, 365
  nursing process, 365
  prototype, 364
Redux (dexfenfluramine), 487t
Regitine (phentolamine), 97t, 302t
Reglan (metoclopramide monohydrochloride monohydrate), 338t
Regular insulin, 410, 411
  nursing process, 411
  prototype, 410
Relafen (nabumetone), 493t
Renese-R, 285t
reserpine, 303t
resorcinol and sulfur, 200t
Restoril (temazepam), 30t
Retin-A (tretinoin), 201t
Retrovir (zidovudine), 197t
Rev-Eyes (dapiprazole HCl), 487t
ribavirin, 197t
riboflavin, 4t
Ridaura (auranofin), 140–142
  nursing process, 141, 142
  prototype, 140
rifabutin, 187t
Rifadin (rifampin), 187t
rifampin, 187t
Rimactane (rifampin), 187t
rimexolone, 495t
Rimso-50 (dimethyl sulfoxide), 213t
Riopan (magaldrate), 361t
Risperdal (risperidone), 71t
risperidone, 71t
Ritalin, Ritalin-SR (methylphenidate), 16, 17, 18t
  nursing process, 17
  prototype, 16
ritodrine HCl, 93t, 420–422
  nursing process, 421, 422
  prototype, 420

Index

ritonavir, 496t
Robaxin (methocarbamol), 128t
Robigesic (acetaminophen), 34, 35
Robinul (glycopyrrolate), 108t, 362t
Robitussin (guaifenesin), 251t
Robitussin A-C (guaifenesin and codeine), 250t
Robitussin-DM (dextromethorphan hydrobromide), 248, 249, 251t
Rocaltrol (calcitriol), 400, 401
  nursing process, 401
  prototype, 400
Rocephin (ceftriaxone), 161t
Roferon-A (interferon alfa-2a), 238t
Rogaine (minoxidil), 305t
Rolaids Antacid (dihydroxy-aluminum sodium carbonate), 360t
Rondec (carbinoxamine and pseudoephedrine), 245t
Ronigen (nicotinyl alcohol), 331t
Roxanol (morphine sulfate), 38, 39
Rufen (ibuprofen), 132, 133
Rythmol (propafenone HCl), 281t

Salazopyrin (sulfasalazine), 182t
salicylates, 37t, 135t
salicylic acid, 200t
salmeterol, 257t
Saluron (hydroflumethiazide), 284t
Sandostatin (octreotide acetate), 349t
Sanorex (mazindol), 19t
Sansert (methysergide maleate), 491t
saquinavir mesylate, 496t
sargramostim, 233–237
  nursing process, 233, 235, 237
  prototype, 236
scopolamine hydrobromide, 110t, 380t
Sebulex (salicylic acid), 200t
secobarbital sodium, 25t
Seconal Sodium (secobarbital sodium), 25t
Sectral (acebutolol HCl), 96t, 280t, 296t
sedative-hypnotics, 22–31
  barbiturate, 22–27
  benzodiazepine, 28–31
  nonbenzodiazepine, 31t
  piperidinedione, 31t
Seldane (terfenadine), 245t
selegiline HCl, 119t
Semilente insulin, 412t

senna, 353t
Senokot (senna), 353t
Septra (sulfamethoxazole-trimethoprim), 178–180, 208t
  nursing process, 179, 180
  prototype, 178
Serax (oxazepam), 75t
Serentil (mesoridazine besylate), 65t
Serevent (salmeterol), 257t
sermorelin acetate, 390t
Seromycin (cycloserine), 486t
Serophene (clomiphene citrate), 440, 441
  nursing process, 441
  prototype, 440
Serpasil (reserpine), 303t
sertraline HCl, 81t
Serzone (nefazodone HCl), 493t
Silvadene (silver sulfadiazine), 200t
silver nitrate, 200t, 382t
silver sulfadiazine, 200t
simvastatin, 327t
Sinemet (carbidopa-levodopa), 116, 117
Sinequan (doxepin HCl), 78t
Sinex (phenylephrine HCl), 252t
Slo-bid (theophylline), 260–262
Slo-phyllin (theophylline), 260–262
sodium bicarbonate, 361t, 447t
sodium biphosphate, 353t
sodium nitroprusside, 305t, 460, 461
  nursing process, 461
  prototype, 460
sodium phosphate with sodium biphosphate, 353t
Solganal (aurothioglucose), 143t
Solu-Medrol (methylprednisolone), 408t, 450t
Soma (carisoprodol), 124, 125, 127t
  nursing process, 125
  prototype, 124
somatrem, 390t
somatropin, 390t
Somophyllin (theophylline), 260–262, 263t
Sorbitrate (isosorbide dinitrate), 272t
sotalol HCl, 280t
Sparine (promazine HCl), 64t
spectinomycin HCl, 177t
Spectrobid (bacampicillin HCl), 151t
spironolactone, 292t
spironolactone and hydrochlorothiazide, 293t
Sporanox (itraconazole), 190t
SSD (silver sulfadiazine), 200t
SSKI (potassium iodide), 251t

Index

Stadol (butorphanol tartrate), 46t
stanozolol, 439t
Staphcillin (methicillin), 152t
stavudine, 496t
Stelazine (trifluoperazine HCl), 65t
steroidal estrogens, 431t
Stimate (desmopressin), 391t
Streptase (streptokinase), 318, 319
streptokinase, 318, 319
   nursing process, 319
   prototype, 318
streptomycin sulfate, 173t, 187t
streptozocin, 219t
Sublimaze (fentanyl), 47t
succinimides, 55t
succinylcholine chloride, 129t
Sucostrin (succinylcholine chloride), 129t
sucralfate, 368, 369
   nursing process, 369
   prototype, 368
Sucrets (dextromethorphan hydrobromide), 248, 249
Sudafed (pseudoephedrine HCl), 92t, 253t
Sufenta (sufentanil citrate), 43t
sufentanil citrate, 43t
Sular (nisoldipine), 493t
Sulcrate (sucralfate), 368, 369
sulfacetamide sodium, 496t
sulfadiazine, 181t
sulfamethizole, 181t
sulfamethoxazole, 182t
sulfamethoxazole-trimethoprim, 208t. See also *Septra (sulfamethoxazole-trimethoprim)*.
Sulfamylon (mafenide acetate), 198, 199
sulfasalazine, 182t
Sulfasol (sulfamethizole), 181t
sulfinpyrazone, 146t, 317t
sulfisoxazole, 181t
sulfonamides, 178–183
   nursing process, 179
   prototype, 180
sulfonylureas, 414–417
sulindac, 136t
sumatriptan succinate, 21t
Sumycin (tetracycline), 166, 167
Suprax (cefixime), 161t
suprofen, 383t
Surfak (docusate calcium) 356t
Surmontil (trimipramine maleate), 79t
Symmetrel (amantadine HCl), 118t, 196t
Synkayvite (menadiol sodium diphosphate), 317t
Synthroid (levothyroxine sodium), 394–396
Syntocinon (oxytocin), 424, 425, 426t

t-PA (tissue-type plasminogen activator), 320t
Tacaryl (methdilazine HCl), 247t
Tace (chlorotrianisene), 431t
tacrine HCl, 101t
Tagamet (cimetidine), 366t
Talwin (pentazocine lactate), 44, 45
Tambocor (flecainide), 278t
tamoxifen citrate, 231t
Tapazole (methimazole), 398t
Taractan (chlorprothixene HCl), 70t
Tavist (clemastine fumarate), 245t
Taxol (paclitaxel), 226t
Tazicef (ceftazidime), 161t
TDM (therapeutic drug monitoring), xxvii–xxxii
Tebrazid (pyrazinamide), 495t
Tegison (etretinate), 201t
Tegopen (cloxacillin), 152t
Tegretol (carbamazepine), 55t
Teldrin (chlorpheniramine maleate), 244t
Telechlor (chlorpheniramine maleate), 244t
Temaril (trimeprazine tartrate), 244t
temazepam, 30t
Tempra (acetaminophen), 34, 35
Tenex (guanfacine HCl), 298t
teniposide, 228t
Tenormin (atenolol), 96t, 272t, 296t
Tensilon (edrophonium chloride), 102t, 122t
Tenuate (diethylpropion), 19t
Tepanil (diethylpropion), 19t
terazosin HCl, 302t
terbinafine HCl, 191t
terbutaline sulfate, 93t, 258t, 423t
terfenadine, 245t
Terramycin (oxytetracycline HCl), 169t
Tesamone (testosterone), 434, 435, 436t
Teslac (testolactone), 229t, 439t
Tessalon (benzonatate), 250t
Testex (testosterone propionate), 436t
testolactone, 229t, 439t

521

Index

testosterone, 434–436, 437t
  nursing process, 435, 436
  prototype, 434
testosterone cypionate, 437t
testosterone enanthate, 437t
testosterone propionate, 437t
Testred Cypionate 200 (testosterone), 438t
  nursing process, 435, 436
  prototype, 434
tetracycline, 166, 167, 201t, 382t, 384t
  nursing process, 167
  prototype, 166
Tetracyn (tetracylcline), 166, 167
tetrahydrozoline HCl, 253t
Theelin (estrone), 431t
Theo-Dur (theophylline), 260–262
Theophyllin KI (theophylline), 260–62
theophylline, 21t, 260–262
  nursing process, 261, 262
  prototype, 260, 261
theophylline ethylenediamine, 263t
therapeutic drug monitoring (TDM), xxvii–xxxii
thiabendazole, 496t
thiamine, 4t
thiethylperazine maleate, 336t
thioamide: propylthiouracil, 398t
thioguanine, 225t
thioridazine HCl, 65t
Thiosulfil Forte, 181t
thiotepa (triethylenethiophosphoramide), 220t
thiothixene HCl, 65t, 71t
Thorazine (chlorpromazine HCl), 60–62, 336t
  nursing process, 61, 62
  prototype, 60
thrombolytics, 318–320
Thyrar (thyroid), 397t
thyroglobulin, 397t
thyroid hormone replacements and antithyroid drugs, 394–398
thyroid, 397t
Thyrolar (liotrix), 397t
thyrotropin, 390t
Thytropar (thyrotropin), 390t
Ticar (ticarcillin disodium), 154t
ticarcillin disodium, 154t
ticarcillin-clavulanate, 154t
Ticon (trimethobenzamide HCl), 338t
Tigan (trimethobenzamide HCl), 338t
Timentin (ticarcillin-clavulanate), 154t

timolol maleate, 97t, 297t, 376t
Timoptic (timolol maleate), 376t
Tirend (caffeine), 20t
tissue-type plasminogen activator, 320t
tobramycin sulfate, 173t
tobramycin, ophth, 497t
Tobrex (tobramycin), 497t
tocainide HCl, 279t
tocopherol, 5t
Tofranil (imipramine HCl), 79t
tolazamide, 416t
tolazoline HCl, 97t, 302t, 330t
tolbutamide, 416t
Tolectin (tolmetin), 136t
Tolinase (tolazamide), 416t
tolmetin, 136t
Tonocard (tocainide HCl), 279t
Toradol (ketorolac), 139t
Torecan (thiethylperazine maleate), 336t
Tornalate (bitolterol mesylate), 253t
torsemide, 288t
Tracrium (atracurium besylate), 128t
tramadol HCl, 497t
Trandate (labetalol HCl), 305t
Transderm-Nitro patch (nitroglycerin), 270, 271
Tranxene (clorazepate dipotassium), 53t, 74t
tranylcypromine sulfate, 81t
trazodone HCl, 81t
Trecator-SC (ethionamide), 487t
Trental (pentoxifylline), 331t
tretinoin, 201t
triamcinolone, 409t
triamcinolone acetonide, inhal, 497t
Triaminic (phenylpropanolamine HCl), 92t
Triaminicol (phenylpropanolamine HCl), 92t
triamterene, 290, 291
  nursing process, 291
  prototype, 290
triamterene and hydrochlorothiazide, 293t
triazolam, 31t
trichlormethiazide, 285t
tricyclic antidepressants, 76–79
tridihexethyl chloride, 362t
Tridil (nitroglycerin), 447t
Tridione (trimethadione), 55t
triethylenethiophosphoramide, 220t
trifluoperazine HCl, 65t
triflupromazine HCl, 64t, 336t,
trifluridine, 382t
Trihexy (trihexyphenidyl HCl), 111t

Index

trihexyphenidyl HCl, 111–113, 111t
  nursing process, 113
  prototype, 112
Trilafon (perphenazine), 64t, 334, 335
  nursing process, 335
  prototype, 334
Trilog (triamcinolone acetonide), 497t
trimeprazine tartrate, 244t
trimethadione, 55t
trimethobenzamide HCl, 338t
trimethoprim, 206t
trimethoprim and sulfamethoxazole, 178, 180, 386t. See also *Septra (sulfamethoxazole-trimethoprim).*
trimetrexate glucuronate, 229t
trimipramine maleate, 79t
Trimpex (trimethoprim), 206t
tripelennamine HCl, 245t
triprolidine HCl, 247t
triprolidine and pseudoephedrine, 246t
Trobicin (spectinomycin HCl), 177t
trolamine polypeptide oleate-condensate, 384t
tropicamide, 107t, 380t
Trusopt (dorzolamide HCl), 377t
tubocurarine Cl, 497t
Tums (calcium carbonate), 12, 360t
Tylenol (acetaminophen), 34, 35
Tyzine (tetrahydrozoline HCl), 253t

Ultralente Insulin, 413t
Ultram (tramadol HCl), 497t
Unasyn (ampicillin-sulbactam), 151t
Unipen (nafcillin), 152t
Univasc (moexipril HCl), 491t
Urabeth (bethanechol chloride), 212t
uracil mustard, 218t
urea (Ureaphil), 289t, 378t
Ureaphil (urea), 289t, 378t
Urecholine (bethanechol chloride), 98–100, 212t
  nursing process, 99, 100
  prototype, 98
Urex (methenamine hippurate), 207t
urinary analgesics, 210, 211
urinary anti-infectives, 204–209
urinary stimulants and antispasmodics, 212, 213t
urine, drugs causing discoloration of, xxiv
Urispas (flavoxate HCl), 213t
Urodine (phenazopyridine), 210, 211
urofollitropin, 442t
urokinase, 321t
Urolene Blue (methylene blue), 209t
Urozide (hydrochlorothiazide), 282

valacyclovir HCl, 497t
Valium (diazepam), 54t, 74t, 126t
  nursing process, 73
  prototype, 72
valproic acid, 56t
Valtrex (valacyclovir HCl), 497t
Vanceril (beclomethasone dipropionate), 407t, 485t
Vancocin (vancomycin HCl), 165t
vancomycin HCl, 165t
Vansil (oxamniquine), 493t
Vantin (cefpodoxime), 160t
Vascor (bepridil HCl), 274t
Vasodilan (isoxsuprine), 328, 329
vasopressin, 392t
vasopressin tannate/oil, 392t
Vasotec (enalapril maleate), 308t
Vatronol (ephedrine sulfate), 252t
V-Cillin K (penicillin V potassium), 151t
vecuronium bromide, 129t
Veetids (penicillin V potassium), 151t
Velban (vinblastine sulfate), 228t
velnacrine, 101t
Velosef (cephradine), 159t
venlafaxine, 81t
Ventolin (albuterol), 89t, 256t
VePesid (etoposide), 226t
verapamil HCl, 275t, 280t, 310t, 447t
Vercyte (pipobroman), 220t
Verelan (verapamil HCl), 275t
Vermox (mebendazole), 491t
Vesprin (triflupromazine), 64t, 336t
Vexol (rimexolone), 495t
V-Gan (promethazine), 244t
Vibramycin (doxycycline hyclate), 168t
Vicks (ephedrine sulfate), 252t
vidarabine monohydrate, 197t, 382t
Videx (didanosine), 196t
vinblastine sulfate, 228t
vincristine sulfate, 228t
vinorelbine, 228t
Vira-A (vidarabine monohydrate), 197t
Vira-A ophthalmic (vidarabine), 382t

Index

Virazole (ribavirin), 197t
Virilon (testosterone), 428t, 434–436
  nursing process, 435, 436
  prototype, 434
Viroptic (trifluridine), 382t
Visken (pindolol), 97t, 297t
Vistaril (hydroxyzine HCl), 74t, 244t
Vitamin(s), 2–5, 479, 480
  A, 2–3, 5t
  B, 4, 5t
  B complex, niacin as, 5
    pathothenic acid as, 5
  C, 5t
  D, 5t
  E, 5t
  fat-soluble, 479
  K, 5t, 317t
  nursing process, 2, 3
  prototype, 2
  water-soluble, 479, 480
Vivactil, 79t
Vivarin (caffeine), 20t
VM-26 (teniposide), 228t
Voltaren (diclofenac sodium), 139t, 383t
Vontrol (diphenidol HCl), 337t
Voxsuprine (isoxsuprine), 328, 329
VP-16 (etoposide), 226t
Vumon (teniposide), 228t

warfarin sodium, 312–314
  nursing process, 313, 314
  prototype, 312
Warfilone (warfarin sodium), 312
Wellbutrin (bupropion HCl), 80t
Winpred (prednisone), 404
Winstrol (stanozolol), 439t
Wyamine (mephentermine sulfate), 491t
Wycillin (penicillin G procaine), 150t
Wytensin (guanabez acetate), 298t

Xanax (alprazolam), 74t
Xylocaine (lidocaine), 279t, 444, 445
  nursing process, 445
  prototype, 444
xylometazoline HCl, 253t

Yutopar (ritodrine HCl), 93t, 420–422
  nursing process, 421, 422
  prototype, 420

zalcitabine, 197t
Zanosar (streptozocin), 219t
Zantac (ranitidine), 364, 365
  nursing process, 365
  prototype, 364
Zarontin (ethosuximide), 55t
Zaroxolyn (metolazone), 285t
Zebeta (bisoprolol fumarate), 296t
Zefazone (cefmetazole sodium), 159t
Zerit (stavudine), 496t
Zestril (lisinopril), 308t
zidovudine, 197t
Zinacef (cefuroxime), 160t
Zithromax (azithromycin), 164t
Zocor (simvastatin), 327t
Zofran (ondansetron HCl), 338t
Zoladex (goserelin acetate), 230t
Zoloft (sertraline HCl), 81t
zolpidem tartrate, 31t
Zosyn (piperacillin-tazobactam), 154t
Zovirax (acyclovir sodium), 194, 195
  nursing process, 195
  prototype, 194
Zyloprim (allopurinol), 144–146, 146t
  nursing process, 144, 145
  prototype, 144
Zyrtec (cetirizine), 247t

PROTOTYPES

Minerals and Electrolytes
  Vitamin A: fat-soluble
  Antianemia, mineral: iron
  Electrolyte:
   potassium
   calcium

Central Nervous System Stimulants and Depressants
  CNS stimulant: methylphenidate HCl (Ritalin)
  Sedative-hypnotic, barbiturate: pentobarbital (Nembutal)
  Benzodiazepine: flurazepam HCl (Dalmane)
  Analgesic:
   aspirin
   acetaminophen (Tylenol)
  Narcotic:
   opiate: morphine sulfate (Duramorph)
   synthetic: meperidine HCl (Demerol)
   agonist-antagonist: pentazocine lactate (Talwin)

Anticonvulsants
  Hydantoin: phenytoin (Dilantin)

Antipsychotics, Anxiolytics, and Antidepressants
  Antipsychotic,
   phenothiazine: chlorpromazine (Thorazine)
   nonphenothiazine: haloperidol (Haldol)
  Anxiolytic, benzodiazepine: diazepam (Valium)
  Antidepressant, tricyclic: amoxapine (Asendin)
  Antimanic: lithium carbonate (Eskalith)

Neurologic and Neuromuscular Agents
  Sympathomimetic: epinephrine HCl (Adrenalin Chloride)
  Adrenergic blocker: propranolol HCl (Inderal)
  Parasympathomimetic: bethanechol chloride (Urecholine)
  Parasympatholytic: atropine sulfate
  Anticholinergic: trihexyphenidyl HCl (Artane)
  Dopaminergic: carbidopa-levodopa (Sinemet)
  Cholinesterase inhibitor: pyridostigmine bromide (Mestinon)
  Skeletal muscle relaxant: carisoprodol (Soma)

Anti-inflammatory Agents
  Anti-inflammatory,
   nonsteroidal antiinflammatory drugs (NSAIDs): ibuprofen (Motrin)
   gold: auranofin (Ridaura)
   antigout: allopurinol (Zyloprim)

Anti-infective Agents
  Antibacterial,
   penicillin: amoxicillin trihydrate (Amoxil)
   cephalosporin: cefaclor (Ceclor)
   macrolide: erythromycin (E-Mycin)
   tetracycline (Achromycin)
   aminoglycoside: gentamicin sulfate (Garamycin)
   quinolone: ciprofloxacin HCl (Cipro)
   sulfonamide: (Bactrim)
    Antitubercular, isoniazid (INH)
    Antifungal, nystatin (Mycostatin)
    Antiviral, acyclovir sodium (Zovirax)
    Antiinfective, topical: mafenide acetate (Sulfamylon)

Urinary Agents
  Antibacterial: nitrofurantoin (Furadantin)
  Antipruritic: phenazopyridine (Pyridium)

Antineoplastic Agents
  Aklylating: cyclophosphamide (Cytoxan)